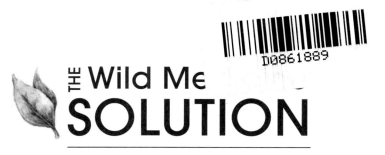

THE Wild Medicine SOLUTION

"A twenty-first-century herbal filled with the wisdom of authentic herbalism. Not only are vital skills of herbalism imparted in a friendly and grounded way, but the book is brimming with insights and wisdom from an herbalist who truly walks his talk."

DAVID HOFFMANN, FNIMH, RH, MEDICAL HERBALIST
AND AUTHOR OF *MEDICAL HERBALISM*

"In *The Wild Medicine Solution*, Guido Masé presents a beautiful tapestry of writing that weaves together the colorfully rich tradition of herbal medicine around tonics and bitters, which are among the most important classes of botanicals for human health. Great information. A delightful read. The real solution to the health care crisis!"

ROY UPTON, RH, DOCTOR OF AYURVEDIC MEDICINE,
EXECUTIVE DIRECTOR OF THE AMERICAN
HERBAL PHARMACOPOEIA

"There are those who incorporate everyday plants into their diet, knowing this is herbal healing at its best. Guido Masé goes one step further. Here's the science that makes clear why direct plant medicine rocks. Tonics, bitters, and aromatics enliven our meals as well as stimulate our life force. Read this book and dare to be healthy!"

MICHAEL PHILLIPS, AUTHOR OF *THE HOLISTIC ORCHARD*
AND *THE APPLE GROWER*

"Whether you are an aging boomer looking for the best ways to stay healthy; a prepper worried about the end days; a sage femme guiding women toward wholeness during pregnancy, birth, and menopause; or a surgeon curious about integrative medicine, you will find ideas here that may overturn your current conceptions of health. This book is a short course on a deep matter, with plenty of practical, do-it-now examples to support your own health and engage in true preventive medicine. It is a gift of green blessings to us all."

SUSUN S. WEED, AUTHOR OF *HEALING WISE*
AND *A WISE WOMAN HERBAL*

"Since ancient times we have been told that bitter and aromatic herbs can improve our health and well-being, but most Westerners avoid these beneficial herbs. Guido Masé, on the other hand, gives us convincing historical and scientific reasons for using them as well as simple recipes to help us enjoy them."

DAVID WINSTON, RH, AUTHOR OF *ADAPTOGENS: HERBS FOR STRENGTH, STAMINA, AND STRESS RELIEF*

"In *The Wild Medicine Solution* herbalist Guido Masé elegantly weaves human history and biology with the history of herbal medicines, offering readers compelling reasons to reharmonize with nature and reintegrate herbs as medicines into their lives. A good read and a beautiful presentation."

AVIVA JILL ROMM, M.D., HERBALIST, MIDWIFE, AND AUTHOR OF *VACCINATIONS* AND *NATURAL HEALTH AFTER BIRTH*

THE Wild Medicine
SOLUTION

Healing with Aromatic, Bitter, and Tonic Plants

GUIDO MASÉ

Healing Arts Press
Rochester, Vermont • Toronto, Canada

Healing Arts Press
One Park Street
Rochester, Vermont 05767
www.HealingArtsPress.com

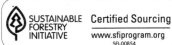

Text stock is SFI certified

Healing Arts Press is a division of Inner Traditions International

Note to the reader: *This book is intended as an informational guide. The remedies,
approaches, and techniques described herein are meant to supplement, and not to be a
substitute for, professional medical care or treatment. They should not be used to treat
a serious ailment without prior consultation with a qualified health care professional.*

Library of Congress Cataloging-in-Publication Data

Masé, Guido, 1975–
　The wild medicine solution : healing with aromatic, bitter, and tonic plants /
Guido Masé.
　　p. cm.
　Includes bibliographical references.
　ISBN 978-1-62055-084-7 (pbk.) — ISBN 978-1-62055-151-6 (e-book)
　Summary: "Restoring the use of wild plants in daily life for vibrant physical,
mental, and spiritual health" — Provided by publisher.
　1. Materia medica, Vegetable. 2. Medicinal plants. I. Title.
　RS164.M287 2013
　615.3'21—dc23

2012032804

Printed and bound in the United States by Lake Book Manufacturing, Inc.
The text stock is SFI certified. The Sustainable Forestry Initiative® program
promotes sustainable forest management.

10 9 8 7 6 5 4 3 2

Text design by Virginia Scott Bowman and layout by Brian Boynton
This book was typeset in Garamond Premier Pro with Caslon and ITC Avant
Garde as display typefaces

To send correspondence to the author of this book, mail a first-class letter to the
author c/o Inner Traditions • Bear & Company, One Park Street, Rochester, VT
05767, and we will forward the communication, or contact the author directly at
www.vtherbcenter.org or **aradicale.blogspot.com**.

For Uli

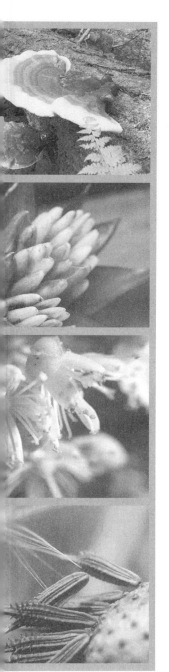

Contents

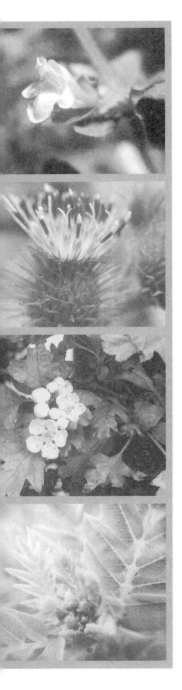

Acknowledgments

I am grateful for Jovial, whose endless support and enthusiasm are always welcome and who loves the plants, looks to the stars, and works hard on the front lines.

I am grateful for Rosemary, who provided encouragement at the beginning of this project, helped point me in the right direction, and has always been a friend.

I am grateful for the editorial staff at Inner Traditions • Bear & Company, all of whom have been a pleasure to work with, professional, and dedicated.

I am deeply grateful for my colleagues, students, friends, and clients at the Vermont Center for Integrative Herbalism, where we work together and learn together every day. Gratitude goes particularly to Rachel, who provided crucial help in compiling the first manuscript and bibliography, and most especially to Betzy, Larken, and Laura for everything they do in service of others—both plants and people.

Finally, I am most grateful for my family. Joe and Mary Anne and Michael and Mary Clare have always done everything in their power to support my work. I would not be who I am without my father, Gigi, the scientist; my mother, Carolyn, the humanist; and my sister, Lisa, the culinary poet. And with a full heart I am most grateful to my wife, Anne, who first knew me when I was young, and my daughter, Uli, who helps me in so many ways. I love you.

Introduction

These days, almost any store that sells food also offers a large selection of pills, extracts, powders, and other combinations that are neither medications nor food. Marketed as dietary supplements, the sheer variety of these compounds, while perhaps intimidating, often rivals that seen at nineteenth-century fairgrounds in the United States. Generally speaking, they contain substances that may be extracted from plants and food (or maybe not), they are perhaps concentrated to a certain degree, and they purport to address dietary and physiological deficiencies. Or they may have some form of nonspecific therapeutic effect that is due to their special processing.

There seems to be a great need both to identify what is missing from what we eat (and, to a larger extent, what is missing from our lives in general) and to employ the most recent discoveries in bioscience to drive that investigative journey (to say nothing of attempts to profit from those discoveries, which is a whole other story). We are learning more and more details about our physiology almost daily, and it is exciting to think that the latest advances represent a potent and effective way to help us feel better, more whole, more comfortable.

Of course, this is usually not the case. It takes years to develop a framework and context for any discovery and, even then, effective therapy may never materialize. Additionally, as we have seen with the

Western diet's heavy reliance on highly processed, nutritionally reen-riched foods, it can be problematic to translate laboratory science into safe and healthy ways to feed ourselves. Our food is not cheaper, cannot seem to be produced sustainably, and certainly has not succeeded in making us healthier (or even keeping us as healthy as our parents).

So back in the food store, are supplements that are primarily made from combinations of isolated chemicals really the key to enriching our lives? Can they truly correct the deficit that is making us feel tired, unfocused, sad, empty? After observing the growth in this market over the last twenty years, we might be tempted to answer, "Maybe, but only until the next thing comes along." To me, this is troubling and indicates that we may never understand what promotes "wellness" by pursuing this approach.

How, then, do we get there? Certainly, at baseline, we have to begin by eating real food. There is a growing consensus on this point. In Vermont, where I write as summer begins, farmers' markets and res-taurants bring us real vegetables, meats, eggs, milk, grains, breads, and more every day. This makes it easy, as Michael Pollan asks us, to "eat food, not too much, mostly plants." This is actually happening all over the United States, and the rebuilding of a whole-food cuisine is helping to improve not only our health, but also our culture, our community, and our environment.

But perhaps this is not quite enough, because it seems that the stores selling the most of this whole, local food also have the largest sections devoted to supplements. As we think about creating a new Western diet, we might need to identify whether or not there are any specific components, other than whole sources of protein, fat, and car-bohydrates, that are essential to the healthy functioning of our physi-ology. Admittedly, this is what nutrition science and the supplement industry are trying to do—but I am skeptical that they will ultimately succeed in a comprehensive way.

What might we be missing, and could we add it to our lives in the context of a whole-food, local, sustainable diet? This is the central question of this book. And the answer will turn out to be surprisingly simple, because all traditional cuisines and healing systems have laid it out for us: consume certain kinds of plants, every day or almost every day, sometimes less, sometimes more, as part of your eating and drinking. To be more specific, I will try to define three simple classes of plants that can easily be added to whole-food diets as part of daily life, but that can also be employed in more directed ways for safe, understandable, and effective preventive health. In the end, we may find that a less complex approach to reaching wellness actually turns out to work better.

How can we be certain it is even possible to arrive at a concise summary of how to incorporate plants into our life in an intelligent and effective way? After all, around the planet there are thousands of species that are employed "medicinally," or with an eye toward preventing or treating disease. The subject matter may seem daunting. The first chapter of this book will provide a framework and rationale for the idea that there are only three broad classes of plants human beings require consistently. To do so, I will draw on ideas from traditional herbal medicine and from an analysis of patterns of interconnection in human physiology.

Those who work with plants for improving health (typically called herbalists) are an interesting lot, representing a diversity of interests and cultural backgrounds. Some spend days exploring wilderness and gathering herbs; others have amazing gardens where they harvest raw materials; still others may dispense precise blends to clients or improvise flu remedies for the neighborhood kids. There are storytellers, mystics, scientists, and naturalists. And in every herbalist there is probably a piece of each of these, and more.

Practicing herbal medicine is a generalist's pursuit. The ability to hold knowledge of botany, pharmacy, physiology, and medicine alongside mythology, spirituality, psychology, and ecology isn't simply useful— it's a necessity. As an herbalist with a particular attraction to the flora of the Northeastern United States, I have had the opportunity to work with living botanical medicine in the forest and field, as well as in our community clinic. I have learned how to grow, harvest, prepare, and administer these herbs, and have explored the physiology of the people, plants, and environment in this area. Thanks to a lifelong interest in myth and magic, I have seen how the stories human beings have always shared weave their way through both the ancient and modern aspects of what I have learned. Perhaps the stories, still so applicable today, are a living expression of the generalist's art. They cut across disciplines and, in doing so, may reveal more than a specialist ever could.

This is important in the day-to-day—when I sit in my office with a client, talk about her health, observe her, and feel her wrist pulse or listen to her breath. I have found that being well-versed in the language of myths and dreams helps me put the process of healing into context for myself and my clients, giving it meaning and approachability. But the herbalist's interdisciplinary style has even more to offer: in a world where information is almost limitless but knowledge is increasingly fragmented, we may need more people who choose to slowly deepen a broad range of knowledge. In health care as in other fields, system and network theories are showing us that we may also need to shift our attention from the pieces of the puzzle to the connections between them.

Traditional herbal medicine plays a crucial role here by identifying some important ingredients: whole plants, a long history of safety (for the most part), and extremely simple preparation. This framework provides an immediately accessible alternative to the endless quest for the next supplement. It features plants that have been in people's kitchens for a very long time, and which are usually considered weedy or at the very least ridiculously easy to grow. All these elements will help us find plants that are safe, have a track record of usefulness, and can be easily and sustainably brought into our lives. Simple preparation techniques will provide clear ways to employ them in the kitchen: cooking daily meals as the chef; creating teas and spirits as the bartender; and crafting more complex formulations as the alchemist.

Each subsequent chapter of this book will include practical examples of how to use the plants we examine. In the kitchen, recipes will focus on using them as part of meals, not only as seasonings but also as central ingredients in soups, stocks, salads, and grain dishes. For beverages, there will be formulas for simple teas and for fresh herbs preserved in alcohol (tinctures). And the alchemist will discuss blending and dosing the plants for when a little more than just daily use is required.

To pick our specific plants, I will attempt to isolate key elements of how we work by exploring simple patterns in our physiology. Herbal medicine has something to contribute here, too, but I will primarily rely on concepts from system and network theory, coupled with modern biochemistry and physiology, to observe how we work on a more general level (though not necessarily a more macroscopic one). This broader perspective will help us identify key "hubs" in activity and interrelationship: places and processes in the system where good function is crucial because if something goes wrong, many other areas become affected in turn. It will come down to the level of activity and tension in our nerves and muscles, the functioning of digestion and food metabolism, and the expression of genes deep inside the nucleus of every cell in our bodies.

We are constantly exposed to influences that, through our organs of perception, can have a substantial impact. Stress can result. Over time, ongoing pressure and overstimulation (or lack thereof) alter our behavior, emotional patterns, and perhaps more. Nerve-to-muscle feedback changes the overall level of tension across our bodies, in our organs, in our minds. While consistent, vigorous movement seems to be the most important way to balance these signals between nerves, muscles, and hormones, there may be some plants that can help as well.

I contend that digestion, which includes the liver's function of chemically altering individual molecules once they've been broken down and absorbed, may be the most directly understandable physiological hub: we all have an intimate relationship with our bellies. Additionally, the importance of healthy digestion, absorption, and metabolism in preventing and reducing inflammation throughout the body cannot be overstated. Much like a clean-burning furnace, strength in this system reduces by-products and irritants, smoke and smolder.

While we've known for some time about DNA and its role in providing the instructions for almost everything that our cells do, we are just recently beginning to understand how different subsets of these instructions can get turned on and off, and the implications appear to be far-reaching. There are connections to inflammation, aging, regeneration, and cancer. And as we learn more, it seems that plants are uniquely attuned to adjusting how the instructions are read, helping us unlock the right pieces for survival and control our own self-destructive power. This isn't a coincidence, and it isn't a result of laboratory analysis. We came of age as a species in a plant-filled world; our genetic instructions are what they are partly because of the influence of consuming lots of plants daily. We will see that some plants have a distinct ability in this area, and consuming them should probably become a daily habit once again.

Based on these key areas in human physiology, we will take another look at traditional herbal medicine and identify what kinds of plants might fit the bill. Oftentimes, systems of healing that have been around for a long time use the idea of taste to classify their medicines, and our approach mirrors this. Ultimately, three kinds of plants will emerge: the aromatics, the bitters, and the tonics (which can be both sweet and sour).

Aromatic plants usually contain oils that enter the air as vapors and reach our noses, providing a unique aroma. Certainly these have been forever prized as spices and are one of the first kinds of plant that children will spontaneously identify as interesting and perhaps medicinal. These same oils generally have a relaxing quality on organs or tissues that are in spasm, tight, or irritated, but they can also stimulate an overly sluggish or depressed situation (think of ginger, for example). What may be less obvious is that balance in this general level of tension can also mean balance in mental and emotional health—and employing this effect could perhaps buffer key aspects of the "modern malaise" syndrome. Aromatic plants open and relax us.

Bitter plants turn on the digestion, at all levels, and improve the metabolic function of the liver. As such, they may stoke a fire in the belly, but they actually reduce inflammation in the rest of the body. Additionally, they provide an important missing element to the Western diet: a challenge. Since industrialization and the centralization of food processing, we have been trying to make our food easier and easier to taste and consume. We'll see how this has led not only to overconsumption but also to stagnation, lethargy, and diminution of overall health.

Tonic is a concept unique to herbal medicine. It presupposes that you might be interested in doing something to enhance your health, even when you're not feeling any obvious symptoms or reading concerning test results. All these plants can normalize how our cells process the instructions in our DNA. Additionally, they seem to impact the way the immune system works and how it handles potential threats. And because changes in these systems take time to manifest, we will find that habitual use of tonics is vital. Thus tonics are generally nutritive and usually consumed with food or during mealtime.

In focusing on bitter, aromatic, and tonic plants in daily life, some may argue that I am overlooking the salty, mineral-rich greens and seaweeds that are often important components of traditional cuisines. I set these aside primarily for two reasons. First, the Western diet may be lacking a lot, but it certainly isn't lacking in saltiness. Second, a whole-food approach to eating usually contains a good measure of green, leafy vegetables, which tend to be the preeminent examples of the salty flavor in herbal medicine. My goal is not to provide general guidelines for eating, as I believe this is being well addressed already. Rather, I advocate for some of the flavors and plants that might be overlooked as we develop new ways of cooking and eating. In addition, I strive to provide an understanding of why you see plants one might call bitter, aromatic, and tonic in the recipes of almost all traditional cuisines. This is not a coincidence: these are plants we are meant to be eating, tasting, and benefiting from. Our physiology matured in the context of consuming them.

Plants that provide us with healthy oils are another important subset that may seem to be conspicuously absent. The right balance of fats in our diet is now recognized as an important factor to consider when thinking about inflammation, heart disease, mental health, and more. At the very least, we as a culture are becoming less afraid of fat and this gives me hope that healthy, plant-based oils and animal-based fats already have a growing place in the new Western diet. For this reason, I will set aside that discussion (with the understanding that we may not yet have heard the end of it).

In conclusion, this book is not designed to provide a guide for curing complaints, nor is it designed to be a compendium of medicinal herbs (though you will certainly find a lot of them within its pages). Rather, it strives to define a clear and understandable framework for using plants mindfully in daily life, based both on thousands of years of safe use and also a reasoned argument that draws on modern understanding. It focuses on what is easy and safe, and on what brings us to a state of more vibrant health while also connecting us to the world all around us. It seeks to provide ways to build and nourish, for prevention rather than for treatment. Therefore, it does not mention many of the "famous" plants on store shelves today. For these important additions to the three basic classes, see your local herbalist or other botanically minded health care provider. But, hopefully, if aromatics, bitters, and tonics feature prominently in your kitchen and garden, this will be a more infrequent occurrence.

The final point I hope to make is that the exploration of how plants work in our bodies may help us regain some trust in our skeptical lives. Certainly, a skeptical posture has served us incredibly well, and I do not mean to say that our first reaction to a new experience should not be a questioning one. What I will try to convey is an appreciation for how the interconnections found in nature have shaped us and a renewed acceptance of some of what our ancestors determined was important for a happy, healthy life. So skepticism, yes—but tempered somewhat by a heart willing to consider some of the old ways of doing things. This attitude may yet open our eyes to valuable knowledge as we probe deeply into the workings of medicine, physics, and ecology. But, in the short term, it can make for some exceptionally tasty and enlivening kitchen alchemy.

1
A Cuisine for Medicine

The challenge we face today is figuring out how to escape the worst elements of the Western diet and lifestyle without going back to the bush.

MICHAEL POLLAN, *IN DEFENSE OF FOOD*

While I was growing up in Ferrara, Italy, my father would pick up my sister and me from school almost every Wednesday in a small, yellow Fiat 500. This was usually right before lunchtime (school days were short in Italy, but you didn't get Saturday off). We would bump along cobblestone streets for a while and then stop outside a small shop that sold fresh-made pasta. I remember the smell of flour, and you could see some cooks in big white aprons mixing it with oil, eggs, and a little water to make noodles, lasagna sheets, or hand-shaped *cappellacci* ("bad hats," usually filled with squash). Others were grinding whole cuts of prosciutto to mix with herbs and parmesan cheese. This would serve as the filling for *cappelletti,* a delicious dumpling similar to tortellini that was a local specialty. It was for these we had stopped. We would pick up a pound or so, wrapped in waxed paper, take it back to the car, and head home.

For lunch, the cappelletti were cooked in a vegetable stock my mother had prepared ahead of time (she taught English on Wednesdays) by simmering carrots, celery, onions, and garlic. Sometimes we'd eat the leftover vegetables—soft and juicy, barely holding together, but delicious and salty—as part of the meal. Other times, we just ate the pasta in a steaming bowl of broth, seasoned with a little grated parmesan. There would often be a salad, and my dad might have a glass of wine. Dessert was a cup of sweetened chamomile tea. We would talk or listen to the radio and all clean up together. All simple things, really—but very meaningful. Nothing too special, either: variants on this ritual were taking place all over the city.

Cuisine means "kitchen." Kitchen, as opposed to restaurant. Kitchen, as opposed to supermarket. Kitchen, as opposed to gas station (where all too many find their food these days). By extension, cuisine is a set of kitchen habits that yield meals—meals usually prepared from simple, whole ingredients. Cuisine has matured over thousands of years and connects us to food, family, and our environment as few other things in life do. It is heartening to see a powerful movement in the United States that, at the beginning of the twenty-first century, seeks to reawaken (and reinvent) a strong, rooted cuisine that marries old ways of cooking with great new ideas on food production, distribution, and preparation.

One of the strongest voices articulating the case for a plant-centered, omnivorous cuisine in the United States is Michael Pollan. In *The Omnivore's Dilemma* he explores how we manufacture what we eat, visiting farms that embody the pinnacle of modern industrialized agriculture and also farms that offer a much more diversified, organic vision of how to produce and consume food. His analysis gives us clarity: in order to achieve good health, we need not focus on the complexities of food refining, processing, and nutritional reenriching (based on what Pollan calls "nutritionism"). Rather, we need to eat real food and prepare it in real ways, ways that involve simple recipes with simple ingredients. In the end, we get to health without overthinking, because, as we've found out, when it comes to nourishing ourselves, overthinking the process hasn't been at all helpful. And once we build a cuisine back into our lives, all sorts of other things change as well. You can't find the best tortellini without getting to know the shopkeeper. The best vegetables come straight from a farmer at a market stand, not from a regularly misted cooler. You've got to spend some time hanging out and talking with your kids while you make and share a meal. All these changes foster relationship and connection, and the results become evident in our environment, in our villages and neighborhoods, and in our homes.

I am particularly keen on this analysis because it comes from someone whose perspective includes the idea that, somehow, plants are driving human behavior and culture. One cannot read Pollan's account (in *The Botany of Desire*) of the tulip craze that swept Holland in the 1630s and not marvel at how these organisms, which have no feet and certainly no brains (as we know them), have employed us to serve their ends. They harness our desires. So when Pollan advocates for plants as a major, important component of cuisine, it's coming from a person who knows that they are our active partners and not just commodities. Again, we see a relational view of the world.

The "Slow Food" movement (proposed as an alternative to a common type of restaurant) began in Italy and has become another leading voice advocating for a real cuisine. Carlo Petrini started this global phenomenon by standing up to McDonald's in an effort to prevent it from opening a restaurant in historic, downtown Rome. Since then, the idea of regional food that celebrates traditional cuisine and is prepared with care has swept the Western world. In the United States there are myriad local chapters of Slow Food USA. They share recipes, gardening tips, and dinner-party schedules. At a national level, the organization is active in shaping legislation that affects food, such as the farm bill. It is a tangible manifestation of a shift that is happening in modern Western cuisine.

Another conscious food choice many people are making involves where their food is grown and made. The locavore movement seeks to support local agriculture and production, both for fruits, vegetables, meats, and grains and for value-added products, such as breads, sauces, cheeses, and beverages. Part of the concern here is the heavy investment in petrochemicals that centralized food production entails. But local food doesn't just have a smaller carbon footprint. If you support local production, you support smaller farms, farmers' markets, and local employment. You foster a community that comes together in the central square instead of the big-box-store parking lot. You might even get to know your farmer personally—or start raising chickens in your backyard. Nourishing ourselves with the plants and animals that breathe the same air, drink the same water, and walk on (or grow in) the same land as we do might have crucial repercussions for our individual health, too. Ultimately, the locavore movement strives for connection between people, land, and food—relationship-based eating at its best.

Our culture's understanding of the importance of real, whole food and where it comes from is increasing, and a new cuisine is being born. But I also hope to convince you that we might need to use some of these same ideas in our approach to achieving health and treating disease. Why do so many folks who buy all their food at the farmers' market also purchase dietary supplements that are packaged in plastic and shipped from far-flung corners of the country (or the world)? To say nothing of the centralized, industrialized production of conventional medication.

Our food certainly is the foundation of medicine, to paraphrase Hippocrates. But throughout history, human beings (and animals, too) have supplemented their diet with a range of substances to prevent illness, treat disease, and feel vibrant, inspired, and connected. It's sometimes hard to draw a line between what we eat and the medicines we use. Was that cup of chamomile tea at the end of lunch part of the meal or was it a therapeutic intervention? If you know anything about chamomile and its power to calm kids down, you might lean toward the latter categorization, but that's not necessarily a given. Other times the distinction is clearer. No one would consider a simmered pot of willow bark tea, perhaps used to treat arthritis, to be food or even a pleasant addition to a family meal. And it might even be lethal to approach a substance such as acetaminophen (Tylenol) with the same relaxed attitude on dosing that we see with carrots.

These, then, are my questions: Might there be a cuisine for medicine? Can the kitchen serve as a pharmacy, a place where we cook up what keeps us healthy alongside what keeps us fed? These are not unreasonable questions, nor do they imply that modern medicine is something we need to eschew. I support local food systems, but I still love a well-made cappuccino. So while a good meal is the foundation of health, I think that we can take the concepts of whole foods, organic foods, and local food production and apply them to medicine as well. In so doing, we might uncover safe, effective, and easy strategies for managing the malaise of modern life, empower ourselves to become more involved in our well-being, and discover local, whole remedies we can grow and prepare ourselves instead of consuming a machine-manufactured pill.

TRADITIONAL HERBAL MEDICINE

Of course, such a "cuisine" for medicine already exists: it is called herbalism. This practice of using whole plants as medicine is actually the dominant form of primary care around the world. Three-quarters of the global population relies on herbs to treat disease.[1] Modern innovations, such as surgical procedures and pharmaceutical agents, are useful complements to this age-old way of doing things, but in the United States they have supplanted it almost completely, much as the Western diet has supplanted real food. I think we can, and should, strive for a model where modern health care technology is used to supplement, rather than replace, traditional plant-based "slow medicine."

On every populated continent, there are ways of healing that are driven by the local flora, and they are as diverse as the cuisines with which they share a kitchen. Some have coalesced into nearly monolithic systems, though every valley still has its own variant on the classic recipes. Even in Europe, where, in the sixteenth century, Paracelsus began applying solvent extraction techniques to plants and may thereby have started us down the path to modern pharmaceuticals, traditional whole-plant remedies are still widely used. So modern medicine is not simply today's version of traditional European herbalism; it is a completely new and different phenomenon.

In the short term, contemporary medicine is unrivaled. Powerfully life-threatening imbalances, infections, and trauma are tended to systematically and effectively in ways that would have seemed magical or miraculous in Paracelsus's time. The process of research associated with modern medicine continues to generate new insights into and understanding of physiology, biochemistry, and pathology—all the while providing the tools for the effective management of more long-term, deadly diseases, such as cancer, HIV, and advanced heart disease. Babies born prematurely, some weighing less than two pounds, can survive and go on to full, healthy, engaged lives. Diseases such as polio have been eradicated—*eradicated!*—from vast sections of the planet. I cannot comment on the long-term ecological implications of these changes, but no one can doubt that their public health impact in the twentieth century has been huge.

The purpose of incorporating traditional herbal medicine into modern life is to try to find an accessible system for addressing much more common (and less scary) complaints, a system that is understandable and can be easily implemented. As we shall see, herbalism satisfies these criteria while also positing a relational approach to healing and, more importantly, to health itself. In this sense, it is much more like cooking: something we all can learn, something that connects us to the garden. Pharmaceuticals are often like sledgehammers swatting mosquitoes; I am simply proposing that there may be a point to the techniques of more traditional medical models. For some of the more complex diseases of twenty-first-century life, these techniques may offer real solutions where modern medicine all too often lacks a gentle enough touch.

People will always desire some measure of involvement in their health. Even the most uninterested among us still practice basic hygiene (mostly). I hope to convince you that simple herbal medicine offers an effective way to enhance health and that when it is used this way it poses no risk, while yielding real benefits. These qualities make it useful as a model for the modern consumer desiring health care empowerment. It reconnects us to a whole-plant ecology and provides clarity in a sea of "nutritionism"-based (to borrow Pollan's term) supplements, megadose vitamins, and druglike extracts. Its remedies stem from plants. They are real, they grow out of the soil, and they are alive. As we explore these plants, it will be worth examining the folk traditions to see what they have to say—both to get some guidance on how to best employ the herbs and also to see if traditional applications resonate with our modern understanding. In so doing, we might get some new ideas about what health really means.

One of the key strengths of a traditional medical system is the simplicity of the preparations that are used. Sure, there are some exceptions—just as there are in cooking. But crafting a simple distillation apparatus to make herbal spirits is just about as complex as it gets and certainly requires neither a chemistry lab nor analytical tools. A good soufflé might actually be more difficult to execute (at least for me). This immediately makes such a system accessible to a wide range of folks. You can grow, or often find wild, many of the remedies you might need for simple home care. And after you harvest them, it is very easy to prepare them for use.*

First and foremost, herbal medicine is interwoven into cuisine itself. Thyme, often used to season fish and seafood, warms the digestion and improves the "feel" of the meal as we assimilate it. Chicken

---

*Full details are beyond the scope of this work. See *Rosemary Gladstar's Herbal Recipes for Vibrant Health*.

soup with a lot of extra garlic supports the body when it's struggling with a respiratory infection. The roots of *Astragalus* and burdock, along with mushrooms, can be simmered into that same soup stock along with chicken bones and vegetables to promote resilience and help speed recovery from illness. And chocolate is divine taken hot in water, with a little local honey, and perhaps a pinch of cayenne pepper. Are these medicines or foods? Both! These few examples give us a feel for the role that medicinal plants have played in food preparation and should immediately give food lovers a new and exciting frontier to explore: recipes for our favorite dishes can be amended to include ingredients that have an application in keeping us healthy, vibrant, and inspired. Beyond that, it might be interesting to those who are passionate about their heirloom recipes to find that there is a strong physiological and medicinal basis for using the spices and combinations those recipes feature. It's not just about flavor.

Though I've been lucky enough to sample some tasty lemon balm–lavender cookies, these plants are usually reserved for another type of preparation that sits in the gray area between food and medicine—the infusion, or tea. More than just a beverage, tea can have profound effects when taken habitually, week after week.* This is another incredibly simple way to bring plants into your life. Herbs are harvested and dried, or purchased dry, and four or five tablespoons are steeped in a quart of hot water, covered, for anywhere from five minutes to five hours (it depends what you're going for). The infusion is then strained and taken with or without a little honey, hot or iced. Couldn't be easier—and many of the plants I'll explore in detail make delicious tea.

A more medicine-like preparation, though still quite simple, is the tincture. From the Latin *tingere,* meaning "to turn color" (the root of our word *tint*), it is simply an infusion that uses high-proof spirits instead of water. Herbs are steeped in 100 proof vodka and sealed

---

*One of my favorite arguments for the herbal infusion is from Susun Weed's *Healing Wise*. This book contains discussions for specific infusions throughout, but general thoughts start on page 261.

tightly in a mason jar for three or four weeks (herbalists usually wait one full cycle of the moon). Then they are strained out, the fluid is retained, and it is taken at doses that range from a few drops to a teaspoon or so. This is certainly a little closer to a pharmaceutical (and just one hundred years ago, that is precisely what it was). But these preparations still cross over into cuisine, primarily behind the bar, and we are starting to see them used in custom "medicinal" liqueurs and cocktails that claim to be useful for digestion, mental health, coughs and colds, and even spring allergies.*

All these simple ways of using plants can be incorporated into daily rituals that are performed in the kitchen. A drink before dinner may be custom-blended from a homegrown apothecary to suit the mood and complaints of the day. Afternoon tea may be a medicinal experience. And family meals can do more than simply nourish us with vibrant, local foods. With just a little attention to the recipe, they can help restore health and keep us well, using special ingredients that grow side by side with the tomatoes. It isn't hard to do, nor, as we shall see, is medicinal activity tied only to one rare, exotic, magical plant. There is broad crossover between species, and this fact leads us to one of the central arguments of this book: even if you only learn to use one of each kind of plant (an aromatic, a bitter, and a tonic), you will experience benefits. Though the full science and art of herbal medicine may be quite complex, it is also incredibly simple to get started and begin to see results.

Just as cuisine brings friends and family together and gathers threads of local food production, *terroir* (the unique flavor of the place where food is grown), and history, using herbal medicine opens up a relational view of health and well-being that ends up changing how we see the world. For example, it is hard to go back to store-bought produce once you've tasted a caprese salad made from your garden.

---

*Again, full details are beyond the scope of this book. See *Rosemary Gladstar's Herbal Recipes for Vibrant Health*. For a more recent take on the use of tinctures in medicinal cocktails, see Proville and Blunts', "Spring Medicinals."

Tomatoes still warm from the summer sun, hand-picked whole basil leaves, and thick slices of an almost-sweet, juicy, fresh mozzarella make all else pale by comparison. Experiencing this food makes you more mindful about future food choices, and once you've tasted homemade pasta dumplings in vegetable broth, it's hard to swallow the dehydrated, processed tortellini on the grocery store shelf. Similarly, once you've experienced better digestive health from the regular use of bitter plants, it starts to seem a little strange to use antacids, laxatives, or weird pink syrups to address the same symptoms.

Once you adopt a real food cuisine, your attitude toward food begins to change. How important then to start using medicine that is also based on traditional methods. There is a cultural (and biological) wisdom to these practices that has evolved over millennia to keep our day-to-day lives running smoothly. This wisdom also necessitates personal involvement, just as real food does. If we could get more involved in promoting our own health, the repercussions would be dramatic. I envision less stress on our overburdened primary care system; a greater range of preventive and curative strategies for the chronic diseases of modern life; and rich, abundant gardens where we cultivate both food and medicine. We can make this vision a reality by adopting strategies that are time-tested, often clinically studied, and effective. And instead of relying on "flavor-of-the-month" supplements, we can do it all using local, wild, easy-to-grow plants we've gotten to know personally—truly a cuisine for medicine.

WHAT KINDS OF PLANTS AND WHY— A SYSTEMS-BASED CONTEXT

Herbal medicine may have its strengths, but just because it's been around for thousands of years doesn't make it inherently valid. Certain examples come to mind—such as the use of kidney-toxic aristolochia[2]— which remind us that we can't just assume that traditional ways of doing things are automatically safe and effective. But my goal is not to use herbalism as a starting point for our investigation of plants; rather, I hope to use it as a touchstone for putting some of the botanicals in the following pages into context.

All in all, aside from a few cases (some of which involve adulteration or inappropriate use), herbal medicine is extremely safe. As Simon Mills and Kerry Bone, English and Australian medical herbalists, respectively, note: "Considering the vast usage around the world of plants as medicines, it is remarkable that there is so little epidemiological or clinical evidence that this is a harmful activity."[3] Indeed. Beyond this, I have chosen the safest examples to explore in this book, with only one (wormwood) being contraindicated in pregnancy. All the others are extremely benign plants—so you can begin working with them, confident that they will cause no harm.

But what about the overall efficacy of plants as medicine? This is a more difficult question. In order to arrive at an answer, I propose to start with physiology. Plants, after all, are complex, living systems interacting with the complex living system of the human being. This interaction takes place at multiple levels and is difficult to quantify completely using the tools of modern biochemistry (such as drug-receptor effects, for instance). If we can organize human physiology into broad patterns, we can see if plants might have an impact by examining how they interact with those patterns. We would thereby try to answer the question of efficacy by taking a relationship-based approach. This makes sense for a system of medicine that is so akin to cuisine.

How can we even hope to describe a broad system whereby herbs relate to human physiology? The sheer number of chemicals in a single plant, let alone all the plants used as medicine, is overwhelming. The genetic instructions, enzymes, cellular processes, organic functions, and integrative pathways in the human being are equally complex and, in many cases, appear disorganized or disconnected to our limited understanding. So what to make of this vastness? Let's start by examining an insight from Warren Weaver, a mathematician, scientist, and scholar of probability and complexity, writing in 1948.

What makes an evening primrose open when it does? Why does salt water fail to satisfy thirst? . . . What is the description of aging in biochemical terms? . . . [These] are all problems which involve dealing simultaneously with a sizable number of factors which are interrelated into an organic whole. They are all, in the language here proposed, problems of organized complexity.[4]

The system as a whole has an organization, a quality we can understand, that emerges from the interrelationship of its individual components. We may not fully grasp how each piece works, but that may not be absolutely necessary. This insight into how to understand complexity underpins a branch of scientific research now known as systems theory, which is essentially a study of reality based on broad patterns of interaction and interconnection in an ecosystem. Right around the same time, in the mid-twentieth century, Ludwig von Bertalanffy articulated the mathematical and theoretical underpinnings of systems theory as we know it today, in his classic paper titled "The Theory of Open Systems in Physics and Biology."[5]

Theoretical physicist Fritjof Capra studied in Austria but has lived in Berkeley, California, for many years. The deep level of both interconnection and uncertainty evident in the world of subatomic physics led him to seek new ways of understanding; as a result, he has become one of the world's leading systems thinkers. His articulation of systems theory is one of the clearest I have encountered. In essence, it describes a way of looking at a living ecology that allows us to more quickly grasp the important patterns of Weaver's "organized complexity": how to describe and predict its behavior without knowing all its individual parts. This is a departure from the driving thrust of human inquiry. Since we started using the scientific method, we've most often tried to break an ecosystem down into individual pieces to figure out how the whole works. In *The Web of Life*, Capra's model of systems theory offers a different view.

First, a system shows what are called "emergent" properties, qualities that cannot be predicted by its individual parts. We often refer to this quality in our daily experience as "synergy," and that underscores the importance of taking a step back and looking at the broader system. Without doing so, we might miss key features.

Second, all systems have multiple levels of organization. A city, for example, has a pattern of daily activity, with its inhabitants moving around in predictable ways, inputs flowing in, and waste and heat flowing out. But an individual neighborhood has its own pulse, too. It has particular centers where the community gathers, hubs of activity. And, of course, a home is its own little system, both in terms of its structure and its inhabitants. Individuals are distinct ecologies, too. You get the idea—organization exists at both the macro and micro levels. This fact, coupled with the mathematical counterpart of fractal geometry, which shows that systems exhibit similar patterns of organization at all levels,[6] comes together in the concept of holism: there exist complex, self-similar structures and relationships at all levels of life. When we look at life on a small scale, it looks and behaves in a remarkably similar fashion to life on a grand scale. This is actually a very old concept, though somewhat forgotten, perhaps best articulated by the hermetic philosophers. As rendered by Sir Isaac Newton, it goes something like this: "That which is below is like that which is above."[7]

Third, as we saw with cuisine and herbal medicine, systems theory focuses on the relationship and connection between components of a system. As Capra puts it, "In systems science every structure is seen as the manifestation of underlying processes."[8] A city is what it is because of how its inhabitants organize themselves into neighborhoods and how those communities interact with one another, more than because of its buildings and streets. The literal shape and structure of its buildings and streets is a reflection of those patterns of interaction. This firmly shifts our understanding of urban ecosystems into a fluid concept of life, rather than an abstract, fixed framework. This is evident in new urban planning ideas. No longer do we segregate our living and working arrangements into separate districts: downtown, shopping malls at highway exits, and residences in the suburbs. Mixed-use, walkable neighborhoods that focus on the patterns of daily life are now in vogue.[9]

One of the classic examples of systems-based thinking is the Gaia hypothesis, developed by James Lovelock and Lynn Margulis. In a seminal paper published in 1974, titled "Atmospheric Homeostasis by and for the Biosphere," they advance the notion that "early after life began it acquired control of the planetary environment" (page 1)—truly a radical notion at the time! The argument that the long-term control of atmospheric oxygen and temperature is due to a global web of microbes and algae was hard to swallow. It implied that there is a greater and more powerful biological "organism" at work on planet Earth than the human being, and that our very survival is contingent on this being and its ongoing health. Drawing in part on systems theory, Lovelock and Margulis examined the gaseous composition of Earth's atmosphere, going back billions of years,* and noted that levels of greenhouse gases (such as ammonia) fluctuated based on solar energy output in just the right ways to maintain conditions favorable for life.

Thus Gaia exemplifies the qualities of a complex, self-regulatory system as defined by Capra (and others). First, if taken as a whole, it has an emergent property. It can control atmospheric temperature and oxygen balance (not obvious when we examine its components—bacteria and blue-green algae). Second, it possesses multiple levels of organization, from the individual microbe and its cellular respiration to tidal pools, oceans, and the planet as a whole. Third, it is the response of the biological components to different temperatures and gas concentrations that truly defines the system, more than any absolute amount of either one. As ammonia and CO_2 levels go up, temperature rises and microbial metabolism decreases. This balance, this relationship, is the crucial point more than the bugs or the gases themselves.

---

*Lovelock's previous research had focused largely on the complex soup of atmospheric gases and what we can learn from altering it. For instance, see Lovelock and Giffen's "Planetary Atmospheres."

Another interesting application of systems theory is in the field of economics, where it is used to analyze and explain events that at first blush might appear unrelated. Some of the more interesting examples were collected by Albert-László Barabási, a physicist and systems theorist who has worked at Notre Dame and Northeastern University. Barabási takes systems theory one step further by using mathematics to analyze the systems themselves, delving into the relationships between their components. His focus is on the network of connections between the components of a system, and his research uncovered an important characteristic of such life webs.[10] Essentially, he proves that networks in systems like the living cell, ecosystems, cities, economies, and even the World Wide Web are characterized by a few, highly connected elements ("hubs") and lots of pieces that have only one or two links ("outliers").

Two interesting implications of this research relate to the global economy in recent years and how systems and networks function.* Right off the bat, it is easier for hubs to get "more"—more connections, more information, more resources. This process quickly snowballs. In our society, we see this embodied in a simple principle: the rich get richer. Not only do the rich control the vast majority of capital resources (they are hubs in the financial network, where the rest of us are outliers), their connections allow them to accumulate more resources at a much greater rate than everyone else.†

Additionally, a threat to a hub, which at first might seem to be of limited concern, can have much wider implications due to the high degree of interconnection the hub has with the rest of the network. A case in point is the bankruptcy of Lehman Brothers in September 2008. Here we have an extremely wealthy financial institution disappearing, essentially, from the ecology in which it was a major player. And while, rationally, one might have expected it to be dissolved in

---

*For details on network theory applied to economics, see Gabaix et al.'s "Theory of Power-Law Distributions."
†As evidenced in the story of Vernon Jordan, retold in Barabási's *Linked,* pages 202–4.

an organized fashion, exactly the opposite happened. Its collapse sufficiently disturbed the network to cause global repercussions in bankers' ability to move money and finance business. Immediate ramifications were felt from North America to Hong Kong. Long-term effects resonated for years across the financial markets worldwide.

As with Gaia, these are also examples of living systems. Economies behave in a complex fashion and display elements of synergy (witness, for instance, the corporate merger). They have self-similar (as above, so below) organization at all levels, from individual finance to families, corporations, sectors, and the world. And the importance of the connections over the components is clearly evident in events like the banking crisis of 2008. But when we look at these systems more closely, we see that they also exhibit the network characteristics described by Barabási. There are crucial hubs and, if something goes wrong—even if it seems like something small (a rumor on the stock exchange, say)—it reverberates throughout the network.

The point I want to make is that human physiology, which comprises the set of processes and functions that constitute the living human being, is a networklike system. It has all the characteristics of the open systems described by Weaver and von Bertalanffy. It has emergent qualities, such as consciousness (we still have no idea where that comes from);[11] it is broadly self-similar and highly organized at all levels, from the whole person to the individual cell; and it is all about the relationship between functional subsets, such as brain and heart, or liver and food. Most likely, physiology also demonstrates networklike behavior, where certain hubs are more connected than others. And, as is the case with nature itself, it exhibits characteristics of all living systems: spontaneous "breakthroughs" into new levels of complex emergent properties (so evident, I feel, in the development of young human beings) and sensitivity to small, habitual, insidious perturbations (such as those from diet).*

---

*Capra summarizes this well in *The Web of Life,* pages 192–93.

Some physicians and researchers have already begun to develop models of the human being as a system, seeking to address disease by looking at processes and patterns of activity, rather than the static anatomy of the body. One example is put out by the Institute for Functional Medicine.[12] It stresses the importance of identifying the context in which the patient lives, the processes (such as assimilation and metabolism, defense and repair, and communication between subsets of the system) that take place, and "personalizing factors" (such as sleep, exercise, nutrition, and relationships) that modify the way the processes behave. From these factors, we can see some disease as emergent qualities of a complex system, and attempt to intervene using gentler "perturbations" that might have safer, longer-lasting results.

Of course, one need not look to twenty-first-century science to find a description of the human being that relies on function and broad patterns of activity, rather than a dissection of our anatomical components. This has, in fact, been the language of traditional medicine all along. It speaks of moisture and dryness, of a fire in the belly both burning our food for energy and circulating vitality through our core, of tension and tone across multiple organ systems, of ecological context. This is a language of weather, of seasons, of flux and change. It speaks in allegories that may actually be amazingly accurate descriptions of process-based emergent qualities in the organized chaos we call life. And, crucially, it proposes an idea that is absent from a system of medicine based on disease analysis: that health, and life, can be fostered, encouraged. Through this lens, well-being is not a state that exists in the negative, occurring once all disease is removed. Rather, well-being is the result of positive nourishment. It is something we can, and should, work to create.

THREE KEY PHYSIOLOGICAL "HUBS"

If the human being comprises a networklike system, what are its crucial nodes? Traditional systems of physiology have some interesting notions.

For instance, the Galenic four humors, based on Hippocratic ideas and evolving into four "temperaments,"[13] are energies, or states of being, that can commingle and whose balance affects personality and physiology. Similar fluid- or energy-based models are also used in Ayurveda, a system of healing from the Indian subcontinent.[14] Paracelsian alchemy reduces life to three basic processes: the sulfur, a kind of personality/ soul; the salt, our physical organs, muscle, bone, and sinew; and the mercury, the common thread uniting the whole. There are numerous animist healing practices around the world that rely on spiritual powers being present in places, plants, waters, and more—and through their interactions, fostering well-being.* And classical Chinese medicine relies on five processes, which also represent states of change, to summarize the human system.[15]

What's most intriguing to me is that we can even devise such a simple way of viewing the human being. After all, medical understanding is extremely broad and deep, and superficial knowledge can be extremely dangerous. You have to know how all the details interact before you can proceed safely. The complexity of physiology makes it seem unapproachable to the layperson.

Yet perhaps this isn't really the case. There are a few problems with the whole notion. The first issue is that we will never know *all* the details of human physiology. Wide areas of understanding, ranging from consciousness and thought to the expression and regulation of our genome, are still elusive. No matter how complex the description, it will always remain incomplete. Traditional, systems-based understandings aren't any simpler (lifetimes are spent on the details, just as in biomedicine), they just have a better-characterized top-level network. The second issue is that danger only seems to arise when you take a single, isolated substance and apply it at a specific level of the physiological system. Traditional herbal medicine has never had this option (aside from a few well-known poisons, of course). It has always

---

*For an ethnobotanical overview of many of these traditions, see Grossinger's *Planet Medicine.*

employed complex chemical cocktails (i.e., plants) to treat the complexity of human physiology. Could this be part of the reason behind its safety? Ironically, the tools of biomedicine might be more dangerous because they get *too* deep into a piece of the network.

To illustrate, consider the example of the yohimbe tree, *Pausinystalia yohimbe,* which grows in West Africa. Its bark is traditionally used as an aphrodisiac, and an alkaloid it contains, yohimbine, has been extensively researched clinically and found to be quite effective.[16] It works by dilating the arteries and improving blood flow to erectile tissue—but biomedicine clearly warns us that it also "turns off the brakes" on our adrenaline response. Under the right circumstances, this might raise heart rate and blood pressure. This could be dangerous in someone with heart disease—and you'd never be aware of this fact unless you took the time to understand "the nature of the hypothalamic response to alpha-2-receptor antagonism." This, at least, is the basic argument.

Traditional herbal medicine has a two interesting responses, and both show systems thinking at work. First, you'd be unlikely to give someone yohimbe if he already had heart disease, even without knowing anything about alkaloids, receptors, or blood pressure. The medicine from the yohimbe tree, so the story goes, is like an August afternoon—hot, potentially oppressive, sweaty.[17] It's not going to mix well with a person who is red, maybe angry, overstressed, with a fast and full pulse. You might choose a range of other aphrodisiacs, thus avoiding any potential danger, thanks to a crude, energy-based assessment of the situation. Second, even if you did decide to use yohimbe (some people with high blood pressure are cool, quiet, and have weak pulses—though in my experience such an individual is rare), it would be administered as a whole plant, not as the isolated constituent. The bark you'd use has a wide range of other chemicals in it, including the alkaloid ajmaline,[18] which reduces high blood pressure while calming and steadying the heartbeat.[19] I'm not trying to say that all plants are danger-free, though, certainly, the vast majority are. This example just serves to illustrate how using systems theory in our approach to physiology and treatment might uncover useful, safe, and—most important—understandable methods.

Now, rather than borrowing a traditional system for our exploration of how to define a "cuisine for medicine," I'd like to take what we've learned from our exploration of systems theory, networks, and their applicability to health and come up with a very basic, top-level organization for biomedicine. Once we have a solid but straightforward framework in place, we can assess how medicinal plants fit in to the modern perspective on physiology. It comes down to this: we need a simple network that describes Western physiology (and pathology) in crude enough terms so that we can begin to see how a crude plant might fit into it. And what we'll find, ultimately, is that looking at the kinds of plants people have always used frames the physiology fairly well. System to system, we can tame complexity and reveal useful information along the way.

The first hub in our physiological network is the ongoing balancing act known as *neuromuscular tone*. This refers to the collection of processes that occur in our body and mind and relate to how tight our muscles are and how active our mind is. Too tight, and we literally get tension, spasm, blockage, and poor circulation. Too loose, and we have sluggishness, fatigue, and poor motor and mental response. Interestingly, because nerves from the body connect to the brain, tension and laxity are reflected in the mind as well—producing anxiety in the former case and depression in the latter.

I propose that, when taken as a whole, the nerves and muscles of the body act as a sort of "pacemaker" of activity, helping us respond effectively to the world's changes by adjusting internal tension as needed. Making sure this hub is functioning well is extremely important. Not only does an imbalance in neuromuscular activity impact physical tension and mental health, but through our hormonal system it exacerbates chronic pain, poor digestive function, blood pressure disorders, and heart disease. And we can all relate to how powerfully our mood plays into everything we experience.

Neuromuscular tension is, ultimately, about how we deal with stress. How we process and internalize stress ultimately makes the difference in how we feel. Exercise may be the best intervention for rebalancing this hub of physiological activity—it improves mental health but also addresses cardiovascular disease.[20] Additionally, key botanicals can play an important role as well. The hope is that by addressing the level of tension in our body and mind, we can buffer the impact of stress on our physiology, and perhaps reduce our reliance on antidepressants, anti-anxiety drugs, stimulants, and sedatives, the use of which has become so pervasive in our society.

The second hub in the physiological network is digestive and metabolic activity—the combined set of processes that deliver nutrition and energy from what we eat to our cells. There are many components to this hub, starting with digestion but involving other organ systems along the way—most notably the liver and the pancreas, key chemical processing centers and balancers of blood sugar. We will find that there are important connections between all these constituent parts and that the whole process of digestion, absorption, and metabolism weakens other areas when it's not functioning well. For instance, big swings in blood sugar figure prominently in type 2 diabetes; elevated blood sugar levels lead to inflammation in blood vessels and cause premature hardening and dysfunction of our arteries.[21]

I propose that what has been called *metabolic syndrome*—a combination of high blood pressure, obesity, and diabetes[22]—is an imbalance in the function of this physiological hub and that the imbalance begins in the digestive system, its rate of movement, and its secretions. It continues in and is perpetuated by dysfunction in the liver and pancreas. Obviously, dietary modification is the key intervention in this area, and here the efforts of Pollan as well as chefs like Alice Waters of Chez Panisse in Berkeley, California, have helped enormously. There is also an important and storied class of plants that positively affects all the elements of digestion, absorption, and metabolism. Here, we will see how everyday digestive complaints (for which modern medicine has little to offer) and blood sugar imbalance are buffered by botanical medicines. They can allow us to live in a more toxic world, surrounded by petrochemicals and processed foods, without our physiology suffering. As a result, good food and some key plants might reduce the massive impact that metabolic syndrome has on primary care in this country—all in the context of the kitchen.

The third and final hub in our physiological network is a bit harder to describe, as it involves functions and activities taking place in each cell of our body. In essence, it is the collection of processes that takes our genetic instructions (encoded in DNA) and turns them into reality. We are becoming increasingly aware that our genetic blueprint is by no means set in stone. Rather, its translation into the phenotype (our physical structure and, by extension, all the emergent properties that come with it) is quite flexible and intimately connected to the surrounding environment.

This hub of the network, though evident at a smaller scale, has the most profound and wide-ranging macroscopic impacts. Most notably, the regulation of gene expression ties in closely to immune activity and inflammation, key components in the etiology of cancer but also the perpetuation (or resolution) of chronic inflammatory diseases. Tissues, made of cells, respond as a whole and behave according to how each cell behaves—so alterations in gene expression are visible in such disparate organs as respiratory mucous membranes, bone marrow, and the brain. Again, diet plays a key role in balancing this hub, too, but the dietary elements that seem to be involved appear to come from more wild plants than, say, potatoes or tomatoes. Chemicals, such as bioflavonoids and other polyphenols, are getting a lot of attention as regulators of gene expression, and they are abundant in medicinal herbs.

By examining these botanicals, we will find a deep connection with the natural world that reverberates through our entire physiology, from the tissue to the cellular nucleus (and probably beyond—we just haven't explored those levels yet). The hope here is that their reintroduction will lower cancer rates, address immune dysfunction, and minimize the impact of chronic inflammatory disease (from "simple" ailments, such as osteoarthritis, to more complex conditions, like lupus). These plants resonate through our history as a clear tone rings through an open space, and bringing them back into our lives may be one of the best ways to deal with (or prevent) the mysterious ailments that continue to haunt us, and for which modern medicine has, at best, palliative drugs and, at worst, outright poisons.

How can we be sure that these three "hubs"—neuromuscular tone, digestive/metabolic activity, and genetic expression—are truly a comprehensive enough "top-level" description of the human physiological network? In a practical sense, the answer to this question makes no difference. If anyone could propose a viable system that would positively impact stress and mood, diabetes and metabolic syndrome, cancer, and chronic inflammatory disease, then I would respond with a resounding "Let's get started!"

Taken together, these diseases have a huge impact on modern productivity and quality of life. They are also the areas where modern medicine, despite its stunning successes elsewhere, has fallen short—which is not surprising, given how hyperspecialized the discipline has become. We are ready for new (or is it old?) ideas to come into play.

These three hubs cover most of the areas of health that a layperson could hope to treat safely at home. Massive infection—forget about it. Broken bones—take me to the emergency room. Kidney disease and pneumonia—though a skilled herbalist might have something to offer, both of these are relatively rare conditions nowadays, and areas where modern medicine excels. Given how strongly immunity and inflammation figure in all disease processes, adjusting the function of our third metabolic hub might help in these more dire cases, too. One final area that may be an exception is fertility and reproductive health. There are interesting options in traditional plant-based healing modalities that might have a role to play here as well. I do not address them specifically, not only to maintain simplicity and clarity, but also because the rebalancing of our second hub—metabolic function (vis-à-vis the liver)—affects reproductive hormone status. If you are interested, there are numerous resources available.*

This simple, three-part network provides a way to understand and relate to physiology that is accessible and practical, and one with which we can all identify because we see and feel its effects daily. Additionally, it offers a context within which we can assess the effectiveness of traditional plant remedies by highlighting their strengths: systems interacting with systems. So, in the end, the case to be made is that these plants, which are simple to grow and prepare and yet quite complex in their nature, can affect these three physiological hubs in powerful, predictable, and consistent ways. I hope to show you that such a case can successfully be made, and that the implications underscore the importance of bringing traditional medicine back into the cultural mainstream in order to cope with the vicissitudes of modern life.

Taking up our wild weeds, let us walk into the field and forest together, mindful that, when we return to our homes and communities, we will be changed, more entangled, more infused with the green blood of our botanical companions. What this will do to our culture I cannot predict, but I hold great hope that the benefits far outweigh the risks.

---

*Among the best are DeLuca's *Botanica Erotica* and Green's *The Male Herbal*.

2
Aromatics

Open and Flow

Let the fragrance of the Eye of Horus adhere to thee.
Fire of incense.
O Pharaoh, I have come, I have brought to thee the Eye of
Horus,
That thou mayest equip thine face with it, that it may
purify thee,
That its fragrance may [come] to thee.

THE PYRAMID TEXTS,
"RITUAL OF BODILY RESTORATION OF THE
DECEASED, AND OFFERINGS,"
LINES 18D, 20A, 20B CA. 2300 BCE

In darkness, or perhaps faint candlelight, deep in the vaults of the pyramid, an Egyptian royal embarks on the journey to the afterlife. His priest—who has already overseen the elaborate preparation of the ruler's body through ten weeks of disemboweling, bathing, curing, and anointing with highly scented plants—has lit the incense and a warm smoke begins to rise in the cavernous space. The recipe for this incense has been closely guarded for many years, a precise mixture of pine resin and honey, frankincense and myrrh, juniper, cypress, calamus, and cinnamon.* It is everyone's hope that, after the priest utters the spells of reanimation, the pharaoh will take his place in the underworld and continue his rule under the influence of Osiris. As the smoke from the aromatic plants permeates the hall, memories are evoked, consciousness is shifted, and all participants begin to occupy a space that is not just physically, but also psychically, different. Without being intoxicating, the incense nevertheless has an effect.

The smells in this ritual are carefully orchestrated for the express purpose of evoking this shift in consciousness. They serve as a message to the gods above (smoke always rises) as well as those of the underworld. They tap into deep-seated patterns of association, linked to a unique fingerprint, while relaxing the body and focusing the mind on the task at hand. For the pharaoh, the aromatic oils and resins used in mummification literally ensure near immortality (of his physical tissue, at least) by sterilizing his body and helping to preserve it for thousands of years.

Later, after everyone has left through narrow, tortuous passageways, the participants of lesser rank will speak in hushed tones about the experience and about the indescribably magical air—its feel, its smell—as the pharaoh embarked on his journey. The entire ritual will be forever embodied in the aromatics, and a chance waft of calamus reed and spices in the marketplace might immediately bring them back to it, if even for a moment.

But before beginning his ceremony, the priest may have consumed a special brew made with many of the herbs he used to prepare the incense, steeped perhaps in a little of the best wine. I can imagine the same aromatics first entering his stomach, where they are warmed and, like the incense, try to rise upward. Finding nowhere to go, they make their way onward through the narrow, tortuous passageways of the

---

*There are many recipes for this famous incense blend known as *Kyphi*. For example, see Manniche's *Sacred Luxuries*.

small intestine and into the priest's blood, through the tangle of the liver, to the heart, and, from there, finally, to the cavernous chambers of the lungs. Here, as the rooms shrink and expand in a great, synchronized, rhythmic pulse, the aromatics find an outlet, rise up and out of the warm blood, mix with the great and swirling winds, and rush out on the breath.

Is the use of plants necessary to bring one to the trancelike, fluid state of consciousness so often sought in traditional rituals and religious ceremonies? Certainly not. Many of the same effects can be achieved through meditative practice, either using the mind, the body, or both. Zazen achieves this. Martial arts achieve this. Running achieves this. The list goes on and on. But it has always been fascinating to me that traditional cultural systems feature some form of smell, some use of aromatic herbs, in their most important rituals. Frankincense will forever be associated in my mind with the high, vaulted cathedrals of Catholic Italy. Native people of the Western Hemisphere employ *Artemisias* (sagebrush), cedar, and other highly scented plants in their ceremonies. In East Africa, citrus peel and cinnamon are mixed for nerves and palpitations.[1] Aboriginal culture in Australia often uses aromatic plants, especially in rituals to drive away "evil spirits" and evil influences. Eastern cultures, from India through Indonesia, China, and Japan, feature elaborate incense blends that employ the abundant resinous and aromatic plants found locally.* Oftentimes, some or all of these blends are also consumed as part of meals or special brews. What we will find is that there are very good reasons for this similarity of use across the world and that it often comes down to dispelling harmful influences on the mind and body, helping to relax and attune people who consume them to the flow of events around and within them.

Ceremony marks change, marks transition. We set milestones in

---

*For an excellent overview of aromatherapy, consult Lis-Balchin's *Aromatherapy Science*. The first two chapters provide a brief overview of the history, definitions, and traditional ethnobotanical uses of scent in many cultures.

our lives not only to remember important events, but perhaps even more to acknowledge that our existence is changing, moving into a new phase. So we pass into adulthood, marry, celebrate the birth of our children, ritualize the deaths of our forebears, and perform countless other ceremonies, both in our community and in private. They range from the very simple (a cup of tea on a bright, cool morning and an intention set for the day's work) to the elaborately complex (I've been to some incredible weddings). Something special happens during these times, something akin to the shift experienced deep inside the pyramid, something that attunes us to the flow of events around us. We turn to ceremony during these peak times because attunement to the flow of events simply makes us feel better, more connected, and more at peace with the tumult of change. And we almost always include aromatic plants in these ceremonies.

It's a good thing that we have learned to do this, because in nature we see constant tension. One could argue that our entire environment is in a near-permanent state of change, pushing and pulling between poles of flux. The Chinese, among others, recognized this long ago, detailing the interactions of yin and yang, the one growing, wrestling, struggling, and eventually changing into the other. Seasons move from cold and dry to hot and moist, with transitions characterized by rapid oscillations between the extremes of each and usually accompanied by intense winds. Inside us, different levels of tension and tone characterize different periods of our lives: waking and sleeping, activity and rest, adolescence and senescence. The whole of our internal milieu is a living ecosystem in and of itself. We have our own tensions, seasons, and fluctuating populations. Big upheavals in our lives are reflected in this internal environment. Just like storms and hurricanes in meteorology, traditional systems of medicine liken these upheavals to a sort of inner "wind," often troubling the mind and the belly, or manifesting as areas of shifting tension in the body.

Instinctively, plants with strong smells seem connected to wind, or at least to the air. Their presence may be noticed on the breeze before you even see them. So perhaps they could have a connection to the internal "wind" that arises during times of tension and change, and this might help explain why we so often turn to them in our ceremonies of transition. The Chinese text *Neijing* (*The Yellow Emperor's Classic of Medicine*; I recommend Maoshing Ni's translation), which was most likely composed between 400 BCE and 200 BCE, tells the story of Huang Di, the yellow emperor, a mythical figure who was well-known as a child prodigy and brought ideas about divination, Taoist philosophy, and medicine to the empire. He is found in his court, or outdoors near rivers and in the forest and countryside, looking at tortoise shells and discussing matters that relate to life, health, and balance with his ministers and advisors.

One day Huang Di asks Qi Bo, one of his most trusted counselors, what the secret of preserving health is. Qi Bo, in his usual piercing wisdom, replies: "Every individual's life is intimately connected with Nature. How people accommodate and adapt to the seasons and the laws of Nature will determine how well they draw from the origin or spring of their lives. . . . When one can manage the polarity changes of the Universe, one will have clarity and not be confused by any disorder."[2] But how might we go about measuring how well we are managing? How can we quantify our state of internal tension, so we can see how aromatic plants might affect it?

HEART RATE VARIABILITY, OR THE CASE OF THE HAPPY FETUS (AND THE HAPPY HEART)

The method of divining people's internal physiological state by listening to their hearts or feeling their pulses has a long and storied history. In China again, pulse reading has been elevated to a fine art.* Other

---

*For an accessible and clear description of pulse assessment in traditional Chinese medicine, see Ted J. Kaptchuk's *The Web That Has No Weaver*. This book has lots more there than just pulse diagnosis, but it's one of the most easily understandable ways to approach this subject without actually holding the wrists of hundreds of people—and it includes a great story of a Tibetan pulse-reader making an accurate diagnosis on the cardiac ward.

branches of Asian medicine have also valued more about the pulse than simply its speed. Ibn Sina (more commonly known as Avicenna), the brilliant eleventh-century Persian doctor who brought European medicine out of the dark ages and gave us the concept of clinical trials, wrote extensively on the pulse in his *Canon of Medicine,* emphasizing how it changed and moved in response to different stimuli.[3] Beyond the historical context, one hears recurrent stories of traditional practitioners holding a patient's radial artery for five, fifteen, or thirty minutes and obtaining the same, accurate diagnoses that require lab and imaging work costing thousands of dollars in a hospital. While I make no such claims in my practice, I often examine the character and quality of blood flow in my clients. When I feel the pulse coursing through someone's wrist, I note its obvious characteristics first, but then "settle in" for a while and try to get a feel for how it changes, moment to moment and minute to minute, in an attempt to get a handle on its variability. All these exemplify traditional ways to gauge a person's internal state of tension, her attunement to and comfort with the changes that are molding her life.

European medicine has its own history of exploring how the heartbeat varies moment to moment, and what this may mean. The biomedical model has actually become quite sophisticated in its ability to assess the internal state of health and psychological tension in an individual by examining the heart rate. As usual, however, it's a bit late to the party and relies on mathematics and machinery rather than a visceral understanding. But the results are no less fascinating or important. The story begins in Europe.

Eighteenth-century England was a time and place of great intellectual ferment: James Watt was developing steam engines to drive the mining industry; Erasmus Darwin (Charles's grandfather) was practicing medicine with opium, heavy metals, and newly discovered "alkaloids" from plants as his mainstay pharmacological agents; Josiah Wedgwood was creating new kinds of pottery based on techniques brought from China; and poets, such as William Blake, were documenting the spirit of this romantic era. Widespread, methodical scientific discovery was in its infancy, and advances from this time (such as the recognition that air was made of multiple gases) would end up powering the industrial revolution. Additionally, the state of understanding was such that "generalists" (those who dabbled in many fields of research) could still make substantial breakthroughs. It was an exciting time in European history—a period when the potential and promise of scientific inquiry was burgeoning.*

In this environment Stephen Hales, a parson, chemist, plant and animal physiologist, and inventor (many were inventors at that time), performed his research on the changes in heart rate observed in animals; horses in particular. His experiments were very simple and certainly crude by today's standards; nevertheless, he provided us with the first scientifically documented example of a heart rate variability (HRV) pattern. That is to say, he came up with the first description in Western medicine of how the changes in beats per minute of the heart mirrored other physiological processes consistently and predictably. His discovery has been expanded on substantially but remains important today.†

Hales documented what is now called "respiratory sinus arrythmia" (RSA), which basically means that he observed pulse rates in horses increasing when they are breathing in, and returning to a normal baseline when they are exhaling.[4] This happens consistently and is something you can easily observe in yourself. Feel your pulse for a few seconds, just to get an idea of your "normal." Then take a big, deep breath. Your pulse rate will increase, reach a peak just before your lungs fill completely, and come back down again. This fluctuation occurs in most mammalian species and may not seem like much of a revelation. If you are like me, you may immediately think that there is a simple explanation for what is happening, something along the lines of extra

---

*See *The Lunar Men,* Uglow's thoroughly entertaining and personal glimpse into mid-eighteenth-century England.
†For a biography of Hales, see Clark-Kennedy's *Stephen Hales.*

pressure in the chest "squishing" the heart and making it beat faster when the lungs are full of air. But it turns out that the real answer is a bit more elusive and interesting.

Medical science began work on what would be three separate fronts, attempting to characterize what was occurring during RSA: (1) the physiological research front tried to explain the causes for the effect; (2) in the clinic, physicians began to explore what types of illnesses might be related to the same physiological basis; and (3) eventually, those interested in mental health focused on what this all might mean for mind and mood.[5]

Franciscus Cornelius Donders, the youngest of nine (and the only boy—much to his parents' delight, though probably not his), was a physiologist who began his professorship in 1847 at the University of Utrecht, in the Netherlands, at age twenty-nine. His research focused on how the brain connects to the rest of the body: how blood nourishes it, how long it takes for nerve impulses to travel up to it, and, crucially for our discussion, how it and the nervous system might link heart rate to respiration. In 1868 he identified the vagus nerve, a long, twining fiber that leaves the skull and connects to the salivary glands, lungs, heart, and gut, shuttling signals and information between them, as the probable "relayer" in the case of RSA.[6] It seemed that information on respiration was being sent up to the brain on the same bundle of nerves that carried heart rate information and that these signals were possibly integrated ("talking" to each other and modulating each other) somewhere in the brain stem (all of which has been repeatedly confirmed, even through today).* As the research progressed into the twentieth century, it became clear that the greater, more regular, and more frequent the shifts in heart rate noticed during RSA, the greater the amount of "tone," or activity, in the vagus nerve bundle.

---

*See, for instance, Grossman and Kollai's research, detailed in "Respiratory Sinus Arrhythmia."

This point is worth reemphasizing because it is the central idea that physiological research has brought to the understanding of HRV: the heart rate itself varies, yes, but the *way* it varies (that is, the pattern in the variations) changes depending on how much activity is occurring along the vagus nerve. So when the vagus nerve is more active, the variations in heart rate noticed during RSA become more substantial and somewhat more frequent, and, also, apparently, a bit more regular. In other words, when changes in HRV become more regular and oscillate from one peak to the next over the period of about seven to ten seconds (or about 0.15 Hz to 0.1 Hz) it is safe to assume that the vagus nerve is more active. But if the changes in HRV are less regular, or oscillating at lower frequencies (if any regular pattern can be detected at all), it usually indicates that other forces are at work.

So take this example: you are sitting quietly, breathing normally, and hooked up to a device that gives you your instantaneous heart rate (by very precisely measuring the time between heartbeats, and translating that to a beats-per-minute figure). If you've ever used a heart rate monitor in the gym, then you know what I'm talking about (though you may not have been sitting quietly). Let's say your beats-per-minute count starts at 65. Over the course of five seconds or so, it gets up to 70. Then, over the next five seconds, it goes back down to 65. And the cycle of up and down keeps repeating itself, roughly every ten seconds. You are experiencing a recurrent change in heart rate: your HRV pattern is clearly visible and repeats regularly about every ten seconds. Then, the cat knocks over that same flowerpot again. So much for that . . .

This line of physiological inquiry has brought us to the concept that, by measuring the patterns of change in heart rate, we can divine something about what's happening internally,[7] especially as it relates to the vagus nerve and its level of activity. This nerve is the messenger of the "rest-and-digest" side of our system, the countervailing current to the "fight-or-flight" response, the yin to our yang. So perhaps these regular, ten-second fluctuations in heart rate might tell us that we are in a state that is relatively less "fight-or-flight," relatively less stressed, relatively less tense. Now we're getting somewhere.

But we can't draw any firm conclusions until we examine a bit of the research on the clinical side of things. To get a handle on whether measuring changes in heart rate variability can tell us anything about what a person is truly experiencing, what his level of distress (or peaceful appreciation) might be, we need to be able to track the HRV fluctuations, while at the same time monitoring a disease process or any other type of life-changing event. If aromatic plants have an effect on our internal state of tension, helping us move more peacefully with the flow of events all around us—as I contend—we need to first make a clear link between HRV and that internal state of tension. If this two-way link is conclusively established, then we might set out to see whether aromatic plants have an effect on HRV fluctuations. The whole reason we are even discussing HRV is to arrive at a more objective assessment of inner stress than is given by answering the question "How's it going?"

It turns out that the first clinical observations on the significance of HRV fluctuations were conducted by obstetricians.[8] Makes sense, right? Not only is birth perhaps the first (and maybe most dramatic) life-changing event, but a fetus has precious few variables to disrupt its HRV fluctuations. Either it is getting what it needs or it isn't. Worldly concerns do not trouble it (yet). It cares about the nutrition it's getting, how Mom is doing, whether that umbilical cord is out of the way, and, once labor begins, how those contractions are going.

Scientific monitoring of the fetal heart rate, including discussion of its variability, began with Edward Hon, an obstetrician who was working at Yale in 1958. His first insights centered on heart rate decelerations— periods when the fetus's heartbeat slowed down considerably.[9] This would usually happen during labor but sometimes even during routine prenatal observation. As you can imagine, he quickly found that these drops in heart rate could be bad signs. Furthermore, once a series of pronounced decelerations occurred, things were usually pretty far along in the bad direction. Dr. Hon needed a little more warning. He began to notice that regular fluctuations in the fetal heart rate would start to "flatten out," or disappear, before the big decelerations started, and he began to find that a loss in fetal HRV was associated with a distressed state.[10]

Dr. Hon was monitoring his patients using a modified electrocardiogram (the machine that measures the electrical activity of the heart using electrodes strapped to the body). This gave him useful information and allowed him to glimpse how the ups and downs of the fetal heart rate might indicate how well things were going inside the uterus. But it was Konrad Hammacher, an obstetrician and researcher in Düsseldorf, Germany, who took it to the next level.

On most evenings, after his long shifts at the Women's Hospital in Düsseldorf, Dr. Hammacher returned to the medical school and worked on developing a machine that might record patterns in fetal heart rate and also the contractions of the laboring mother's uterus. Usually contractions brought on a slight fetal heart rate deceleration at about the same time, but a more pronounced deceleration shortly *after* a contraction was associated with a more dangerous situation. So it would be useful to have a machine that could record both the heartbeat of the fetus and the contractions of the uterus at the same time. That way, an obstetrician could see the fetal heart rate, its variability, its accelerations and decelerations, and how they related to maternal contractions all on one strip of paper. He decided the best way to do this was to have his machine listen for fetal heart sounds (rather than electrical activity) and measure pressure coming from the mother's abdomen (which increases as the uterus contracts). By continuously recording these two measurements on paper at the same time, and later teaming up with Hewlett-Packard to mass-produce the device he came up with, Dr. Hammacher invented the modern cardiotocograph, or electronic fetal monitor, which is a crucial tool in the practice of obstetrics today. In effect, watching its output over time is much like holding a person's radial artery pulse, and equally as fascinating: we get a deep appreciation of her internal state.

Doctors today describe the ideal output from these machines as showing a fetal heart rate between 110 and 160 beats per minute, with "moderate" variability (the line is squiggly), and no "late decelerations" (slowdowns that occur after the uterine contractions).[11] One of the worst signs to witness: the fetal heart rate trace loses all variability, and turns from a squiggly, ever-changing, ever-adapting tightrope walker to a flat, smooth curve. That indicates that the living system of the fetus is losing its capacity to adapt to and integrate with the changes in its environment. In other words, it is dying.

Most traditional cultures burn aromatic plants, or strew them about, during labor and birth. Monks in Lhasa use local cedar and wormwood. In India and Persia, frankincense is burned for forty days and nights, starting the night of a birth, to honor mother and child and "dispel evil." This practice is echoed in the New Testament story of the birth of Jesus. Roman culture used floral incenses and waters (featuring lots of rose) in preparation for, during, and after labor. And while some have talked about the antiseptic qualities of most aromatic plants as being the "original reason" for using them in the context of birth, as well as an explanation for their power to "dispel evil" (that is, germs), or simply to cover the sometimes unpleasant odor of childbirth, I contend that their principal use stemmed from the plants' ability to modulate both maternal and fetal stress and tension.[12] These represent the "evil" traditional cultures are attempting to dispel. Thus it is not surprising to me that modern research shows that exposure to aromatics reduces maternal and fetal stress, evidenced by an increase in high-frequency heart rate variability patterns—waves peaking every seven to ten seconds. As a tightrope walker might tell you, more frequent adjustments are better.

In the fetus, the complete loss of heart rate variability is one of the strongest clinical signs of fetal distress. But going back to the physiological research on HRV, recall that the "low-stress" state was characterized by a roughly six-to-nine cycles per minute oscillation in heart rate (equivalent to a maximum heart rate occurring every seven to ten seconds). Once these cycles start to disappear from the fetal heart monitor's strip, it can presage distress to come. Not as bad as a complete loss of variability, but nevertheless an ominous sign. Clinical research in adults has focused on this six-to-nine cycles per minute frequency (often termed the "high frequency," or HF, band of heart rate variability). You may remember that, based on the work of Donders at the University of Utrecht in the late nineteenth century, this HF band of oscillations is associated with increased activity in the vagus nerve, the main channel for "rest-and-digest" parasympathetic activity in the nervous system. Perhaps, when we're in the HF band, we are more relaxed and at peace with our surroundings (fetuses certainly seem to be). What could this mean for the heart muscle itself? It is likely that the longer one spends in the HF band of heart rate variability, the less stressed the cardiovascular system. After all, the vagus nerve speaks gently to our hearts, encouraging slow, measured strokes and suppressing the secretions of vessel-constricting chemicals. If this is the case, we might expect that a loss in heart rate variability and a decrease in time spent in the HF range might be linked with greater rates of heart disease, high blood pressure, maybe even heart attack and death.

Starting in the early 1990s, this link became clear to clinical researchers who focused on heart disease and heart attacks. David Ewing, at the University Hospital in Edinburgh, Scotland (on the site of the Royal Infirmary), was one of the first to notice that some patients, after a heart attack, had poor HRV and lost those high-frequency fluctuations.[13] During the 1980s, others observed decreased vagus nerve activity preceding episodes of a bad heart rhythm disturbance, known as ventricular tachycardia (spasmodic, irregular jerking of the heart muscle that often precedes a heart attack). Research linking low HRV and heart disease was progressing.[14] But it was Ewing who first began to use HRV as a way to predict whether heart attack mortality was more likely before a second heart attack happened. He reported that his patients with poor HRV and reduced HF fluctuations following a heart attack had "long term survival . . . considerably reduced, independent of other risk factors."[15] A few years later, he found that observing a decreased HRV, obtained from twenty-four-hour heartbeat monitoring, was enough to accurately separate individuals who had angina (chest pain related to poor blood flow to the heart) from normal individuals.[16] In another strong piece of research that followed over 560 individuals for almost three years, he teamed up with Italian scientists to assign a risk factor for heart attack to those with poor HRV. Having fewer fluctuations meant a roughly 3.5 times greater risk of having a heart attack and dying.[17] All this sounds a lot like sophisticated pulse diagnosis to me.*

Numerous studies followed up on this initial research during the first decade of the twenty-first century, and the results generally fall into line. As the variability of the heart rate decreases, the risk of heart attack goes up, as does the risk of death. A summary of these studies, which merged the data of almost 3,500 cases, found that a reduction in variability of the heartbeat meant a fourfold greater chance of dying within three years.[18] This is greater than the risk posed by smoking.

Research conducted in 1998 by examining the participants in the Framingham Heart Study surveyed over two thousand patients at the Massachusetts clinic and recorded their HRV and blood pressures.[19] They tracked them for four years and found that those with poor heart rate variability were consistently more likely to have high blood pressure (true for both men and women). High blood pressure is itself another risk factor associated with heart disease. The Framingham researchers concluded that people with poor heart rate variability probably were experiencing a nervous system problem, an imbalance and dysfunction of their vagus nerve signaling, and the heart was suffering as a result.†

---

*And that is precisely what Chin-Ming et al.'s study, "Radial Pressure Pulse and Heart Rate Variability in Normotensive and Hypertensive Subjects," confirms, using a mechanical pulse-reading machine—a fascinating read.

†In the study "Reduced Heart Rate Variability and New-Onset Hypertension," J. P. Singh and colleagues commented: "A noteworthy finding in our study was that the LF [low-frequency] component of HRV in men was observed to be a stronger predictor of hypertension than body mass index, a measure of obesity" (page 296). In conclusion, "The presence of reduced HRV in hypertensive subjects and the association of LF with new-onset hypertension are consistent with the hypothesis that dysregulation of the autonomic nervous system plays a role in the pathogenesis of hypertension" (page 296).

In sum, what we have discovered clinically from our exploration of heart rate variability in humans before, during, and long after birth is that it can provide a clear measure of health in the heart muscle itself. So losing variability may be one of the starkest warning signs of that all-important cause of death in the modern society: cardiovascular disease. As the heart loses its ability to adapt to ever-changing circumstances, its rhythm becomes rigid, stubborn, tense. As Qi Bo might have said, that vital muscle loses its ability to "respond to the polarity changes of the Universe." Not particularly good.

HEART RATE VARIABILITY, STRESS, AND MOOD: HAPPY IS THE SUPPLE HEART

Having poor variability in your pulse is a warning sign for high blood pressure, heart disease, and heart attack. This seems connected to the level of activity in the vagus nerve, a key messaging bundle for our autonomic nervous system, the relay for many of our "gut feelings." But does a defect in the heart cause the vagus nerve to become less active or is it the other way around? If we are under constant stress, and don't indulge the "rest-and-digest" side of our physiology enough, could that somehow damage the heart and lead to death, like a heart literally breaking from too much stress? I suspect that, like so much of how human physiology works, nerves and heart participate in a feedback loop where one leads the other farther down a dangerous path. As the nervous system experiences stress, as it retreats from relaxation, the heart hardens. This makes the cardiovascular system less able to endure and respond to stress; thus, the nervous system swings more wildly at every near-miss. And onward the cycle repeats itself. But I also think that the changes in cardiac function evidenced by poor HRV most likely have strong roots in the nervous system because even transient changes in mood and perception have dramatic, powerful, and measurable effects on HRV. Though these effects dissipate, they may become cumulative if experienced over and over again, day after day, year after year. This has been the focus of the psychiatric arm of research into heart rate variability. What does it mean for our mood, our happiness, our level of internal stress?

Clinical researchers and physicians who deal with behavioral and emotional disruptions (such as anxiety and depression, but also poor response to stress and patterns like compulsive disorders) began to notice connections between emotional state and HRV around the same time as cardiologists were discovering its connection to heart disease and heart attacks.* Some of the earliest psychological investigations into HRV came from exploring the link between major depressive disorder, panic disorder, and cardiovascular death. A connection was already becoming quite clear.† Mental health researchers began to wonder if a decline in HRV could be predictive of the disease states they were observing. After all, if major depression and fatal heart attacks are linked,‡ and loss of HRV (especially the high-frequency oscillations) is also linked with fatal heart attacks (as we have just seen), then perhaps major depression and other imbalances are also characterized by similar changes in HRV.

Let us take a moment to think about this. It is not a given that emotional state and mental functioning, heart health, and the variability of the heart rate are necessarily connected. Depressed, anxious, or stressed-out individuals could have a different chemical makeup that somehow adversely affects the heart muscle independently of how

---

*See, for instance, Lacey's 1967 study, "Somatic Response Patterning and Stress," or Kalsbeek's 1963 study, "Scored Irregularity of the Heart Pattern." These early efforts largely left the significance of HRV unrecognized, but a correlation was emerging nevertheless.
†Of course, the heart-mood connection has long been recognized. It is an intuitive one. Some of the earliest research includes observations that, when the heart is damaged or defective, abnormal psychological states may result. For example, see Maholick and Logne's 1949 study, "Psychosomatic Aspects of Heart Disease," or Benedict and Evans's 1952 study, "Second-Degree Heart Block and Wenckebach Phenomenon Associated with Anxiety."
‡This topic has become extensively researched and the association is well established. For some of the pioneering work see Anda et al.'s 1993 study, "Depressed Affect, Hopelessness, and the Risk of Ischemic Heart Disease." Almost twenty years later the understanding of the topic has become much more complete. See Fiedorowicz et al.'s 2011 study, "The Association between Mood and Anxiety Disorders with Vascular Diseases."

variable the heartbeat is; after all, reduced HRV is not the only connection to death from heart disease. But if this link truly existed, then beyond connecting reduced HRV to our mental/emotional state, it would also provide a powerful piece of evidence that the mind and the body, and, in particular, our emotional-processing centers and our cardiovascular system, are not really separate entities.

Further, this would give much greater weight to HRV as an indicator of balance between individual and environment, between the internal organs and the mind. As you can imagine, already in the 1990s, research was confirming this three-way link between the brain, the heart, and HRV.[20] But in terms of internal balance—or internal "coherence," as it is now termed—even deeper and more far-ranging implications were just over the horizon. These implications would come to define a state of being in which humans, and presumably many animals, experience deep appreciation and satisfaction, highly creative and adaptive thinking, and feelings of strong connection to their environment. This state, as we shall see, can be elicited by a variety of practices, including the use of aromatic plants. Some have called it "being in the flow." Huang Di, the yellow emperor, would have called it simply "health."

One of Rollin McCraty's first contributions to the research on connections between HRV and emotional state was published in the *American Journal of Cardiology* and consisted of a tidy experiment in which a couple dozen individuals were either asked to elicit feelings of anger or feelings of genuine appreciation toward an individual or situation they had experienced.[21] Changes in heart rate variability were monitored during the process. McCraty had trained his subjects in a technique called the "freeze-frame method," which teaches you to reset your emotional state and refocus it on the requested emotion. Training had taken at least three months (but up to two years in some cases). Regardless of the amount of training the subjects underwent, the results were clear: recalling anger or frustration consistently decreased

HRV and moved any regular heart rate oscillations out of the HF band. Conversely, experiencing appreciation increased variability of the heart rate, and the variations took on the characteristic, recurrent seven-to-ten-second pattern we've seen is associated with increased activity in the vagus nerve. These results alone are pretty remarkable: if you spend your time angry or frustrated, your heart behaves like the heart of someone who is four times more likely to die of a heart attack. Not only that, but with just a little mindfulness training, you can control your heart rate variability fairly easily and put yourself in a state that seems associated with less cardiovascular disease.

McCraty published his results from the lab at the Institute of HeartMath in Boulder Creek, California. He has since continued to expand on this original discovery, exploring how music, exercise, and spiritual experiences affect HRV and connect back to this state of appreciation and creativity.[22] His results document that anxious, depressed, chronically stressed, and obsessive individuals experience declines in their HRV.[23] But his more recent research, conducted through the first decade of the twenty-first century, substantially expands the lines of connection between mind and body.

In short, McCraty and his colleague Doc Childre identify a state they have termed "internal coherence."[24] Remember that six-to-nine cycles per minute variation in the heart rate that indicates relaxation, appreciation, and less heart disease? It is a state where the beats per minute (bpm) of the heart are fluctuating between two regular extremes, say 65 to 70 bpm, and hitting that maximum of 70 bpm every seven to ten seconds. It turns out that when this is happening, other vital rhythms of the body are fluctuating at similar rates, or at least multiples thereof. This means that for every ten-second-long heart rate fluctuation cycle, you are also going through two complete breath cycles. The electrical activity in your brain is cycling at a similar frequency. Even the pulsing of digestive secretions is falling into line. If you're exercising, you may be going through four or five complete breath cycles for every ten-second HRV cycle, but this is coordinated with the cycles of muscle firing in your thighs. In short, your entire physiology is hitting the same downbeat, and while some cycles may hit that beat only once every measure, all of them are in sync. They positively reinforce one another. Running becomes easier, because the heart is sending blood to the legs in rhythm with their contracting muscles' requirements. Breathing becomes easier, because the diaphragm is contracting in sync with the core, which is supporting the contractions of the legs.

To get a rough understanding of this effect, try jogging using random, unsynchronized arm motions. It's tough. Then jog naturally, and notice how your arms swing in sync with your legs, and how much easier that is. While you're at it, notice your breathing. You may be going through six, or four, or even two stride cycles per breath (that last one would be a good solid effort), but whatever it is, your breathing and your legs are not disconnected; their pattern of activity is coherent. When all this coherence is occurring, we feel comfortable, at peace in our skins and with our surroundings. We are the opposite of anxious, frazzled, scattered, or depressed. We are in the flow.

So decreased HRV is associated with states of stress, tension, anger, frustration, anxiety, and depression. All this also seems linked, not only through HRV but also on its own, to increased heart disease. This state of decreased HRV has a counterpart, the "healthy" HRV pattern, in which the heartbeat varies in cycles of six-to-nine cycles per minute and other physiological rhythms begin to express coherence, or patterns of change synchronized with HRV. Emotions even out. Stress is reduced. But what is happening in the nervous system? How does this relate to our ability to adapt to stressful situations, to perform better, in short, to function better in our day-to-day lives?

Julian Thayer knows about synchronizing downbeats. He plays upright jazz bass and has recorded with a variety of musicians. He continues to perform live in the United States and Europe. He also composes, and leads ensembles from behind his bass in pieces that I would characterize as complexly layered and, when you first hear them, arrhythmic. After listening a few more times, however, I notice overlaying lines between instruments recurring at intervals that, though hard to pin down, have some degree of spiraling regularity. The music is very organic—perhaps reflective of an appreciation of our own internal music and rhythms.*

In addition to his jazz career, Thayer is also a professor of clinical psychology at Ohio State University. His focus there is—you guessed it—heart rate variability. He is attempting (successfully) to describe a model of mental process and function that incorporates the rest of the physiology and uses HRV as a benchmark measurement of each individual's internal state.† His approach is to analyze behaviors and, using techniques of brain imaging such as functional magnetic resonance imaging (fMRI), link these behaviors to specific areas of the brain and to patterns of heart rate variability.

Thayer and his colleagues have presented a detailed description of a web of brain structures, based on the model of the central autonomic network, or CAN (a network first described by Benarroch in "The Central Autonomic Network"), which accomplishes two tasks that are crucial to the day-to-day activity of a successful organism.[25] First, the CAN connects to areas in the cortex of our brains (the outer layers, often called the "gray matter") and helps to activate those cortical structures involved in the retention of working memory. Working memory is where we store details of a particular place and time we are currently experiencing so as to better integrate and process changes in our surroundings.[26] For instance, it is very difficult to participate in a good discussion unless you can quickly recall and integrate the

---

*An album of Thayer's original compositions, called *Zakú*, was released in 2007.

†Thayer has published extensively in the field with various colleagues. His more recent work includes confirmation of the brain/heart/HRV connection in 2010, "The Relationship of Autonomic Imbalance, Heart Rate Variability and Cardiovascular Disease Risk Factors"; the role of anxiety and stress on decreasing HRV, also in 2010, "Effects of Momentary Assessed Stressful Events and Worry Episodes on Somatic Health Complaints"; music and its positive effects on HRV, with R. J. Ellis in 2010, "Music and Autonomic Nervous System (Dys)function"; marital discord and its effects on HRV in 2011, "Matters of the Variable Heart"; and smoking, depression, and HRV, also in 2011, "Depression and Smoking."

points that framed the conversation. This is where working memory comes in—it allows us to link our brain's "output" with a whole line of "inputs" that we feel are pertinent. Since outputs become inputs almost immediately, the cortical structures involved in this type of processing require a substantial measure of flexibility and adaptability.

The second major function of the CAN is to bring signals from the heart, lungs, internal organs, and emotional centers to bear on the matter of successfully negotiating the present reality.[27] That is, the CAN takes in information relayed through structures such as the vagus nerve and emotional content passed through the limbic system, lays out that information for the cortex to examine, and helps to integrate it into the whole experience. It links autonomic input, feelings and drives, and working memory and processing centers into a single state of being. This is something we actually do every day, and it runs in both directions. Fear can be deeply felt in the belly, but nausea also has strong effects on our mood and decision making. You can feel love and longing strongly in your chest, right over the heart, but conversely the constriction of blood vessels that can sometimes come with high blood pressure can also make us more close-minded, less open, less loving.

Between these two functions, the CAN (and its associated emotional-processing centers in the limbic system) literally acts as a bridge between mind and body. It is a loosely structured network, which can actually rearrange itself based on the types of situations we encounter most often.[28] It thus seems to be a major, central structure involved in keeping us on top of day-to-day changes, especially unexpected sources of stress. As such, it is crucial to successful performance in response to a wide range of social and cultural demands.

The first step in Thayer's research involved taking pictures of blood flowing to the areas that are part of the CAN. Using this technique (the fMRI mentioned above), he connected increased activity in the network (as measured by blood flow) with an increase in heart rate variability, especially in the high-frequency range.[29] Recall that the HF range of HRV is an indicator of overall heart health, more stable mood, and greater activity along the vagus nerve (an important part of the "rest-and-digest" parasympathetic nervous system). So this network integrates signals from the body with emotions experienced in the limbic system and sends them to the perceptual framework currently stored in our working memory. When it is humming along well, sensing and adapting as it is meant to do, heart rate variability increases and shifts into the HF band. Our heart is happier for it, presumably, and we certainly feel less anxious, stressed, frazzled. Based on Thayer's findings, it seems the CAN is crucially important for getting—and keeping—us in the flow of events. And, by looking at HRV, you can tell how well it's working.

Ultimately, the model Thayer proposes goes something like this: When we are in the flow, working efficiently and effectively on a task, the CAN is efficiently shuttling information from the body and the limbic system to the cerebral cortex (specifically the prefrontal cortex). It is also integrating current memories of the task at hand and generating an ongoing, adaptive framework for our behaviors. Crucially, it seems the CAN is also inhibiting our fight-or-flight response, which is very good at what it does but gets in the way if we're trying to do something other than fighting or fleeing. If the CAN is active, it literally feels good inside, and our heart rate variability increases.

What is left to examine is whether folks with high HRV, and especially high-frequency HRV patterns, are actually better able to perform executive-function tasks under pressure than those with poor HRV.* If this is indeed the case, it tells us that having a high degree of HRV means we are better adapted to our circumstances, more effective in our decision making, and overall a lot happier and less stressed about everything we are doing. In short, it means that a high degree of HRV indicates that we are in a state of internal coherence, that the levels of tension and communication between our internal organs and our brain are well balanced

---

*For a definition and description of *executive function* and the areas of the central nervous system believed to be involved, see Shimamura's "The Role of the Prefrontal Cortex in Dynamic Filtering."

and well synchronized. We have also seen that being in this state means less heart disease and fewer heart attacks, as well as less of a range of psychological complaints. So what did Thayer and his colleagues discover?

From his research, it would seem that those with high HRV at baseline consistently perform better on tasks involving executive function, that is, tasks where ongoing focused attention is required. For tasks that involve programmed responses to stimuli (where the individual doesn't have to make a lot of decisions, like a simple one-step task), low HRV folks do just as well. But when observing the results of a battery of tests over the first decade of the twenty-first century, Thayer consistently found improved reaction times, fewer false-positive responses, and greater overall accuracy (summarized in Thayer's 2009 study, "Heart Rate Variability, Prefrontal Neural Function, and Cognitive Performance"). In some tests, he threatened subjects with electric shock for giving inaccurate answers[30] (though no shocks were actually delivered). Even when threatened, high-HRV people consistently did better. High-HRV individuals had lower levels of the stress hormone cortisol coursing through their veins.[31] They also demonstrated better and more adaptive situational awareness.[32] The bottom line seems to validate our thesis on the importance of heart rate variability: it is a crucial marker of a highly adaptive, efficient, low-stress individual. It is a marker we should all be pursuing in this current cultural context, as it shows us how to be more comfortable in our lives and find a way out of the malaise and overstimulation so often encountered in the general population. If we can get our heartbeats to vary in a pattern of six-to-nine cycles per minute, we will essentially be walking through our lives more ready, more creative, and much happier (and our hearts will be much happier, too).

Once Thayer established the HRV-CAN performance connection, his attempts to improve his subjects' HRV centered on physical training programs, and he got excellent results putting people through eight-week exercise regimens designed to increase their HRV.[33] But since this is a book about plants, my proposal to you is that, even though exercise is invaluable for defusing stress and making us happier and more creative (it should be pretty clear by now why this is), aromatic plants are uniquely suited to improving our HRV and bringing us back into the flow. Ultimately, I propose that this is why humans have so often turned to aromatic plants during peak experiences in their lives. They help us perform better and integrate the lessons of these moments more efficiently into our individual and collective stories.

Cultures that figure this out are more likely to succeed, and hence the universal use of aromatic plants in cultural rituals and ceremonies such as those tied to religion. But we don't use the aromatics to make the church smell nice, or to cover up the body odor of sweaty hunters who return with a kill. We used them, and can use them still, to help us move through life's changes more effectively, to learn our lessons more clearly and gracefully, to make decisions more effectively, and to be happier about our choices. The key brain structures involved in this process have been identified. The body is also intimately involved. Their interplay is evidenced by the degree of heart rate variability. Now, before we get too far ahead of ourselves, we need to confirm that aromatic plants actually can substantially improve HRV.

AROMATIC PLANTS, HEART RATE VARIABILITY, AND NEUROMUSCULAR TENSION

I want to start by examining the link between aromatic plant consumption and an increase in high-frequency heart rate variability (HF HRV). If we can find such a link, we could draw the conclusion that the consumption of, or exposure to, aromatic plants can help to keep us adaptable and "in the flow," largely by improving our ability to integrate moment-to-moment changes both around and within us. Aromatic plants might have beneficial effects on our focus and decision making, and in the end might have a strong role to play in protecting us from heart disease. Once we find that aromatics increase HRV, we can explore what traditional herbal medicine and modern pharmacological research have to say about these plants. I would like to conclude by offering the idea that our bodies and cultural systems are well tuned to experiencing aromatic plants directly, every day (or at least fairly often). This is because aromatics have been around since before human beings emerged on the planet (chimpanzees, for example, seek out strongly scented herbs for a lot of reasons that don't have anything to do with killing bacteria), and they have been featured in the rituals of successful cultures for a long, long time. They are an important part of who we are.

Research on aromatic plants has focused on a unique subset of their chemistry: the volatile, or essential, oils.* These complex blends vary considerably from botanical species to botanical species, but they have one universal quality: the small size of their component molecules makes them very easy to vaporize. Even at room temperature, you can quickly detect the essential oils of an aromatic herb. In studying their effects (beginning in the 1920s), researchers tried exposing both animals and humans to a wide range of different plants. Early experiments involved, among others, valerian, asafoetida, lavender, sandalwood, roses, violets, and incense gums, such as olibanum. Almost immediately two broad classes started to emerge: some plants seemed to have sedative effects, while others were stimulating. Some had dual effects, depending on the experiment.[34]

As research continued, more plants with aromatic essential oils came under scrutiny. Among them were pine and spruce; neroli, lemon, and bergamot; rosemary, peppermint, and basil; frankincense and myrrh; chamomile, clove, and many, many more.† The odors still appeared to be either sedative or enlivening, with some exhibiting both qualities. However, herbs such as lavender were starting to be regarded

---

*For a comprehensive summary of the research and an excellent aromatherapy reference, see Lis-Balchin's *Aromatherapy Science.*

†Again, for a review see Lis-Balchin's *Aromatherapy Science.* For examples of individual research papers, see Torii et al.'s "Contingent Negative Variation and the Physiological Effects of Odor" and Manley's "Psychophysiological Effects of Odor."

as universally calmative, whereas others, such as rosemary, seemed stimulating in all circumstances.[35] Research on mental performance was indicating that perhaps rosemary improved results, compared to lavender, but the latter, though considered more sedative, still caused a rise in performance compared to no scent at all, and participants felt pretty mellow throughout the process.[36] When examining aromatics from the perspective of traditional herbal medicine and aromatherapy, I will spend a little more time talking about the concept of "warm" and "cool" aromatics. For now, suffice it to say that there seem to be some important differences in the various strongly scented plants we know.

Interestingly enough, however, this appears to have no bearing on our discussion of heart rate variability. Warm or cool, stimulating or sedating, plants with aromatic qualities consistently increase HRV, enhancing the adjustments the heart muscle makes to the frequency of its beats. When exposed to any herb from a wide range of aromatics, people experience physiological changes very similar to those experienced by runners, meditators, and music lovers.*[37] This means that, regardless of the immediate effects on the mind of any essential oil, the mere fact that we are interfacing with a strongly scented plant puts us into the flow of events and increases our capacity to adapt to stress and change.

Lavender, traditionally a calmative oil,† has been studied in situations of both acute and chronic anxiety; in general insomnia and insomnia of menopause; among students and teachers; even in performance of night-shift nursing staff.[38] In all cases heart rate variability increased in those either exposed to the smell, given the plant by mouth, or both. Bergamot, which, depending on whom you ask, is either sedating or stimulating,[39] increased HRV in students and teachers.[40] Spruce, often regarded as stimulating, prevented an excessive stress response after

---

*Combining music and aromatics is certainly a good way to improve HRV. See Peng, Koo, and Yu's "Effects of Music and Essential Oil Inhalation on Cardiac Autonomic Balance."

†See, for instance, *Culpeper's Complete Herbal*. The original dates to 1653 and has much to say about the use of aromatic plants and their extracts.

subjects had been forced to stare at a computer screen—and increased the HRV of all participants.[41] Bay laurel, peppermint, lily of the valley, and more are linked to an increase in HRV,[42] and especially the high-frequency band of HRV. Even the fragrance of coconuts shows this effect.[43] In Japan, there is a practice known as *shinrin-yoku* or "forest bathing," where long sessions of deep inhalation are conducted in the forest. A host of benefits comes to its practitioners, and greater HRV is one of them.[44] In fact, researchers investigating forest bathing found that just sticking your nose in woodland moss improves your heart rate variability.[45] Though the human research is still beginning (the concept of HRV as a measure of comfortable adaptability is still relatively new), I suspect the results will continue to show that strongly scented plants consistently enhance HRV in those who smell them, and especially in those who consume them. We can be more relaxed and at ease, or more focused and creative, or both. But in any event, since our heart rate variability increases after using aromatic plants, they will enable us to better adapt to the changes of nature.

THE TRADITIONAL APPROACH

To further make the case that aromatics attune us to changes and make us function more efficiently and calmly, let's examine the use of these plants in traditional herbal medicine. Having discovered that consuming them has the immediate impact of increasing our heart rate variability (and promoting all the good effects that go along with that), we can make this prediction: it is likely that traditional systems of healing use aromatic plants to address conditions of stress, mental health, and perhaps also cardiovascular disease. Let us see if this is the case by first examining what types of plants are used for mental health and then investigating the various uses of aromatic plants.

Herbalists in the Western tradition tend to classify herbs used for mental health under the action of *nervine*, meaning they have an effect on the nervous system. Within this classification we find sedatives, anxiolytics, antidepressants, hypnotics, and more.* Generally speaking, these herbs are somewhat calming, to different degrees, and fairly safe until you get into the stronger members of the Papaveraceae family (the poppies). Those stronger ones are most often reserved for emergency situations (at least theoretically). What about the plants that are more of an everyday habit?

One botanical family, the Lamiaceae, or mint family, has a lot of members in it that are considered "nervine." Peppermint may help with focus and alertness[46] but also is well known historically as a relaxer of tension and spasm, especially in the abdomen but in the mind as well.[47] It is used to treat headaches, either internally or rubbed on the temples.[48] Lemon balm is another mint that makes a delicious tea used to relieve sadness and darker moods. There are other, more subtle mints as well, such as motherwort and scullcap, which, at first blush, may not seem incredibly aromatic but contain rarefied but effective volatile oils that contribute to their effects: motherwort is used to treat anxiety and heart palpitations, while scullcap features in many remedies for convulsions and tremor, anxiety, and stress. As we saw above, classic Lamiaceae, such as lavender and rosemary, have a long track record of use and research in the area of balancing mood and mental health. One of the more exotic mints—holy basil, or tulsi—is revered in India as a physical manifestation of the Divine. Planted in front of many homes to protect inhabitants from evil influences, it also serves as a main ingredient in teas that claim to confer long life, calmness of spirit, and endless vitality.[49] Almost all the mints are strongly aromatic.†

Other nervine plants come from a diversity of botanical families.

---

*For lists of herbal "actions," references can be found that are relatively old. From the turn of the twentieth century, see Petersen's *Materia Medica and ClinicalTherapeutics.* For a more recent classification, see Hoffmann's *New Holistic Herbal.*
†For references to many of the herbs listed above see Hoffmann's *New Holistic Herbal, Rosemary Gladstar's Family Herbal,* "Dr. Duke's Phytochemical and Ethnobotanical Databases," and Uri and Felter's *King's American Dispensatory.*

Chamomile, an Asteraceae, is a traditional calmative,* especially used in children. (As I was growing up, there was always a cold and somewhat sweetened bottle of chamomile tea in the fridge.) Linden is a tree in the Malvaceae family that makes one of my favorite teas, relaxing but not sedating (see Uri and Felter's terse but precise account of linden's activities in *King's American Dispensatory*). It is milled and blended into soaps across Provence, France,[50] where it is regarded as a fragrance second only to lavender. Mimosa, or *Albizia*, a member of the Fabaceae family also known as silk tree, has wonderfully aromatic blossoms that smell like a light combination of citrus and rose. Called the "tree of happiness," it is used as a remedy for depression, anxiety, insomnia, and discontent.[51] Valerian, an herb in its own family whose aroma many describe as somewhat revolting, is an important sleep aid[52] that was also used traditionally to relax muscles and improve circulation.†

Then there are the stronger plants, such as kava (in the Piperaceae family), which is an intoxicant, though extremely effective as a treatment for anxiety and tension.[53] (This plant was also given a rating of "Good," based on the quality of evidence for its effectiveness by Singh and Ernst in *Trick or Treatment?*) And Jamaican dogwood, a member of the Fabaceae family, which was traditionally used as a fish poison when its grated bark was scattered on the surface of ponds to act as "bait," does a great job in addressing pain and sleeplessness.[54] There is the whole range of Papaveraceae (including the now-illegal opium poppy): California poppy is used as a gentle sleep aid and pain reliever; corydalis is a sedative and painkiller.[55] We can round out our overview of these nervine plants with another highly aromatic one: the common hop, found (to varying degrees) in almost all products of the beer-brewing industry. It is calmative, reduces spasms and anger, and promotes sleep.[56] These stronger plants have indeed been used for men-

---

*This property of chamomile is referenced in almost every classic herbal text. See, for instance, *Rosemary Gladstar's Family Herbal*. For an interesting application of chamomile in adults, see Roberts and Williams's study, "The Effect of Olfactory Stimulation on Fluency."

†First referenced by Hippocrates, as quoted by Dioscorides in *De Materia Medica*. The Eclectic physicians very much appreciated valerian.

tal health problems in traditional Western herbalism, but less on a day-to-day basis and more for specific, immediate, and usually transient complaints. Nevertheless, the most aromatic one (hops) has certainly found its way right into everyday use, in most cultures.

So, with the exception of stronger-acting plants (which often contain powerfully intoxicating chemicals from the class known as alkaloids), most herbs used for common, relatively mild mental health complaints belong either to the mint family (Lamiaceae), or to a variety of other botanical families (though it could be argued that more than half of all the nervines are mints). Aside from the noted exceptions, these are all very strongly aromatic plants. Traditional Western herbal practitioners tend to use aromatics as their go-to, safe, daily mental health balancers while reserving a few powerful herbs, which don't necessarily have strong smells, for times when you need a little extra kick in your nervine remedy.

Before we expand our view to look at the uses of aromatic plants in general, what about cardiovascular disease? If aromatic plants improve HRV, it seems as if traditional systems of healing would have picked up on this and added aromatics to formulas that treat heart problems. As it turns out, this seems to be true, though they generally play more of a supportive role.* One of the most succinct articulations of this principle is a classic triad developed by English herbalist David Hoffmann. He recommends that all formulas for high blood pressure include hawthorn berry, dandelion leaf (an herb that promotes the flow of urine), and some kind of aromatic plant.[57] Some choices might include crampbark, which smells a lot like valerian due to its similar essential oil profile; yarrow, which has an amazing medicinal smell; ginger, with its warming, spicy aroma; or linden again. The aromatic component of the formula is said to "open up the circulation," helping to dilate blood vessels and reduce blood pressure. This concept is echoed in Chinese

---

*For instance, see the references to the use of the *Leonurus* (motherwort) species in traditional Chinese medicine in Ghorbani et al.'s research, "Ethnobotanical Study of Medicinal Plants," or the highly prevalent use of *Ocimum* (basil) species in Africa in Mensah et al.'s research, "Phytochemical Analysis of Medicinal Plants."

and Ayurvedic medicine,[58] and we will explore it further when we look at the pharmacological effects of aromatics. For now, suffice it to say that many traditional healing systems that use plants employ aromatics as part of a strategy for managing cardiovascular disease, and lean on them heavily if heart disease is coupled with mental health disturbance.

What about broader uses of aromatics in herbal medicine? Before we can proceed further, we have to take a moment to explore the art of aromatherapy (a term first coined in René-Maurice Gatefossé's *Gatefossé's Aromatherapy* in 1937). Aromatherapy is a healing system all its own that employs aromatic plants or their concentrated essential oils. Most often, the remedies used in aromatherapy are inhaled, though you can also find them used topically (as massage oils, for example) and even internally, though this is rare. But since the art of aromatherapy is exclusively focused on the use of aromatics, we should be able to get a pretty good idea of what these plants are used for by analyzing the therapeutic strengths of this modality.

It's hard to say exactly when aromatherapy began to be regarded as its own discipline. Certainly, as we have seen, humans have used strongly scented plants for a very long time. For example, in Egypt the use of incense (known as *senetcher,* or the "divine-maker") has been part of the culture for over four thousand years.[59] The same can be said of China and India.[60] In these historical contexts, the use of aromatics centers around two main goals: reducing infection, and enhancing rituals and ceremonial events (even if the ritual is a simple courtship dance). In Europe during the Middle Ages, aromatics made a strong showing as antiseptic agents as well.[61] I have always been somewhat haunted by the image of the physician during the Great Plague, covered in a long skin robe, a wide hat, and a mask resembling a stork's beak, wandering the wards of the sickhouses. They say the beak of that mask was stuffed with rosemary and mugwort, and that rosemary brews were used throughout to wash floors, blankets, and clothing of the sick, as well as the sores on their plague-ridden bodies.[62] This was all for the purpose of cleansing the "bad air"—presumably, by replacing one air with another, more strongly scented, they would eliminate the contagion.

So aromatic plants have been important allies for helping our species get a handle on infectious agents:* bacteria (but also viruses and fungi) with whom we have always had an uneasy, though not entirely unfriendly, relationship. As the risk of infection began to decrease (with the advent of hygiene and fewer open sewers), this aspect of the aromatics' potential became a bit less important on a day-to-day basis, and this change may have ushered in the practice of aromatherapy as we know it today. This was probably sometime in the seventeenth century,† and may have been best exemplified in Europe by Nicholas Culpeper, the rebel herbalist who dared to publish a book of self-care recipes in English, not Latin (much to the dismay and scorn of the Royal College of Physicians). He was also one of the first apothecaries (pharmacists of the time) to seriously delve into aromatherapy, crafting distillates from aromatic plants and recording their uses.[63]

Some of Culpeper's extracts included elixirs made from the vapors of wormwood, hyssop and all the other mints, rue, chamomile, orange, and lemon. Sometimes those preparations were recommended for use as-is, in two-to-three-drop doses, for "nerves and melancholy," "afflictions of the head," "internal wind" (presumably gas), and asthma and other lung conditions. By mixing these extracts with animal fats and turning them into ointments, he crafted medicines used for the plague, chest rubs for respiratory complaints, and enhancers of circulation (for ailments such as the "dropsy," which we now know is a failure of the heart muscle). In sum, Culpeper's contribution to the art and science of using aroma as therapy involved treating infection, respiratory complaints, intestinal

---

*There are innumerable references to the antipathogenic effects of aromatic plants and their volatile oils. For a representative summary, see Lis-Balchin's "Comparison of the Pharmacological and Antimicrobial Action."

†While hygiene was certainly gaining in prominence, it would be another two hundred years before the urban sewer and sanitation system as we know them were developed on a large scale. See Cosgrove's *History of Sanitation*.

gas, and mental health conditions. It is interesting and worthy of mention that, at least in the mind of a popular English herbalist of the early seventeenth century, aromatics had a huge range of uses for almost any nervous system complaint and, beyond that, were also useful for the three other disease categories mentioned above. This is further evidence that the main applicability of these plants is in balancing the interplay between mind and body, even though they have other strengths. Aside from the antiseptic quality, I contend that the effects aromatics have on lung and intestinal tissue are manifestations of their same tension-taming power, but that is a pharmacological topic we will explore a bit later. For now, let's see if this trend of antisepsis and "antitension" holds for aromatics as history advances.

As I just mentioned, better hygiene reduced the importance of the antiseptic qualities of strongly scented plants. As stronger disease-fighting agents came into use, aromatics fell out of favor as disinfectants. After World War II, when petroleum-based synthetic chemistry made the mass production of antibiotics possible,[64] aromatics were all but forgotten outside of culinary tradition, religious ritual, and Christmas potpourri (arguably, a religious ritual). Unless, of course, you count the entire perfume industry—which had taken off like a rocket since the time of Nicholas Culpeper.

Aromatherapy and perfumery are historically intertwined, and one can argue that perfumery is actually a branch of aromatherapy concerned not only with putting people at ease, but also with increasing sexual attraction between them.[65] So those who would have you scent your body with various combinations of plant (and animal) fragrances are recommending something that affects the mind, and targets many of the same areas we have seen are activated by aromatic plants: those relating to openness, flow, and relaxation. A perfume that puts people into fight-or-flight mode hasn't come onto the scene, and if it were to, I seriously doubt it would do well in the marketplace. Granted, the possibility is there—male pheromones are often quite aggravating to other males of the species.[66] But you don't see that marketed in department stores.

Beyond perfumes and other ritual fragrances, scent as medicine is found in cosmetic preparations (bath salts, lotions) and in specific aromatherapeutic delivery systems (diffusers, room misters, essential oil blends). These preparations are used more and more these days (at least in the United States, where they were much less prevalent before 1970).* But to what end? Is the trend observed by Culpeper still true? Do we still use aromatics mostly for mental health, relaxing tension in the lungs and intestines, and disinfecting?

Clinical research into aromatherapy is relatively new and has a track record that is roughly thirty years old. Pharmacological research has been going on for a bit longer.† If you examine the experiments conducted in both these areas since about 1980, some unmistakable trends emerge. Pharmacological research finds aromatics effective for relaxing smooth muscle in airways, in circulatory tissues in the intestines, and in the uterus. (While some oils are found to stimulate the uterus, this often depends on the timing of administration.) They are great at killing pathogens. And they have noticeable effects on behavior. If you collate all the clinical research to date, aromatherapy is found to be effective in addressing the following areas: dementia, childbirth, epilepsy, insomnia, anxiety, depression, headaches, and nausea (especially nausea related to chemotherapy). Additionally, research finds essential oils to be effective in treating acne, athlete's foot (a fungal infection), and respiratory infection. These sound exactly like the conditions Culpeper was using his aromatics for: mental health, gut tension, and infection. Compiling research on over forty common aromatic plants over the last thirty years, you end up with two basic classes of action: either the plants are stimulating or they are sedating.[67]

This has been the trend throughout recorded history: the remedies used in aromatherapy, which consist exclusively of highly scented plants,

---

*For a summary of the history and patterns of essential oil use in the United States in recent decades see Herz's "Aromatherapy Facts and Fictions."

†Lis-Blachin's *Aromatherapy Science* contains a comprehensive review and critique of clinical and pharmalogical studies of essential oils both inhaled and taken by mouth.

have effects that are couched entirely in terms of nervous system function: they either enliven or they soothe and calm. Sometimes they do both. And while you do hear about their ability to kill pathogens, you rarely learn much about their ability to stimulate digestive function, enhance immunity, or directly affect cellular aging. Their specialty, it seems, is to balance our level of neuromuscular tension and thereby address a range of complaints that stem from being out of sync with life's ups and downs: anxiety, frustration, depression, sleeplessness, compulsiveness. No wonder they have a positive impact on heart rate variability. We seem to be uncovering a pattern that is deep and pervasive, linking the use of aromatic plants to a successful, adaptable, and ultimately happy human being.

Beyond aromatherapy, herbal medicine employs aromatic plants in teas and extracts meant for internal use. Setting aside infectious conditions for a moment (for example, aromatics such as thyme are used for lung infections; juniper for urinary tract infections; oregano for gastrointestinal infections; rosemary for skin infections),[68] and having already discussed the extensive use of aromatics for mental health, what other uses for these plants can we uncover? How might they fit into the hypothesis that humans use them mostly for balancing tension in mind and body and thereby attuning to the flow of change all around them?

In general, aromatics rich in essential oils have three broad spheres of applicability in Western herbal medicine. The first is mental health, where they are employed not only for conditions involving mood disturbance and sleeplessness, but also to promote focus and relieve headaches. The second sphere relates to treating conditions relating to muscle spasm: sometimes externally, but also internally as teas and tinctures (that is, hydroalcoholic extracts). Finally, in the third case, aromatics are often added to hot teas to induce sweating and help break a fever: this time-honored use is one of the principal strengths of an herb like peppermint. We have also seen, as articulated by David Hoffmann, that aromatics can be used as support in cases of high blood pressure—and heart disease, more generally. But I contend that this last use is a special case, in which the aromatics calm muscle and increase perspiration. These are all related to an opening, relaxing function.*

One final area garnering a lot of research lately has been on aromatics' power to reduce inflammation in the body. Resinous plants like frankincense (*Boswellia*) top the list.[69] While I do not mean to minimize the anti-inflammatory powers of these plants, which are very real and useful, this property is hardly unique to aromatics themselves: almost all plants reduce inflammation. This is another reason we should consume them every day. But, as is the case with frankincense, the essential oils themselves do not exert the most profound anti-inflammatory action. Rather, the heavier organic acids of the triterpenoid class (such as boswellic acid, in this case) do the work.[70] I want to stick to actions and characteristics unique to this subset of plants and to their more volatile, vaporous constituents. We have already explored the use of aromatics in mental health. We have also discussed their ability to control infection and reduce inflammation. Let us turn now to their antispasmodic (muscle relaxing) and diaphoretic (fever-breaking) functions, for these relate in very important ways to improving our heart rate variability and returning us to the flow.

Next time you feel uncomfortable in your belly, try a warm cup of ginger tea. Or, for that matter, try some fennel seed or chamomile tea, or even peppermint spirits. You might also consider taking a sip of an anise liqueur. Any of these remedies will yield similar results: relaxing the belly, so greater comfort quickly ensues.† It is certainly not surprising that many of these herbal preparations are taken after meals, sometimes even an hour after a big meal, to help us feel more at ease. Their immediate noticeable effect is to relax feelings of fullness and cramping, and the side effect is sweet-smelling breath. Relaxing the belly has a decidedly

---

*See Hoffmann's *Medical Herbalism* for listings of the aromatic plants that fall under the traditional "action" classes of nervine/sedative/hypnotic, antispasmodic, antiseptic, and diaphoretic (that is, relating to breaking a fever).

†Innumerable instances have been personally observed by the author. A wide range of texts on herbal medicine reinforce these traditional applications; for instance, see *Rosemary Gladstar's Family Herbal*.

positive effect on mood as well, and the aromatic quality of the plants consumed likely contributes to less tension and anxiety in the after-meal conversation. Think of what types of preparations people enjoy after meals: some are bitter—like coffee, for instance—but most often an aromatic tea or cordial features prominently. This is because strongly scented plants are regarded in herbal medicine as gas-dispelling,[71] in this case quite literally calming the internal "wind."

But leave it to traditional systems of cuisine to think one step ahead: aromatics are featured *throughout* the meal in many indigenous cultures. These are the spices and seasonings that have been prized for millennia for enlivening our food and are essential defining ingredients of any "roots" meal. To a certain extent I agree with the characterization that aromatics were used in cooking, in part to disinfect and cover up the smell and taste of spoiling food and thereby to extend its shelf life.[72] However, I also think that their effects on the nervous system cannot be discounted. Taste is in large part a function of smell—as anyone with a cold can tell you—so these herbs also contribute to the enjoyment of the meal. And as the herbs enter the stomach and travel from there, well-warmed, into the intestines, they exert a relaxing, wind-dispelling effect that keeps us at ease.

Additionally, cultural culinary intelligence tells us a lot about the same factors aromatherapy research has uncovered: some herbs and spices are warm, or enlivening, while others are cool, or calming. Since certain foods are considered to have similar qualities, you begin to see pairings of warm meats (lamb, beef) with cool aromatics (spearmint), and cool seafood (fish and shellfish) with warm spices (thyme, ginger). This makes sense from a flavor perspective, but these pairings may have some medicinal value as well. In fact, it is hard to say which goal came first. Most likely the two coevolved. We wanted food that tasted good but also food that "worked"; that is, it made us feel consistently good, nourished, and strong. So we used aromatics to modulate the effects of the meal, and habits became cuisine.

Thus, when it comes to digestion, aromatics tweak the effects that food has on our belly and our mind. They are also specifically employed after meals for "problem situations," relating to bloating, cramping, and pain, and to encourage a calm, convivial atmosphere. All this most likely relates to their ability to relax the muscles involved in digestion. What about other muscles in the body?

Take the uterus. Such a solid ball of contractile fiber you will not find elsewhere in the human frame—with the exception perhaps of the heart, though even this muscle can't squeeze itself into the size of a fist while also stretching out to accommodate a ten-plus-pound mass, a lot of water, and a vast network of blood vessels. Every so often, as it sheds its lining, this muscle initiates a series of spasmodic contractions that, though mild compared to those of childbirth, can still be a source of considerable distress. Invariably, herbal medicine uses two kinds of plants to help with menstrual cramps: aromatics, which reduce the spasmodic writhing of the uterine musculature, and painkillers, which, well, kill pain (we'll leave these aside for this discussion).[73] Warm ginger compresses are applied to the belly and low back. Calendula flowers are taken as tea. Crampbark, with its characteristic valerian-like aroma, is a well-named favorite. Even pennyroyal, which has a bad reputation and is a highly aromatic mint, is used externally to relieve cramping.[74] As with digestion, we see similar effects on the uterine musculature: generally speaking, if it is tense and crampy, aromatics relax it.

The case of the uterus brings us to an interesting alternate effect for aromatics on human muscle: historically, if a woman missed her menstrual bleeding, aromatics were suggested to actually stimulate the uterus to contract (and potentially expel any unwanted pregnancy). Strong aromatics were used to cause abortion—from bitter aromatics such as wormwood, which we'll meet later, to pennyroyal, which I mentioned above.[75] So how could these plants have patently opposite effects, stimulating the uterus in one case but relaxing it in another?*

---

*This was shown in animal experiments conducted during different parts of the menstrual cycle and pregnancy by Lis-Balchin and Hart's study "The Effect of Essential Oils on the Uterus."

The answer, which gives us an important lesson in the nature of aromatic herbs, relates back to heart rate variability; to studies on aromatherapy that found both stimulating and sedating qualities to essential oils, depending on the setting and experiment; and to the state of internal neuromuscular tension. Aromatics, it seems, help to adjust tone, or overall degree of stimulation, along the muscles that line all the internal organs of the body. If tone is high, and there is spasm, aromatics can relax that spasm. If tone is slack, and there is stagnation and sluggishness, aromatics can enliven and gently open things up. I posit that these are actually two sides of the same coin, most clearly exemplified by the antinausea effect of taking gingerroot:* food sitting in a sluggish stomach too long (sluggish due to stress, or due to jostling movements, or age) is met with increased contractions from the gastric musculature, while at the same time the tight valve at the end of the stomach is relaxed and the food can move along. Result: food goes down, not up. The ginger both stimulates and relaxes. Similarly, pennyroyal can relax a spasming uterus but stimulate a sluggish (or pregnant) one.

We see this same effect in the lungs. Here, aromatics are generally used for two purposes (aside from killing pathogens that take up residence there). In conditions of increased tension in the airway muscles, such as asthma, herbs like eucalyptus relax and open the tight passages.[76] Conversely, if there is a lot of chest congestion and fluid, warm and spicy aromatics like elecampane (and ginger again) help to stimulate expectoration, increasing the rhythmic contractions of the airway muscles to get the mucus out.[77] We are seeing the same effects here that we saw in the digestive tract and the uterus.

And while it seems smart to pick a "cool" aromatic in conditions of painful spasm and a "warm" one when the tissue is wet and sluggish, you can get decent results by using peppermint in both cases. Extra tone, aromatics relax. Slack tone, aromatics enliven.

---

*There has been much clinical research on ginger's antinausea properties. Some recent work includes: Ryan et al.'s 2011 study, "Ginger (Zingiber Officinale) Reduces Acute Chemotherapy-Induced Nausea"; Pillai et al.'s 2011 study, "Anti-emetic Effect of Ginger Powder Versus Placebo"; and Smith's 2010 study, "Ginger Reduces Severity of Nausea in Early Pregnancy."

Why is this? I believe this is the crux of the important lesson these plants have to offer. We will explore the why in greater detail in just a moment. For now, suffice it to say that the lungs, the uterus, the stomach, the intestines, the heart, and the brain all have one important thing in common: they are all touched by the vagus nerve. If aromatics can improve heart rate variability, a key marker of activity along the vagus nerve, and the vagus connects all these tissues that are strongly affected by these plants, then perhaps what is happening is that aromatics are helping to balance all the "gut feelings" we receive from our internal organs by increasing or decreasing their tone, as necessary. As was the case with the after-dinner cordial, this can also relax the mind. At the same time, aromatics directly impact the brain and mood. Feelings, by acting through the vagus nerve, have a very real impact on the body—as evidenced by such examples as heart rate variability, butterflies in the stomach, and anxiety-induced asthma. By reducing tension through both the mind and the body, aromatics keep us supple and well balanced—a powerful way to enhance overall health.

In summary, by delving into traditional herbal medicine (and aromatherapy as well, in this case), we have discovered that there might be a good basis for the observed effects of aromatic herbs on key markers of relaxation and adaptability (such as HRV). They are generally used for mental health, and they balance the tone of the muscles that surround our internal organs. These plants affect our conscious mind; they are traditionally used for frazzled and "hyper" states but also for alleviating darker moods. These plants also affect our unconscious mind—those parts of us governed by the gut, the heart, the reproductive organs—keeping them in the right state of tension. Is it any wonder that aromatics promote our internal coherence, that they put us in the flow of events? Aromatics seem to fit perfectly into all the pieces of Thayer's central autonomic/limbic system network: consciousness and the working memory of current perceptions, visceral feelings relayed upward by the vagus nerve, and emotions. We will explore why this is so in the last section of this chapter. But before we do, let us return for just a moment to David Hoffmann's prescription for high blood pressure.

You will recall that Hoffmann suggests a mix of hawthorn, dandelion leaf, and an aromatic to address hypertension. The first two herbs are there to help the heart itself and to get the kidneys to let go of a little fluid, respectively. But why the aromatic? Certainly we can say that, given the positive effects aromatics have on heart rate variability and therefore cardiovascular health, no further explanation is necessary. But an extended part of the answer brings us back to that other traditional use of highly scented plants: they induce sweating and break a fever.* In fact, when taken at the right times (that is, when someone feels cold and feverish), even cool aromatics like peppermint help to encourage perspiration and warmth. Not only are these plants used for bringing down fevers, but they help with a peculiar syndrome called Raynaud's phenomenon[78] where fingers and toes get so cold that they often turn purple, or even lose all color, and can become numb and tingly. This is thought to be a condition of spasm in the arteries that bring blood to the hands and feet. You can probably see where I'm going with this. Aromatics, as we will see in a moment, relax the muscle that surrounds our arteries as well. So more blood flows from the core to the extremities, and we sweat, or at least feel warmer. Our heart is less burdened because the blood it has to pump is flowing through channels that are literally less tight. We are more open, more relaxed, in both mind and body. Circulation improves. Blood pressure goes down. You can read this by plotting graphs of heart rate variability—or you can feel it as you hold the radial pulse.

---

*Mills and Bone's, *Principles and Practices of Phytotherapy* gives a list of aromatics that includes yarrow, elderflower, chamomile, linden, and catnip to manage fever (pages 136–39). Also, they note on page 30, "Infusions of essential oil-containing herbs are often taken as diaphoretics especially during acute respiratory infections."

THE PHARMACOLOGICAL APPROACH

How do aromatics, and their volatile essential oils, actually accomplish all this? Many mechanisms have been proposed and studied. To conclude this introductory section, I would like to review some of the most compelling and discuss their potential implications.

Let us start where we left off: by examining the effects of aromatic essential oils (the primary chemicals responsible for defining the class of aromatic herbs) on the muscle that lines the human arterial system. This musculature, which is very much out of the realm of direct conscious control, is of the exact same type that lines the stomach and intestines, and the bronchial passages of the lungs. It also makes up practically the entirety of the uterus. Human arterial muscle is different from the muscle that we are used to seeing—for instance, our bicep—in that it contracts in on itself, like the shutter of a camera, instead of contracting along a straight line. So it's great for tightening and loosening, but not so good for lifting or pulling. What is interesting for our discussion is that there is an anatomical and functional similarity between the muscles that line our arteries and those that surround all our hollow organs. The muscle is called "smooth" to distinguish it from bicep-type muscle, which has stripes, or striations, in it when observed microscopically. This fact immediately helps explain why aromatics have pronounced effects on all these different tissues. If an herb can modulate the tension in the smooth muscle of the stomach, it will also work on the smooth muscle of the arteries once its essential oils are absorbed and find their way to the heart. From there, it's onward to the tissues of other organs, such as the uterus, and finally to the lungs, where the volatiles are ultimately expelled through exhalation (some come out through the kidneys, too— and effects on the bladder are also possible).[79]

In researching how essential oils affect smooth muscle, scientists have uncovered a few basic mechanisms of action. It doesn't seem that nerves are affected by these oils (at least in the local tissue), nor is the nerve/muscle connection. Neurotransmitter receptors on smooth muscle are left untouched by the volatile oils.[80] In fact, it would appear that these substances work on the muscle itself, by increasing the production of cAMP[81] (an intracellular messenger that reduces the activity of many cells) and perhaps also by limiting the ability of muscle cells to take in calcium,[82] a critical element involved in initiating contraction. For blood vessels, a third mechanism comes into play: essential oils boost the activity of a strongly vasodilative (artery-relaxing) chemical called nitric oxide.

Put this all together, and the research paints a picture of a class of chemicals that can directly affect isolated smooth muscle (which is usually used in these types of experiments). Even without a connection to "central processing"—that is, the brain—aromatics affect the tissue responsible for tension and tone around all our internal organs and our blood vessels. But the pharmacologists have taken it one step further.

Remember the distinction between relaxing, or "cool," aromatics and the "warmer," stimulating ones? This is the distinction between, say, lavender and ginger. All aromatics exert both these actions on smooth muscle, but, depending on the precise makeup of their essential oil cocktails, they can exhibit a little more of one or the other effect. The bulk of the aromatics don't exhibit a preference—they have balanced blends of volatile chemicals. But in some we see a preponderance of slightly heavier, less "airborne" constituents—and these plants are generally more relaxing on smooth muscle, though even they cause a little contraction at first. In others, where the constituents are smaller and lighter, there is a longer period of contraction before relaxation eventually ensues.[83] This is interesting for two reasons. First, it validates some of the subtlety in the traditional understanding and applications for aromatics. Second, it confirms that all aromatic plants have the ability to both stimulate and relax—and that, depending on the context, either effect may be elicited.* When present in and around a

---

*Or, as stated in Lis-Balchin's *Aromatherapy Science:* "Many essential oils show both effects: the spasmogenic effect comes first followed by the spasmolytic phase. . . . The reason for these differences lie in the chemical compositions of the essential oils and the effect of individual components on smooth muscle . . ." (page 45).

functional piece of smooth muscle, they provide the necessary ingredients to help with any imbalance in that muscle's tone. No other plant chemicals seem to be able to do that.

Essential oils from aromatics affect all smooth muscle of the body, regardless of its connection to the brain. But, of course, in a living human being, the brain *is* connected! Since we've seen that the signals coming to the muscle (through the vagus nerve) are unaffected by aromatics, all we can really say is that these herbs modulate smooth muscle tension, and that the vagus relays that level of tension up to the brain (because that is precisely its job—the vagus nerve is a two-way street). However, we cannot forget that aromatics also have a strong odor, and before their chemistry even makes it into our mouths we are pointedly aware of them through our sense of smell. This sense is ancient and very powerful. How might it play a role in the effects of aromatics?

The olfactory mucous membrane, a small area less than a half-inch across and located under the bridge of the nose, is loaded with incredibly sensitive odor detectors. It is thought that we can discriminate between ten thousand different fragrances, each having a unique molecular receptor implanted into that small patch of tissue inside the top of your nose.[84] In some ways, smelling is like tasting—if you lived in the ocean, these two senses would quite literally be one—except that the sense of smell is orders of magnitude more discriminating and sensitive than the sense of taste. We can perceive certain molecules that are put under our noses in such minuscule quantities as two billionths of an ounce. Another important distinction between smelling and tasting is that, once a particular chemical connects with its receptor, it immediately initiates a nerve signal, which, after being amplified by the olfactory bulb, travels directly to the limbic system of the brain. By contrast, when we taste (or, for that matter, when we touch, see, or hear), the signal passes first through a gatekeeper, the thalamus, before it goes anywhere else.[85]

The thalamus is a great censor, responsible for blocking out the vast majority of what our senses perceive. Which is why I can't find my car keys, even though I'm looking right at them. Most of the time this is actually helpful, as we would otherwise quickly be overwhelmed with the huge quantity of sounds and sights we experience. But when we smell, this gateway, this first screening pass, is itself bypassed. The signal generated by smelling travels straight to the limbic system every time.

From Julian Thayer's work, we have found that the limbic system can be seen as a key component of the central autonomic network, that web of brain structures that regulates the efficient processing of high-level tasks (via prefrontal cortex working memory), balances the function of internal organs (via input from the vagus nerve), and connects to our feelings (via the limbic system). It is in the limbic system that we find centers that affect anger, pleasure, and reward, and also memory formation. These structures have been part of the animal brain since before mammals existed.[86] And as part of the central autonomic network, they are crucially involved in modulating our vital pulses, how we deal with the present moment, how we feel our way through life. It would certainly be most advantageous for an organism to be able to tie environmental cues into this system quickly and effectively: such a skill would improve adaptability and survival. So it would seem that we use smell as a "fail-safe," an uncensored link to events all around us. No wonder this sense has such powerful effects.

We come to an image of an aromatic herb, its volatile oils warmed and rising, entering our nasal passages. There, they activate very specific nerve endings whose signals are relayed directly to the feeling centers of the limbic system. Next, nerve impulses link up with structures involved in regulating internal organs, managing stress and our response to it, and making second-by-second decisions on events happening around us. As these structures are stimulated, we become more focused and modulate hormonal cues. Finally, once the smells enter our lungs and from there the blood (or, if ingested, the oils make it into our bloodstream through the belly), the level of tension in our internal organs is directly balanced. These organs send signals back up to the central autonomic network, too. It would seem, therefore, that the actual perception of smell ends up in the same places that are stimulated by the chemical action of the aromatics on smooth muscle deep inside our bodies. One action reinforces the other.

Most likely, aromatics bring us into focused, flowing balance and help us function more efficiently because, in nature, new and strong smells are often a sign of a changing environment or circumstance (after all, we really are only sensitive to new smells; we become quickly accustomed to ones that linger). There may be an evolutionary reason for why having a sense that directly hits the physiology's "autopilot" systems is a good idea. Without needing to think too much about it, a new smell can immediately wake us out of a wandering daydream or calm us out of a panic, helping us deal with the present moment. As we have seen, almost all plant-based smells have these effects. Animal smells (such as musk, urine, sweat, and sexual fluids), on the other hand, tend to get us in a fighting mood or make us want to have sex. It's not that stimulating the receptors on the olfactory mucous membrane yields universally similar results. Animal smells activate our instincts for dominance and reproduction. Plant smells calm, center, and focus our energy.

There may also be a cultural advantage to the effective use of plant smells, and this is where we return to the idea of ritual, ceremony, and the role aromatics play in these social customs. Since the odor-perception areas of the limbic system are so tied into the memory-creation and emotional centers of the brain, we can harness specific scent combinations to elicit not only a state of focused flow, but also a memory/feeling/behavior pattern that is much more specific. Cultures that leveraged this insight could literally bind groups together by using *specific* aromatics from the plant world and thereby influence not only their level of focus but also the *direction* that focus would take. Consider these scents: the smell of morning coffee, the incense in a temple, the rosewater in your evening bath, a lavender sachet, tobacco on the back steps, calamus in the marketplace. These all mean something very real and very specific to me and to countless others, too. For you, the associations may not be the same. But if you know the smells I love, you have the power to control my thoughts.

Aromatics from the plant world have a direct link to ancient and well-connected structures in our brains, areas that lead us to calmer, more focused, more efficient functioning, and awaken very specific stored memories and associations. We have used aromatic plants throughout history because they help us deal better with the constant change that surrounds us, and because they bind cultures together in shared patterns of association. By activating these old, reptilian centers in our brains we find that our pulse rate begins to sway back and forth in a rhythmic dance where the downbeats synchronize with breath, muscular contraction, and the electrical activity of the brain itself. These smells come from the green, wild world around us. We can literally "breathe in" the forest and share in the common "cultural" bond of being an animal. This makes us feel right. But what happens as the forest retreats? What happens when these plant aromatics are lost from the culture or replaced with others whose effects are unknown?

WHY AROMATICS?

Psychologists at the University of Warwick, in England, made some interesting observations about individuals who had either a blunted or completely absent sense of smell (a condition known as *anosmia*).[87] Generally speaking, beyond the immediate recognition that not smelling makes it really tough to enjoy (and therefore seek out) a good meal, the researchers noted increased depression, increased feelings of vulnerability, and increased difficulty coping with stressful situations and environmental change. (They also noticed a substantially reduced sex drive, so those animal smells are important, too.) This all makes sense, of course. Unfortunately, my guess is that anosmic individuals would have higher rates of heart disease because of changes related to being unable to smell. More recent research has begun to link defects in odor processing (including, but not limited to, anosmia) to Parkinson's disease.[88] We are also learning that our ability to smell tends to decrease with age.[89] While you and I may still be able to smell, the palette of natural smells around us is much less colorful than it was ten thousand years ago (or even a hundred years ago), and the nature of the odors we experience has also dramatically changed. In lieu of forest bathing, we have freeway breathing. In lieu of basil, oregano, garlic, and olives, we have something in a spray can that I can't quite pronounce let alone spell from memory (and it smells kind of weird, too). If withdrawing the sense of smell leads to depression, fear, and apathy, then perhaps the gradual withdrawal of plant-based aromatics from our culture is also contributing to a general malaise, poor attention span, and dark moods. Perhaps aromatics spark the spirit, and a soul bathed in scent can actually become "immortal," fly free, and be at peace.

So as the smoke of incense rises in the dark interior of the pyramid, as the steam rises from my cup of linden tea, an ancient ritual repeats itself: we smell, we take volatile plant chemicals into our lungs and bodies, and we thereby connect to what surrounds us. A fresh scent stimulates deep centers in our brains, and our thought processes become more focused, efficient, and relaxed. Our feelings retreat from anger and domination, and stress begins to have less of a hold on our minds and bodies. All the vital rhythms in our internal milieu begin to synchronize in a way that just feels right, feels like flow. We may be drawing on old animal comforts here: walking in a familiar forest, the smells of the season returning us to a timelessness where cares and sadness have a little less power over us. And as we focus, flow, and synchronize, our pulses take on a characteristic pattern. We can feel this in our arteries—a balanced vital rhythm born of a balanced state of internal tension, a skillful tightrope walker under our skin.

It is no wonder that, in all cultures, we use smells during peak times of our lives. We need to be present at these moments. The aromatics bring us there. The aromatics also help us remember, they help us carry the timelessness of being present *now* into our future lives. We can return to the very moment whenever we need to, and that, too, is a great comfort. We can, and should, bring these scented plants into our lives when we feel the weight of the modern world upon us, when we feel disharmony within and around us. They truly can help us buffer the asymmetries of tension and calm the often destructive winds that follow.

As the pharaoh's priest drinks the aromatic herbs, as he burns the incense, he crosses into the spirit world and can usher his ruler's body into the afterlife. He uses smells that bind a thousand-year-old kingdom. He is in a flow that spans generations and, as such, he unburdens himself of all worldly cares, while focusing like a flame on his present intent. It is similar to what the old Taoist sages called immortality, free and easy wandering, doing-without-doing. I can see you on a riverbank, on young green springtime grass, cherry blossoms falling occasionally from the branches above as the sweet air mixes with the vapors from your teacup. Huang Di, the yellow emperor, gently holds your wrist, feels the vitality throbbing within it, and smiles.

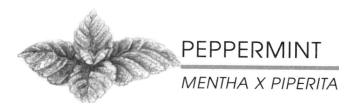

PEPPERMINT
MENTHA X PIPERITA

There is a small pharmacy in Florence, Italy, not more than three blocks east of the great cathedral of Santa Maria del Fiore, that has been processing medicinal plants in almost the same way for eight hundred years. While it has an entrance on the public road, the larger doors in the back of the main apothecary lead to an inner cloistered courtyard, much in the style of Renaissance Italy, with simple columns, terra-cotta tilework, and spare but elegant gardens. This courtyard is at the heart of a small triangle of the city built around the church of Santa Maria Novella (yes, lots of churches), and the pharmacy bears the same name.

This tiny shop was founded by the Dominican friars who set up residence on this block in the thirteenth century, and it became known for extractions of medicinal plants focused on their aromatic, ethereal components. Some of its specialties, used for cosmetic and antiseptic purposes, include rose waters, rosemary distillates, and hand-blended soaps. But the preparation that has always garnered the greatest acclaim (enough to warrant a personal dispensation from the archduke to sell it to the public) is a distillate known simply as "water of Santa Maria Novella." Its only ingredient is the volatile spirit of peppermint, *Mentha piperita*. Peppermint is a classic aromatic, and its high concentration of essential oils make it perhaps the strongest plant in this category.

Remedy Recommendation

The apothecaries recommend taking a small amount of the water of Santa Maria Novella, perhaps ten to thirty drops, in a half cup of water. At this dilution it is light, pleasantly enlivening, and definitely refreshing to the palate. But it can also be taken in more concentrated form to remedy such diverse ailments as fever, headache, tension, stomachache, flatulence, and, of course, "hysteria" (a very interesting term whose Greek root, ὑστερα or hystera, means "uterus").

GROWING, HARVESTING, AND STORING PEPPERMINT

One thing to remember about mints in the garden: they have a wandering way and are difficult to disentangle from areas where they have taken up residence. But despite their hardiness and competitive skills, they do have a preferred set of growing conditions they find most favorable. So, if you have the space, I suggest planting peppermint in a somewhat cool and slightly moist spot, where the sun doesn't shine continuously, and wilting heat is rare—far away from your other herbs and vegetables. If conditions are good, minimal fertility is required and your mint will thrive year after year, mixed among the grasses. I harvest from a great patch on the eastern border of the field, where afternoon sun isn't too hot and the soil stays cool all summer long. Alternatively, containers made of terra-cotta are suitable. Given water and placed in part shade, you can expect multiple harvests if you cut the peppermint back every time it flowers. Grown on a kitchen patio, it can also be used as needed for teas and cooking.

The whole plant is glossy and smooth, and it releases its aroma at the slightest touch. It has a strong and biting quality, almost too strong to eat lots of it directly. Reddish-purple veins continue the purple color of the stem into the small, fine-toothed leaves. It comes up quickly in the spring and is one of the last plants to retreat in the fall; flowering begins anywhere from June into early July and continues throughout the growing season. The inflorescence is a spike of multiple small flowers, with side shoots of blooms all around, arranged in an opposite branching pattern up the stem. Harvest peppermint by cutting the stems and then stripping off the leaves and flowers. These can be used directly, or dried over two to three days and stored for up to a year.

By far the easiest way to establish this herb in your garden is to get a few grown plants from a friend or a nursery. If they have some, most folks are more than willing to dig it up and give it to you. Transplant them into medium-sized holes with a little compost and water them for the first week, if necessary.

USING PEPPERMINT

We have used peppermint as an archetypal aromatic plant for many centuries. It soothes the belly and eliminates cramps and intestinal spasms. It reduces headaches and relieves tension. It can relax airways and improve breathing. In concentrated, tiny doses, it stimulates the mind and improves focus. Its efficacy in controlling fever is legendary. And its flavor, as the Dominican friars found so long ago in Florence, is quite appealing. No wonder so many still turn to it for a wide range of complaints. It's truly a great introduction to the use of aromatic plants in daily life.

 Peppermint Sun Tea

In summer, you can often get a sense of what the afternoon might bring by walking out into the garden first thing in the morning. Sometimes (at least up here in Vermont), in late July or August, the hazy sunrise comes with a certain feel and smell to the moist air. It will be quite hot today, it seems to say, so you'd better get to work before the sun gets any higher.

These are the times you will want to stuff a bunch of fresh peppermint into the biggest glass jar you can find, fill it with water, and cap it tight. Then it can sit in the sun until late afternoon, when evening, just over the horizon, promises relief. The solar energy alchemically converts the heat of the day into a choice brew, rarefied, subtle but strong, its depth and potency belying its easy preparation.

Peppermint sun tea is not nearly as biting as a cup brewed with boiling water, yet it is not timid at all. It reinvigorates the spirit and prepares the body for a magical summer evening. You can even use some to wash your face and neck before dinner: you will feel rejuvenated in no time. After the meal, it relaxes the belly and improves digestion by alleviating bloating and spasm, and stimulating the function of the liver. It is a delicious, simple, and effective way to enjoy this plant when it is most abundant, our ally for the hot days.

The Water of Santa Maria Novella (Peppermint Spirit)

> Dried peppermint leaves
> 100–150 proof vodka
> Home distillation apparatus (see box on pages 87-88)

To approximate the water of Santa Maria Novella, we will require a little more ingenuity. The preparation is essentially a hydrosol, except made from an alcohol infusion, rather than from a tea. We will start with a tincture and, by heating it, separate its aromatic components from the more bitter and fibrous "fixed" constituents. This is perhaps the most elaborate of preparations listed in this book, but it is also one of the most rewarding, as it yields an intense, highly concentrated, and highly effective peppermint spirit that has been crafted using alchemical principles that are almost one thousand years old.

Prepare a tincture from dried peppermint, using a pint mason jar filled with chopped and lightly packed leaves. Cover the leaves with a strong alcohol, preferably 150 proof, though 100 proof will do (between 75 percent and 50 percent alcohol by volume). Close the jar tightly and label it with the date and source of your peppermint. Shake the jar occasionally over the next two to four weeks.

During this time, the alcohol dissolves the volatile essential oils, rich in menthol, from the oil-bearing glands on the surface of the peppermint leaves. Extraction of minerals, chlorophyll, organic acids, tannins, and other nonaromatic constituents is occurring as well.

After a few weeks strain and press your tincture into a measuring cup, rinse out the jar, and pour the strained extract back in. It should be anywhere from bright green to greenish brown, depending on the strength of the alcohol used. But before replacing the lid, you must drill a hole in it to serve as an exit for the aromatic vapors we will be attempting to separate from the tincture.

For the final step, we simply need to heat up the peppermint tincture while the copper coil is connected to the lid (see box on pages 88–89 to create this home distillation apparatus). The safest way to do this is to place the distiller in a pot with simmering water, allowing the copper tubing to hang outside the pot over a measuring cup, ready to receive the distillate. Since alcohol boils at about 185°F, simmering water at 200°F will vaporize it, along with any aromatic constituents, and they will rise up into the copper coil where the temperature will drop, the vapors will condense, and fluid will be recovered drop by drop.

When you're done, bottle up the peppermint spirit and store it in a cool, dark place. It will keep indefinitely and be ready for use either full strength (with caution) or, more often, diluted in some water. Full strength, it is recommended topically, rubbed into the temples for headaches that arise from tension or stress, while internally it's consumed in doses of two to three drops, for an immediate and powerful increase in focus and alertness, or to decongest the airways. The diluted spirit is still used the same way as it was in the Middle Ages: to treat indigestion, bloating, headaches, fever, cramps, and spasms. It is a very powerful regulator of the level of tension in the internal organs.

The alchemical process of distilling peppermint spirit is fascinating, and though it is somewhat laborious, in the end you are also left with a tidy homemade still, which can be used to separate the aromatic fraction of any herbal extract you choose to make (try motherwort or scullcap, for instance). But a much more simple, though no less effective, method of using this herb sticks most in my mind, perhaps because it reminds me so much of childhood: the time-honored peppermint compress.

Making a Home Distillation Apparatus

You will need:

- A small coil of copper tubing

- Gasket (or the rubber bulb on the top of a dropper)

Most copper tubing sold to carry water (think drinking water supply for a refrigerator, for instance) is one-quarter inch in outer diameter. A small coil of this type of food-grade tubing can easily be found at any hardware store. This piece will serve as collector and conduit of the peppermint spirit: one end will fit into the lid of the mason jar, the other will drain out into a suitable receiving vessel.

It's pretty simple to attach the tubing to the lid of the mason jar. Drill a hole through the metal lid with a quarter-inch drill bit. Keeping the bulk of the copper tubing coiled up, gently bend a small section three to four inches long so that it points downward, ready to be fitted into the hole in the metal lid. But before putting it in, slip a gas-

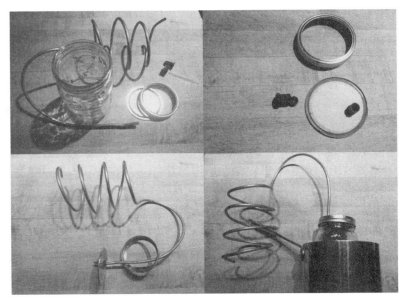

How to assemble your home distillation unit
(Photographs by Guido Masé)

ket around it to secure the seal. Believe it or not, I've found that the rubber bulb at the top of a dropper (found on any bottle of herbal extract) is precisely the right size for this job.

Separate the rubber bulb from the dropper by pulling out the glass dropper itself, and pushing the bulb through the plastic ring that secures it to the bottle. Once you've isolated the piece of rubber, cut the closed end of the bulb off with scissors, essentially creating a rubber tube. This should slide onto the end of the copper coil, and the whole ensemble will fit in to the hole in the mason jar's lid. Tighten everything onto your jar and—presto!—you have a simple home distillation unit.

 ## Peppermint Compress

> Peppermint tea
> Clean piece of cloth

When an illness causes a fever, there is also usually discomfort, headache, and alternating heat and chills. Next time this happens, try this simple remedy to produce sweating, reduce headache, and help "break" the fever to provide relief.

Soak a clean piece of flannel or cloth in a strong, warm cup of peppermint tea. Gently wring out the excess fluid and apply this warm preparation (technically a "fomentation") to the forehead, allowing it to sit there at least fifteen minutes. This process can be repeated every hour or so, until headache and fever are reduced, and sweating begins.

By helping to relax and dilate arteries, warm peppermint tea reliably increases surface circulation in the forehead and temples, helping to radiate off heat and encouraging perspiration. It is ultimately this sweating, or diaphoresis (an effect displayed to a certain extent by all aromatics), that cools the body and brings the internal temperature down.

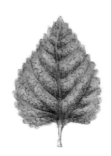

LEMON BALM

MELISSA OFFICINALIS

Virgil was poet to the emperors—the first emperor of ancient Rome, in fact. His epic works served largely as propaganda to glorify the genealogy and exalt the divine status of Augustus who, fresh from repeated military campaigns, had succeeded in consolidating the entire old Republic under his authority. Through glorified language and warlike analogy, the poet's power served his master well.

But at heart Virgil was a lover of the countryside and the bucolic life. In his *Georgics,* published 20–30 BCE, he details the life of farm and garden, devoting an entire volume to the keeping of bees, one of his favorite subjects. He was keenly aware that bees sought out aromatic plants for nectar, for protecting the hive, and, perhaps, for managing their mood. He describes a method for corralling an errant swarm.

> *Burst from their cells if a young troop be seen,*
> *That sails exulting through the blue serene,*
> *Driv'n by the winds, in clouds condens'd and dark,*
> *Observe them close, the paths they steer remark;*
> *They seek fresh fountains, and thick shady bowers,*
> *'Tis then the time to scatter fragrant flowers.*
> *Bruis'd balm, and vulgar savory spread around,*
> *And ring the tinkling brass, and sacred cymbals sound:*
> *They'll settle on the medicated seats,*
> *And hide them in the chambers' last retreats.*

THE ECOLOGUES AND GEORGICS OF VIRGIL (1753),
TRANS. JOSEPH WHARTON

Balm, in Virgil's words, is *melissaphyta,* which literally means "plant of the bees" and is also the root of lemon balm's genus name: *Melissa.* Bees certainly love it, and it may indeed serve to soothe them when a swarm has gone astray—it has much the same effects in humans and animals. Its delightfully citrusy, aromatic quality is rarely if ever bitter and lacks any bite, making lemon balm tea a perfect beverage for any complaint where stress and digestion are fighting it out.

GROWING LEMON BALM

You will want to brush up against lemon balm as often as you can. It is irresistible. Even young children are fascinated by the leaves and rub them to release the fragrance. For this reason, and also because it's a very well-behaved plant (for a mint family member), I like planting melissa as a border to a path, with something taller behind it, like echinacea or butterfly weed. It is also a plant well-suited to container gardening, right at home in a terra-cotta pot on a sunny balcony (provided it has a good amount of water). When dining al fresco on the terrace, you can pick a little sprig for garnishing dessert, ice cream, or sorbet.

Lemon balm is a dry plant: somewhat astringent to chew directly, covered in a very fine down that makes it feel just a little bit bristly, definitely not juicy. It comes up fairly early as the weather warms up in spring, with big, wide, frilly-edged leaves that are quite delicious. Over the course of the warming summer, the leaves get smaller as the plant grows, to a height of two feet or so, and they take on a yellowish hue. This is most often the case in soil that is just a little rockier and less compost-rich, but, in my opinion, these conditions make for a stronger, more deeply scented herb. Flowers start blooming in late June and are white to cream-colored and whorled around the square stem. If you harvest the leaves before the flowering is too far along, they are a bit less astringent. After each successive cutting, lemon balm will grow back quite strong and continue to provide its sweet and sour fragrance well into the frosty months.

It is easy to grow this herb from seed. Three or four of the small, black, oblong seeds per container should do, covered with a little soil and kept thoroughly moist. You may have to wait a few weeks for complete germination, but once the seedlings are established and have gotten a taste of the sun and wind, they can be planted out even in marginal soil. In warmer climates, lemon balm escapes to hedgerows and sunny cracks in the patio, competing very well in the wild and making smaller, but vibrantly aromatic, specimens. Where it's colder, more attention might be required, with occasional weeding to keep out the grasses, and a little compost mulch.

USING LEMON BALM

As an important aromatic herb, lemon balm (also known simply as "balm") is both soothing to the nerves and uplifting to a dejected spirit. Its traditional uses generally focus on mood, as does the modern research: short-term anxiety support, with effects from a single cup of tea lasting many hours; long-term reduction of stress after daily use; even an ability to calm the confusion associated with the dementia of old age. Depressive or, more appropriately, irritable conditions are also soothed by all preparations of this plant. But its uses don't stop there.

Melissa may be one of the more appropriate choices for so-called butterflies in the stomach—the feeling of impaired digestion, perhaps even accompanied by a bit of nausea, that comes when stress and anxiety overtake us. Now, indigestion can make us feel anxious, too. But in this case, it's the other way around. Always get symptoms in your belly when eating in a crowded, noisy restaurant? Have you learned not to eat food before a public speaking engagement or a performance? Is eating on the run a recipe for bloating and pain? Try lemon balm, in any and all preparations (tincture-soaked sugar cubes are my favorite).

Another traditional use of this plant relates to its antiviral qualities. It is recommended for cold sores, or herpes virus infections, where it reduces nervous tension (stress is thought to trigger outbreaks) and also directly inhibits viral replication. I have always had the best success treating cold sores with lemon balm essential oil or tincture applied topically, and sometimes combined with licorice root powder. But for general prevention, any preparation will do.

Think of the swarm of bees flying in the summer sun, perhaps a little confused or at least stirred up and not quite pleased about the whole affair. They course through the air looking for a signal to return home, to a place that's safe, a place that makes them glad again. This signal is melissa, an aromatic with a citrus scent that gladdens the garden but also brings happiness to those who consume it, loosening tension in the spirit and in the belly. Of all the aromatics, it is perhaps the most uplifting, though never stimulating—the joy of bees. May it be your joy as well.

Lemon Balm Tea

The infusion of melissa into water is certainly the most traditional approach (if you don't count mashing it up and smearing it all over beehives to both calm and attract their inhabitants). You can certainly use fresh sprigs, steeped in hot water, for an effective and very pleasant afternoon preparation.

But I prefer to gather lemon balm with a knife, cutting sprigs and thereby encouraging new growth, and then removing the leaves from the stems and drying them. The dry leaves can be stored whole in glass mason jars, and a generous pinch can be taken as needed, rubbed together, and infused into a cup of tea. The drying concentrates the essential oils (by removing the water content) and enhances the lemon taste and fragrance.

Even on warm summer days, I like to take this tea hot. And in the evening, as the heat of the day dies down, it can't be beat.

Lemon Balm Tincture

> Freshly dried lemon balm leaves
> 100–190 proof alcohol (the higher the proof the better)

The tincture of lemon balm is made like the tea, but with the freshly dried leaves (not more than a week or so after harvest) and the strongest alcohol you can get your hands on. One-hundred proof vodka is okay, 150 proof is better, and if you can get hold of pure-grain alcohol (190 proof), that is ideal. The plant, though very aromatic, is quite stingy with its essential oil and to maximize extraction we need more alcohol (since alcohol dissolves oils especially well).

Fill a mason jar with lightly packed, crushed, dry leaves, then cover them with your best score from the liquor store and close the lid tightly. Using grain alcohol (or anything above 160–170 proof) will extract a lot of chlorophyll, too, making the tincture a shining emerald-green.

After two to four weeks, strain and bottle.

Remedy Recommendation

Lemon balm tincture can be given in quarter-teaspoon doses, mixed with a little water. Alternatively, a fantastic after-dinner treat (and aromatic digestive) is made by slowly adding five to ten drops of the tincture to a sugar cube or a slippery elm lozenge. You can make a bunch of these at a time and store them for later use.

Lemon Balm Infused Honey

> Dried, crushed lemon balm leaves
> Honey (ideally raw, unfiltered, local honey)

Given its strong historical association with bees, perhaps the best preparation to make with lemon balm is an infused honey. Honey has always been used as a medicine itself, but historically it has also served as a carrier for a variety of medicinal plants. It extracts their virtues fairly well and, being highly antiseptic, preserves them for an indefinite period.

To make an infused honey, start with dried, crushed lemon balm leaves and fill a mason jar half to three-quarters full. Pour honey over the herb until the jar is full. Ideally, this would be a raw, unfiltered, local honey—loaded with vitamins, minerals, fiber, and antiseptic resins and waxes. Cover and seal the jar tightly.

At this point, you have two options. The most gentle, though time-consuming, option involves placing your jar in a sunny window or greenhouse for a couple of weeks, shaking occasionally. The more rapid alternative is to simmer the jar in a hot water bath for a few hours. This latter option is less attractive to raw honey purists, and I understand any reluctance to heat this precious substance. The choice is yours.

Once your honey is ready, and when it's still warm from the sun or the simmering water, strain it through a very coarse steel mesh and store the honey for later use.

A spoonful can be taken as is or placed in the bottom of a teacup and hot water added for an "instant" brew. Another option is to drizzle the infused honey over vanilla ice cream or into plain yogurt. Not all plants impart their flavor to honey very well—but melissa most certainly does.

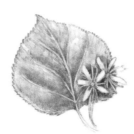

LINDEN

TILIA EUROPEA

Trees make powerful impressions. More than their smaller herbaceous relatives, they hold sway over our imaginations, winding their way into myth and legend, even driving our culture at times. It may be their sheer size, or their longevity, or both—but trees have an ability to link the earth to the sky and to frame natural "cathedrals" for human beings. Legends have always followed certain species—from the apple to the yew—and the linden tree, also known as *Tilia*, is no exception.

This tree has a wild side, to be sure, and it's an important native member of low- to mid-elevation forests across the entire Northern Hemisphere. However, it is also often found planted in villages and cities as a companion tree, because of both its beauty and its amazing fragrance. In Central and Eastern Europe it is held in the highest esteem, serving as the national symbol of Slovenia and the Czech Republic (where it is known as lipa). Here, majestic old lindens served as gathering points for the local community, and villages would hold court under their branches, confident that the tree would ensure justice but also bring about peace and an amicable resolution to conflict. In many villages, this practice continues today.

Brixen, a very ancient town in northern Italy steeped in Germanic influence, sits at the confluence of two rivers—the Isarco and the Rienza. There the linden has always had a strong presence. A medicinal tea is made from the flowers (as is the case everywhere this tree grows), and its wood is sculpted into incredibly elaborate carvings by artisans in the surrounding valleys. Two *Kaiserlinde,* or chief lindens, rumored to be over eight hundred years old, overlook the city from foothills on the eastern and western sides.

Ireland also boasts its share of ancient lindens (here, as in Great Britain, they are called lime trees). I was lucky enough to find a pair of huge ones, their dense shade cooling the grass in a clearing of old-growth forest that was otherwise mostly oak and laurel. They grew side by side, the bases of their trunks touching, forming something of a cradle, or gateway, where we lingered for a while. Burlington, Vermont, is planted with a great many linden trees, lining some of the residential streets that run west, down toward the lake; at the lakefront itself, small-leaved lindens (so different from the native basswoods) create an intoxicating fragrance for summer evening walks. But in Provence, where the same fragrance mixes with the red ochre soil that nourishes lavender and other aromatic herbs, the cult of linden's power is most ritualized. Tilleul, which refers to the tree, a tea made from its flowers, and a perfume distilled from the linden flowers, is firmly embedded in the culture as a remedy for everything from distress and sorrow to digestive complaints, fevers, and high blood pressure.

For the heart, tilia is a great ally—so it's nice to note that its leaves are generally heart-shaped, though this varies a little depending on species (there are over thirty of them). American basswood can have huge leaves, bigger than the palm of your hand, and larger, thicker flowers (due to a second set of sepals). *T. cordata* has smaller leaves, with slightly less showy flowers, though I consider them more aromatic. *T. platyphyllos,* a mostly European species, has medium-size leaves, fragrant flowers, and is considered the longest-living species. The tree is at home in almost any temperate climate, enjoying the balmy Mediterranean basin as much as frigid Vermont. It doesn't mind a little moisture and grows fairly quickly. Its leaves are silvery on the underside and catch the wind easily, much like a cottonwood or aspen. It's fantastic to watch a breeze shake the linden tree, then wait for the smell to drift from across the field.

Walter von der Vogelweide was a medieval German poet who lived during the beginning of the thirteenth century. He may have been born not too far from Brixen, the town in northern Italy at the confluence of two rivers. Regardless, he certainly spent long periods in that valley. Perhaps he even saw the planting of the two *Kaiserlinde* that still overlook it. Here are the opening verses of a poem, "Unter der Linden" (Under the Linden), that he wrote from the perspective of a young girl remembering her beloved.

> *Under the linden*
> *On the meadow*
> *Where last night we shared a bed*
> *I found today—*
> *Great joy to behold—*
> *Crushed flowers and trampled grass.*
> *From the wood and across our vale,*
> *Tandaradei,*
> *In beauty sang the nightingale.*

FROM VON DER VOGELWEIDE'S *DIE GEDICHTE WALTHERS VON DER VOGELWEIDE* (POEMS OF WALTER VON DER VOGELWEIDE), TRANS. BY GUIDO MASÉ

HARVESTING LINDEN

When I harvest linden flowers, usually sometime in the first weeks of July, I take a big round basket up into the tree with me or, if the branches are too dense, up the ladder. At this point, there usually are bees to contend with. If the image is one of waving leaves and the smell a light, bright, sweet fragrance, then the sound is a full, droning buzz from the hundreds of bees gathering nectar for honey. The flower itself is attached to a light-green bract, a long, oblong, leaflike structure that is pierced by the flower's stem. This bract is a very important part of the medicine, so I will harvest it along with the single or double fully opened flower (it's almost impossible not to). You can get a bushel-basket full in a few hours, if it's a good year. Then it's off to dry the flowers as quickly as possible and store them tightly in glass jars, out of the sun.

Though it always happens a bit later in Vermont (and in Eastern

Europe), lindens typically bloom around the summer solstice (late June) in places like Provence. When winter is dark and night is deep, we will come back to those jars, open them, and release a one-of-a-kind aromatic medicine, whose fresh fragrance holds the joy of a midsummer night.

USING LINDEN

The linden tree, sacred in many traditions, offers us a fragrance and a medicine that are soothing, relaxing, opening, and encouraging to love and appreciation. Of all our aromatics, it is perhaps the best suited for the stressed and anxious, or overwhelmed and irritable, personality type—and who among us hasn't felt that way from time to time? Our modern lives are amazingly rich in communication and information, but the barrage of information that assails us every day can have its negative effects. First, the simple volume of data can be overwhelming. But second, it can so capture our attention, and demand so much of us, that we begin to neglect the people and places in our lives that matter most: our families, our friends, our homes and gardens. I feel linden helps me unplug and allows me to appreciate the nourishment and love that's right in front of me. And this is a powerful gift from a strong and beautiful tree.

 ### Tilleul or Linden Flower Tea

Tilleul, the simple infusion of linden flowers, is a subtle but incredibly powerful remedy. It is made by pouring hot water over a few handfuls of the dry, crushed blossoms and bracts stuffed into a teapot. Make sure that the tea steeps covered, or you will lose a lot of the aromatic quality into the kitchen air.

The linden can steep for three or thirty minutes, for it will have none of the astringent unpleasantness of an overbrewed green or black tea. On the contrary: the infusion is round, velvety almost, slightly thickened by simple starches found in the bract. Coupled with its distinctive fragrance, it truly is a luxurious experience for such a simple ritual and is perhaps my favorite kind of tea.

Try it at the end of a day to unwind. It slightly shifts consciousness into a more joyous and calm place, allowing us to relax and appreciate life for a moment. You can also drink it throughout the day, especially if work or family are sources of stress that foster anxiety and frazzled thinking. Taken habitually, it can replace rituals such as alcohol or drug use for breaking away from workday or family stress.

Tilleul is also thought to foster love and an open heart, alleviating impatience and anger as well as high blood pressure. In Europe it is routinely recommended for cardiovascular disease, as it is a safe adjunct to conventional therapy (and it tastes delicious, too). Some will suggest a tincture, or alcohol extract, of these flowers—and while this can be very effective, there's something to the ritual of a cup of tea that makes it the best way to enjoy this herb.

Taken as hot as possible, it is still used frequently for fevers and chills associated with winter illness. This ability to cool the body by stimulating slight perspiration is another reason it's so highly prized in places like Provence, where summer afternoons can become overwhelmingly hot. To this end, a cup is enjoyed after lunch—usually around two or three o'clock—and is often drunk cool and slightly sweetened. It's one of the best iced teas I've ever had.

The postlunch benefits linden offers extend to the digestion, too. Herbalists prescribe a simple tea for many types of belly issues, from heartburn to gas and bloating (though its effects on problems like constipation is less pronounced). The aromatic quality is relaxing to the muscles lining the gut, and the smooth, soothing nature of the tea softens and heals areas of irritation.

Linden Flower Bath

> A few cupfuls linden blossoms
> A washcloth or muslin bag

The tea has a fantastic and well-deserved reputation, but linden's fame extends into the perfume industry, too, where its bright floral notes are sought after in producing eau de toilette, soaps, and creams.

My suggestion is to try turning your bathtub into a giant teacup full of tilleul, then steeping yourself in it for some time. This is easily done by taking a few cupfuls of blossoms and tying them up in a washcloth or muslin bag, then placing it in the tub as it's filling with hot water.

Those who extol the benefits of lavender baths for relaxation would do well to try linden, too—much less biting of a fragrance, and the soothing qualities that make the tea so lovely do wonders for the skin, too. A cup of tea and a warm bath surround you with the vapors from this tree's amazing flowers, and both mental and physical knots untangle, the pores open and the skin cools, and the heart relaxes just a little. While we might not have the time to take a luxurious bath every day, it nevertheless is an experience everyone should try.

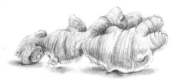

GINGER

ZINGIBER OFFICINALE

I remember ginger best from the time I spent in Bali, Indonesia. The days there start with a warm haze, a quick sunrise over the rice *padi,* and a sultry heat that wafts through the tiled homes with their thick, thatched roofs. Often, the slightly oppressive afternoons are broken by a rain shower—but this does little to refresh the thick air. Flowers are everywhere—from jasmine blossoms, left as offerings on every step, to huge sprays of white, pink, red, and yellow coming from the ginger plants that line the trails between the rice terraces. And the ginger, known as *jahe* locally, is harvested and used in nearly every dish, from the "mixed rice" (a mélange of vegetables, egg, shredded meat, and fried rice that is a lunchtime staple) to candies and drinks. It is also a central remedy for the indigenous system of medicine, called *jamu* in Indonesia, and is found in nearly every formula.

Ginger's energy is warm. It's spicy, though not in the same way as the hot chilies that are also often used in the cuisine of Southeast Asia. Its aroma is more floral, at times almost fruity, and its flavor reflects this. Because of its warmth and the unique accent notes in its palate, for me this aromatic herb will always be associated with tropical Bali, its sacred volcanoes, and its animist religion that worships the spirits of springs, mountains, ancient trees, and hidden valleys. Its immediate effects are a welcome treat on warm and humid afternoons. Ginger can help to induce perspiration, and even though it tastes warm, this action ends up cooling us off nicely. Pretty nifty trick from a cup of tea.

Interestingly, in the cold weeks of November when, back in Vermont, hunters take to the forest in hopes of restocking their freezers with excellent wild venison, this tropical plant can provide amazing support. Long hours are spent in silence, in stillness, in the deer stands or blinds of the leafless forests. Often hunters pick the time between four and six in the morning to stalk their prey—the coldest hours of the day. The temperature, coupled with the lack of movement, can lead to discomfort, regardless of how many layers of clothing the hunter is wearing: fingertips and toes become tingly, muscles lose their responsiveness, and reaction time crucial to success is lost. A mugful of ginger tea, or a few ginger capsules taken beforehand, strengthens the body against the bone-chilling cold. As with so many of the aromatic plants, this root works differently depending on the circumstances: cooling off a body that is overheated and warming up one that is too cold.

GROWING, HARVESTING, AND PURCHASING GINGER

Technically, the underground part of the ginger plant that we use for medicine is known as a rhizome. From this rhizome's fleshy, yellow body rise pointy growing tips that will shoot upward, given the right conditions, into a glossy, reedlike stalk and its smooth and shiny leaves. If conditions are right (meaning, a pretty constant seventy-five-to-eighty-degree air temperature and high humidity), a flower bud that resembles a pink pineapple will emerge and send out yellow flowers from its core. The underground parts of ginger will lengthen and fatten over time and can easily be harvested by cutting and replanting to ensure the next crop. Even if conditions aren't ideal, you can still get the rhizome to sprout a few green shoots—but don't expect it to grow much. In Vermont, even in my greenhouse, ginger has a difficult time.

This is not too much of an issue, however, since this storied spice is available, dry or often fresh and whole, at nearly every grocery store. If you can't find any fresh, stop by a specialty Asian foods store or even a natural foods supermarket or cooperative. While the dry, powdered root is certainly serviceable for medicinal purposes, it can be a bit too stimulating, especially if folks are already feeling a little dried out. It keeps well in the open air of a room-temperature kitchen for at least a couple of weeks, though it will start to dry out after seven to ten days.

My recommendation: purchase it fresh, in small quantities, once or twice a week. If you live in a warm and humid climate with no danger of frost, you can plant it in your garden, usually in part shade and fertile, loamy soil, allowing the green ends of the growing tips to stick a half-inch up out of the ground. But be forewarned: nonorganic rhizomes have often been heat-processed, or even irradiated, and won't grow at all.

USING GINGER

The simplest and most traditional way of using ginger is to cook with it. I peel the rhizome and cut it into thin slices with a very sharp paring knife. These can be added to hot peanut, sesame, or coconut oil and left to cook for two or three minutes before adding more stir-fry ingredients: carrots, onions, mushrooms, burdock roots, or whatever strikes your fancy. Before serving your meal, remove the slices and set them aside (a bit too fibrous to just eat straight). Ginger shares this use with its cousins turmeric and galangal (and cardamom, too, to a certain extent). Eaten habitually, three or four days a week, its aromatic and pungent constituents will gently and safely adjust the subjective feeling of body temperature: a cool constitution will warm up a bit, and warmer folks will overheat less. This latter effect is echoed in the modern research literature, where ginger and its chemistry consistently show anti-inflammatory results—not exactly a temperature issue, but helpful nonetheless as a daily habit.

Ginger's soothing effects on the belly are due to its relaxing aromatic qualities, which quickly relieve nausea and allow food to move down the digestive tract. Its aromatic chemistry also explains why it can warm up cool hands and feet: by relaxing the smooth muscle that surrounds the arteries, warm blood moves from the core to the periphery. If we're hot, this will make us sweat—and sweating leads inevitably to cooling (also useful, as are all aromatics, in managing a fever). But if we're already cool, the extra circulation will remedy cold, numb, or tingly fingers and toes. Raynaud's phenomenon, mentioned earlier, describes an extreme example of cold hands and feet. Cold temperatures, but also stress and tension, can cause those who suffer from Raynaud's to get numb and even have their fingertips turn purple or white. This is thought to be associated with a constrictive spasm of the circulation—and ginger does wonders to relieve the condition, both in the short term and following habitual use.

So from the tropics comes an aromatic that is a useful counterbalance to the relaxing, cooling mint-family plants we've explored so far. Ginger is warm, and its relaxing effects are coupled with a gentle anti-inflammatory action that makes it ideally suited for muscle pain and tension, either taken internally or applied topically as a warm compress. While it is difficult to grow in temperate regions, it is so widely available that you should have no problem adding it to your home medicine kit (and spice rack). And every time you taste it, or feel its relaxing warmth on your back or belly, it will bring you back to its tropical home: warm, relaxed, a place where time moves more slowly and the pace is often more leisurely—a much-needed oasis in our modern lives.

 ## Ginger Tea

> 2 teaspoons ginger powder or 4 slices rhizome
> 12 ounces boiling water

While its culinary uses are well known, ginger has a unique and extremely powerful medicinal effect when taken as a tea. It is strong, so two teaspoons of the powder or four good-size slices of the fresh rhizome can be infused in twelve ounces of boiling hot water for just five minutes or so.

This preparation, while delicious in and of itself and useful for temperature regulation, is specifically powerful in controlling nausea. I've seen it work consistently and in a variety of situations, from the morning sickness of pregnancy, to after-meal indigestion, to motion sickness. In this final application, it seems as effective as technological medicine—and way tastier! I will always be grateful for the little bag of pickled ginger that helped me on a particularly turbulent entry into Tokyo.

Hot Ginger Compress

>3 teaspoons ginger powder or 6 slices of rhizome
>
>1 cup water
>
>A clean piece of cloth

Tense muscles are almost an inevitability of modern life. At some point, we have all seen ourselves holding our shoulders tight when concentrating or under stress. This can lead to soreness, or creep up the neck and morph into a tension headache. Since ginger is so useful at improving circulation and relaxing tension in the muscles of the belly, perhaps it could find an application for skeletal muscle tension, too. In fact, this might be my favorite use for this tropical plant.

Make a really strong tea (three teaspoons of powder, or six slices of rhizome, per cup of hot water) and saturate a clean piece of flannel with the infusion. You can then apply the cloth directly to areas of tension, soreness, or pain. Circulation to the affected area improves, inflammation is reduced, and the tightness dissolves. This application is known by herbalists as a hot ginger compress and is recommended for everything from muscle pain to arthritis.

Massage therapists sometimes use a few drops of ginger essential oil in a base of grapeseed or olive oil to help melt away knots during a relaxing body rub. In Bali, and nowadays throughout the world, women use ginger compresses for the low back and pelvic pain associated with menstruation, as well as the uterine pain that can linger after childbirth. Warm cloths soaked in ginger tea are applied to the low back and belly, and the whole midsection is wrapped up in linen. Leave these preparations on for fifteen minutes or so, then check: you don't want to warm the tissue up too much!

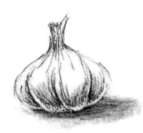

GARLIC
ALLIUM SATIVUM

In the Balkans, the region just north of Greece, mountain folk talk of a strongly scented remedy whose mere aroma dispels all manner of evil, from sorcerers and demons to the dread *upir,* a witch-spirit who, rising from the grave, travels the countryside in search of blood. Its victims slowly lose color and vitality, become depressed, and eventually fade away. It is possible that the term *vampyr,* which evolved into our present-day *vampire* at some point in the eighteenth century, comes from these Central European legends. Regardless, the remedy is the same: the bulb of a stinking lily, cultivated for cuisine but also used as a potent disinfecting medicine. This remedy is, of course, garlic.

Garlic braids and wreaths, so common as a way of curing and storing the bulbs, are still hung in the rooms of small children and sick people to prevent evil influences from taking hold. In this sense, garlic embodies the essence of the aromatic herbs. But it also possesses a great power to enhance vitality, acting as a strong stimulant to those who consume it. In India, where the herb has been used for over five thousand years in similar negativity-dispelling rituals, it is shunned by yogis because of the fire it engenders in the spirit—it arouses passion and *élan vital,* sometimes too much for those engaging in a meditative path. In ancient Egypt it was given in large, daily doses to slaves working on pyramid construction to keep them healthy but also strong and vital (and, perhaps, to keep depression and apathy at bay). In all these uses, garlic transcends its aromatic powers and shows much more of its tonic qualities—previewing the virtues of another important class of medicinal plants.

GROWING, HARVESTING, AND STORING GARLIC

It is quite easy to grow good garlic, and the process is understandable (the seed is huge), straightforward (into the ground it goes), and quite rewarding (one clove becomes a whole bulb). It is an ideal project to help children learn the joys of gardening and its rewards. As the garlic rests over the winter months, children can anticipate the first green shoots of spring, watch the plant's development over the early summer months, and participate in the process of harvesting, cleaning, and curing. How much more delicious is the roasted bulb when you were the one who pulled it from the rich garden soil! So even if you never plan a garden, nor expect to get your garlic anywhere other than the supermarket, I encourage you to try an experiment at least once to witness this magic of growth. The plant takes up little space, and five or six bulbs can be raised in a small planter box on a windowsill.

The first step is finding good "seed." Not a seed-bearing plant, like an onion or leek, garlic propagates from a single clove that grows into a whole bulb. If left untended, this bulb will eventually burst and each of those cloves will try to grow, too—but the plant will quickly lose vitality this way, and become a shadow of its former self. It requires the human hand to thrive. So find yourself a local farmer who has grown garlic for some years in the same soil and environment you have in your garden. Try a farmers' market or natural foods store. Look for the biggest, firmest heads you can find or, better yet, ask if there is any "seed garlic" for sale. Chances are that, starting in late September, there will be lots available. I've found that three or four pounds is an adequate amount to grow for my small family, providing enough to last until May. Talk to your farmer or produce department manager about the differences between softneck (stores well) or hardneck (more pungent) varietals, and make a choice that suits your needs.

The time is late October or early November. Garlic "seed" in hand, make your way to the garden. The one trick for this plant is well-prepared soil with little competition from fast-growing weeds. I make sure that there is a lot of compost in the beds, but I also add a little bone meal (for my acidic Vermont soil) and an organic fertilizer, such as fish emulsion or another concentrated source of nutrition. If your spring and summer tend to be dry, just dig the soil deeply and plant the garlic at ground level. You may need to water the cloves from time to time. Conversely, if your climate is moist, raise your beds six to twelve inches above grade. You can always use a planter box or another container, even planting it among tomatoes and basil in a large ceramic pot. Separate the head of garlic into individual cloves first, and leave the papery wrapper on. Then push each clove, pointy side up, into the loose and fertile soil. Space them about eight inches apart.

Over the winter, your garlic will put out small rootlets that give it a jump on the growing season. Come spring, it will be one of the first plants to emerge, strong and green, quickly sending up lilylike shoots already rich with its characteristic smell. The plant will get bigger and bigger until, usually in mid- to late June, it begins to flower. Now, a garlic flower is a bit different from your usual blossom. In softneck varieties, a swelling begins in the stem that erupts into a cluster of small "bulbils." In hardneck varieties, a snakelike "scape" twists its way upward and forms a similar swelling at its end. The scapes can, and perhaps should, be cut off and either chopped fresh for soup or stir-fry or preserved by canning or pickling. A few weeks after the flowers, when the bottom three to four leaves of the garlic plant have turned yellow and the whole thing is about three to four feet tall, it's time for harvest.

If you wait too long, the new garlic head will burst open and really cut down on storage time (though not edibility). But when you feel the time is right, usually in the middle of July, simply grasp the neck of the plant and pull up vigorously. An entire brand-new head will come up with a tangle of rootlets and soil beneath it. My recommendation is to try this raw form immediately, on a hot day in the garden. Peel a clove and bite into it. It is both milder and sharper than the cured bulb. It

gives an immediate, enlivening spice but little of the long-term burning you can get from aged garlic. Before bringing it in for storage, clip
off the rootlets sticking out of the bottom of the bulb and trim the
neck just below the bulbils for a softneck, or at about eighteen inches
from the bulb for a hardneck. Then tie the stalks into bundles of five
to seven plants and hang them in a room with good air circulation.
Traditionally this meant the barn, but a covered porch or a room with
open windows and low humidity is perfect, too. After about ten days,
you can clean up the bulbs (remove the least amount of wrapper possible), cut the rest of the neck off, and place them in a cool, dark place
for long-term storage.

USING GARLIC

Entire books have been written on the medicinal and culinary uses of
this remarkable plant. In Italy, it is considered a virtual panacea. The
cloves are crushed whole and used as treatments for wounds (excellent and effective), eaten for worms, and given as stimulant tonics to
improve digestion, liver function, and mood. It is one of the first remedies on the list for treating the common cold or influenza, and features prominently in many of the most famous national dishes, from
marinara sauce to bruschetta. There is little doubt that this is a good
herb that is quite good for you, too. So, to conclude our exploration,
I would simply like to offer a brief note on its chemistry and preparation, and the medicinal effects of its aromatic qualities.

First off, you can't swallow a whole garlic clove and expect to get
much out of it. The chemical compounds responsible for its antiseptic and aromatic quality are sulfur-rich molecules known as isothiocyanates, but they don't exist in active form in the clove. Rather, since
they probably evolved to deter browsing animals and insects, they are
synthesized as needed whenever the plant is traumatized. Normally,
inactive forms and the enzyme that converts them into the pungent
spices we know so well exist in two different compartments. When

something (like a knife, or the teeth of an herbivore) break the membranes that separate these compartments, the enzyme kicks into action and the isothiocyanates are born. Now garlic is ready to work its magic. What this means is that, for maximum medicinal effect, the cloves should be chopped and allowed to rest for two to three minutes.

When we eat this garlic, either close to raw or infused into warm olive oil or soup, the pungent compounds are absorbed into the bloodstream relatively quickly. Here they act as all aromatics do: they dilate blood vessels, opening and relaxing the circulation. But garlic also has a dual action on the heart, usually decreasing the strength of its contractions and slowing the heartbeat. Put all this together, and you have a remedy that can contribute to lower blood pressure and a feeling of relaxation. Conversely, if circulation is poor or if the heart is already fatigued, garlic has a decidedly stimulating action, warming the hands and feet (again, by dilating vessels) and perhaps increasing the strength of the heart's contractions.

This latter effect may have been what the supervisors of the pyramid crews were after when they prescribed daily garlic rations to the slaves. Improved circulation and stronger hearts push back fatigue. But that may also underlie the use of garlic in protection against vampires. The pale, deficient, weak individuals who were thought to have been victims of nightly bloodletting would show renewed signs of vigor after consuming the cloves for some time. And while, in the past, weakness and deficiency were dominant concerns, in our modern culture we often see the opposite: heat, stress, and excess often manifest in the heart as high blood pressure, rapid heart rate, and, eventually, heart disease. Like most aromatic plants, garlic helps us find the balance point of tension in our bodies and in our hearts. But few are so easy to add into everyday life, or as enriching to everything from a simple plate of grains to a rich and complex seafood stew. Truly, as they say, garlic is as good as ten mothers.

3

Bitters

Turn On and Challenge

Poison is in everything, and no thing is without poison.

PARACELSUS, CA. 1520

What seems to us as bitter trials are often blessings in disguise.

OSCAR WILDE, 1895

Our tastes are our preferences, literally. Often these preferences favor sweetness, ease, and comfort over bitter trials and provocation: but despite how much we try, there is no avoiding fate's travails. Some lives experience them in small measure. Others are overtaken by them, ending in tragedy. This is the story of an ancient king obsessed with toxins.* It gives us a potent example of the tragic case—and also reveals the secret behind a bitter antidote to all poison.

---

*The primary sources for this story are Pliny's *Natural History* and Justinus's *Epitome of the Philippic History of Pompeius Trogus* (which includes details on Pompey's campaign against Mithridates and his eventual demise). An excellent contemporary appraisal and collection of these primary sources is Mayor's *The Poison King*.

Mithridates Eupator was nearing the end of a protracted, bloody war with a rising power from the west. For over twenty-five years he had resisted the advances of Rome, challenging the warlike republic and often succeeding. But now, under the leadership of a new general and reinforced with fresh armies, Roman centurions had driven him from his native lands, pursued him across the kingdoms of his allies, and backed him into a far northern corner of his realm, where his son Machares was viceroy.

Hoping to rest, regroup, and renew his armies, Mithridates wanted to make a desperate last stand: a counterattack from north of the Black Sea. His pride allowed for no less. He counted himself among the descendants of Alexander the Great. He cherished his kingdom's history: the people of Pontus, in what is now northern Turkey, had long held back both the Persians to the east and the Greeks and Romans to the west. He himself had repelled numerous attempts at his crown (a professional hazard for all royalty at the time), and, now, nearing the end of his seventh decade of life, he was not about to back down peacefully.

His son, Machares, however, had made different plans. Messages took time to travel, but he had been following the course of the war and, being no fool, had realized that the tide was turning against his father. Having secured an alliance with Roman leaders, he didn't particularly wish to jeopardize his long-term fate on a risky gamble. Through compromise, he envisioned a chance to forge a comfortable and possibly lucrative relationship with Rome. A period of peace might allow him to consolidate his holdings, return productivity to the land, and spare lives. He had hoped his father would never return from the battles on the southern shores.

Mithridates was clearly shocked by his son's betrayal. Though historical accounts vary, they lead to the same conclusion: be it through deception and false promises of safety, or perhaps just through simple force, Machares was poisoned and quickly died. The beleaguered king might even have been able to mount his counteroffensive, to test his meddle once more against an old enemy who would not have been expecting such a move. One can only imagine the corrosive rage and sadness that consumed him. But victory was not to be his.

His youngest son, Pharnaces, had been riding north for days with a small but fast contingent and arrived just after his brother's death. Pharnaces had been groomed as heir since he was young and, though he was the last son of Mithridates and his wife, Laodice (also his sister), he had always shown the most promise. He came upon the encampment where his father, sisters, and remnants of the army were stationed. He was able to quickly convince the disillusioned generals that a kingdom under his control, allied with Rome, would be better for everyone concerned. He recruited their aid in a coup to overthrow his father.

Mithridates caught wind of this plot through a few elite soldiers whose loyalty remained steadfast, but by now it was too late. Despairing, he returned to his poisons, always close at hand (some say hidden in his staff), and rapidly crafted an especially strong preparation. Among his cache were true toxins, such as nux vomica beans from far afield, and deadly nightshade berries, grown much closer to home, plus the viciously acrid root of aconite—especially bitter, death-giving plants. He mixed quickly and with a skilled hand. First, his mistress and daughters, including Drypetina, who had loved him and stood by his side for over forty years, were made to taste the poison. It proved remarkably effective, and they all quickly perished. Next, surrounded by the corpses of his family and a few loyal guards, the king briefly contemplated his life of war, struggle, betrayal, and revenge. He took the vial to his lips, closed his eyes, and drank deeply.

The kingdom of Pontus occupied land on the southeastern shore of the Black Sea, an expanse of water surrounded by Turkey, the Balkans, the Caucasus, and Crimea. This land connects the Mediterranean basin to the rest of Asia, and its climate is mild. Being a long strip of coastline, it ranges almost four hundred miles across and is bordered about sixty miles to the south by an impressive mountain range whose eastern peaks exceed ten thousand feet. These mountains slope quickly to the sea and are rich, green, steep, and dotted with clear lakes.

These slopes are still covered by very old forests, which, in the time of Mithridates, would have been even more extensive. The woods at lower elevations are rich in beech, chestnut, oak, and spruce. There are occasional colonies of yew and a storied grove of boxwood, holly, and ivy where the boxwood trees are over thirty feet tall. Proceeding up the mountain slopes from the rocky cliffs of the coast, evergreens begin to dominate, including spruce, Black Sea fir, and Scotch pine. Finally, above about six or seven thousand feet, forest is replaced by wide Alpine fields, and we find great quantities of native meadow herbs: yarrow, gentian, arnica, and lady's mantle, which flower in the summer months; and snowdrops, crocuses, and irises that bloom in the spring.

Traveling back toward the sea, we follow springs and streams to rivers cut deep into the mountains and lined with dense stands of alder. Here there are also rhododendrons, delphinium, monkshood, wild roses, honeysuckle, calamus, cyclamen, and deadly nightshade. All these plants may have played a part in the life of the poison king of Pontus, but we know at least that he experimented extensively with the more toxic ones, such as monkshood and nightshade. He would also include gentian, calamus, iris, parsley, carrot seed, and various tree resins in many of his preparations. The base was always extremely bitter; aromatic plants, such as ginger, cardamom, and rose, came in smaller proportion; and the whole was bound together with resins, gums, or tree sap.

Mithridates began his experiments in poison formulation (as well as his research into antidotes) by collecting plants on his walks in the wild. His studies started early: when he was fourteen, his father was poisoned and control of the kingdom was turned over to his mother (she herself was the prime suspect in the murder) until he or his brother would be ready to ascend to the throne. This was the beginning of a strong interest, some say a paranoid obsession, with poisons and their antidotes. If it happened to his father, he reasoned, it could happen to him as well.

The young prince hit upon an interesting idea: perhaps, if full doses of poison could kill, then smaller doses might strengthen him against death. Simply employing plants that tasted like the poison but were not toxic themselves (like the root of high mountain gentian) might do the trick. Mithridates retreated from palace life for a period and apparently delved deeply into venom brewing and antidote crafting, because when he returned, both his mother and his brother were poisoned and died. The prince became king, married his sister, and set about building an army—all the while looking over his shoulder, fearing the murder in his evening meal, but confident that the regular use of his antidotes would keep him alive.

The work of Mithridates proceeded along two tracks. First, he learned all about the toxic plants and how to prepare and administer them. This was accomplished through experiments on himself (and others, including many animals) both to determine dosage and also to build a tolerance to the poisonous alkaloids found in these herbs. Second, he constantly worked on the perfect antidote, a medicine so powerful it could reverse the effects of poison and thereby preserve life. In these pursuits, he had the assistance of a varied group of poisoners, shamans, and herbalists, ranging from snake charmers of the eastern lands (who taught him how to extract toxins from vipers), to the mushroom eaters who lived in the north (who, experienced with all toadstools, had a special fondness for the white-flecked red caps of the fly agaric). Of all his coconspirators, one stands out for his depth of knowledge and skill in pharmacology: the root doctor Crataeus.

Crataeus was from Pergamon, a storied capital that, roughly one hundred years earlier, had commanded almost all of modern-day Turkey and parts of Greece. As a trained herbalist, he would have had access to the collected knowledge of the time on physiology and pharmacy, which, of course, included extensive information on medicinal and toxic plants. Additionally, as was often the case, he most likely gravitated toward wealthy and influential patrons, so that he might pursue his (relatively) esoteric trade in comfort and have access to often exotic—and expensive—remedies.

Because Mithridates and the kingdom of Pontus had come to dominate Asia Minor and the lands Pergamon had formerly controlled, Crataeus quickly found himself in the court of Sinope, the Pontine capital. He discovered in the young monarch a kindred spirit and a powerful ally, and the two formed a strong bond. Together, Mithridates and Crataeus fine-tuned powerful poisons that killed rapidly without producing symptoms; they discovered new and effective medicinal plants; and they perfected a supposed antidote to all poisons, which became a daily tonic for the toxin-obsessed king. Crataeus, who was equally methodical, kept extensive records and is in fact credited with the first visual compendium of medicinal plants in the Western world[1]—annotated in detail and enriched with his own illustrations of the herbs being described.

This manuscript must have been a fantastic collection. Not only were individual plants outlined and named, their illustrations accompanied by their medicinal uses, but also, the recipes for numerous remedies and tonics (including the famous mithridate, as the universal antidote became known) were recorded along with numerous variations.

Crataeus identified and discussed several "new" plants, too: including agrimony, boneset, and gravel root (all of which he named after his royal patron).* The famous herbal of Dioscorides, published over one hundred years later, copied huge portions of Crataeus's work[2] and has itself been copied by every herbalist since. So, even though the original work was lost, we are still feeling the influence of the palace herbalist of Pontus over two thousand years later.

What was the composition of the mithridate, the mythical universal antidote, that Mithridates and Crataeus formulated so long ago? What made it so powerful, so successful, that physicians revered and copied it for hundreds, if not thousands, of years? There are numerous

---

Eupator, Mithridates's suffix, was the chosen appellation. Agrimony is *Agrimonia eupatoria,* and the genus *Eupatorium* includes both boneset (*E. perfoliatum*) and gravel root (*E. purpurea*).

recorded recipes, starting with Celsus's *De Medicina* (pages 178–79 and also well summarized in Norton's "Pharmacology of Mithridatum"). It seems clear that the antidote itself did not contain poisonous plants but rather was a mixture that included many herbs, both local and exotic, but all nontoxic in normal doses. Some of the king's first attempts at antidotes were straight *kyphi* mixtures (see page 35), sent over by the pharaoh of Egypt: aromatic resins mostly, sacred incenses and gums, which opened the circulation, reduced inflammation, and increased the body's adaptability to the stress (in this case poison) it was experiencing.

But while the aromatic mixtures may have conferred an advantage in withstanding the poison, they were not adequate to prove universally effective against toxins. They may not have known this at the time, but what the king and his root doctor required was a way to improve the processing (metabolism) and elimination of the poisons from the body to make the mixture complete. Since almost all poisons were administered by mouth, any antidote needed to work through the digestive system and its associated "chemistry lab," the liver. By harnessing our own detoxification mechanisms, the mithridate may have blunted the effects of poisonous alkaloids, such as aconitine, strychnine, and atropine, helping the body to neutralize them more quickly and excrete their by-products more effectively.

In examining the ingredients of the mithridate (as best can be determined by the historical record and the flora of northern coastal Turkey),[3] we find a few categories of plants that appear consistently in the many documented variants of the universal antidote formula. First, as mentioned, were the aromatics. These ingredients included Egyptian calamus, cinnamon, myrrh, and frankincense; but also valerian and cardamom. Next, the blend featured a few "special" plants that were highly revered for their ability to heal. Some examples included St. John's wort and saffron. Finally, and perhaps most importantly, Crataeus and Mithridates added a large proportion of roots and leaves whose only common characteristic was their intense bitterness.

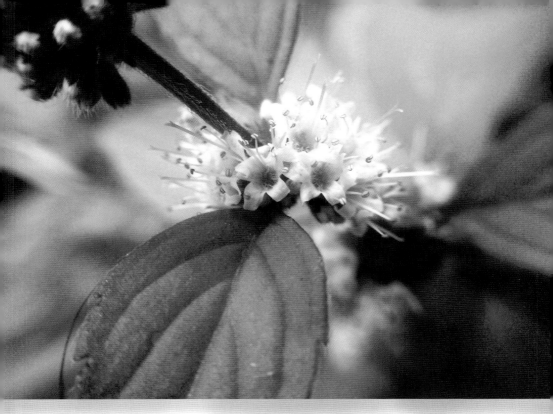

Plate 1. (above) *Mentha x piperita,* Peppermint inflorescence
(Photograph by Guido Masé)

Plate 2. (below) *Melissa officinalis,* Lemon Balm flower
(Photograph by Guido Masé)

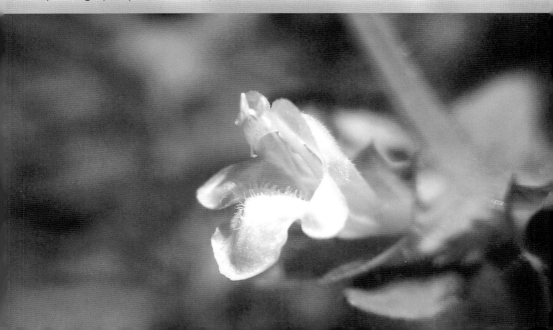

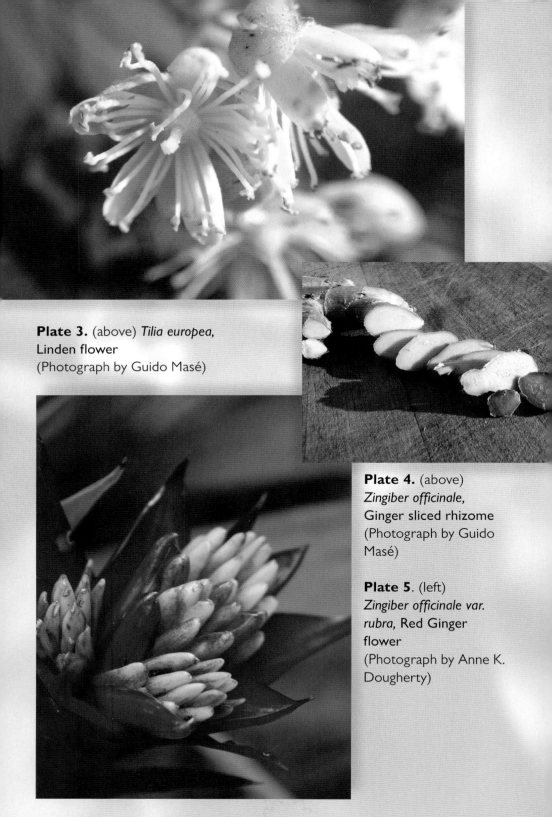

Plate 3. (above) *Tilia europea,*
Linden flower
(Photograph by Guido Masé)

Plate 4. (above)
Zingiber officinale,
Ginger sliced rhizome
(Photograph by Guido
Masé)

Plate 5. (left)
*Zingiber officinale var.
rubra,* Red Ginger
flower
(Photograph by Anne K.
Dougherty)

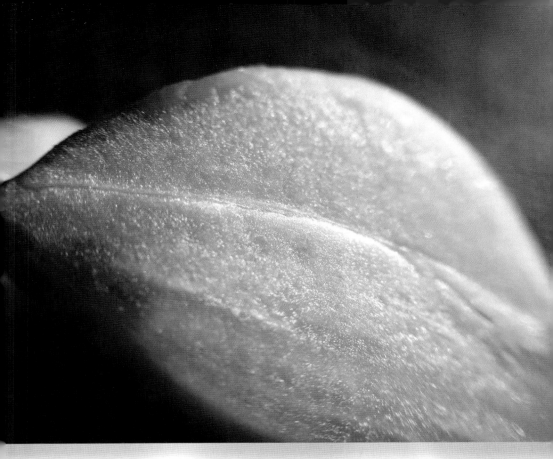

Plate 6. (above) *Allium sativum*, **Garlic clove** (Photograph by Guido Masé)

Plate 7. (below) *Allium sativum*, **Garlic bulb** (Photograph by Guido Masé)

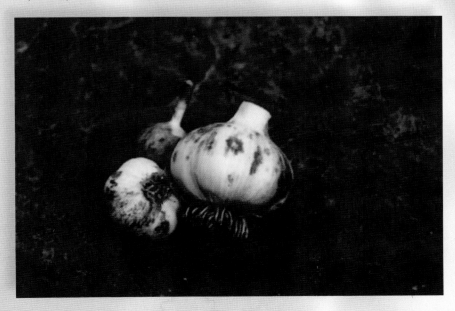

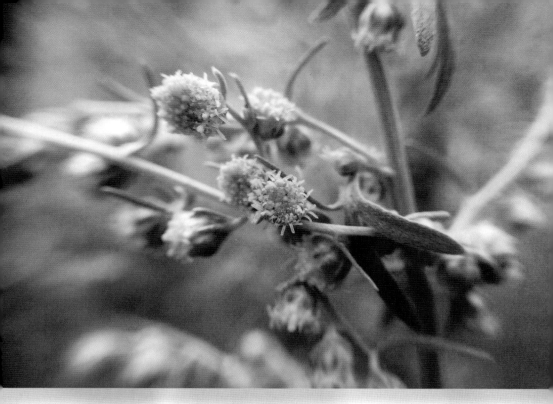

Plate 8. (above) *Artemisia absinthium,* Wormwood inflorescence
(Photograph by Guido Masé)

Plate 9. (below) *Taraxacum officinale,* Dandelion flower
(Photograph by Guido Masé)

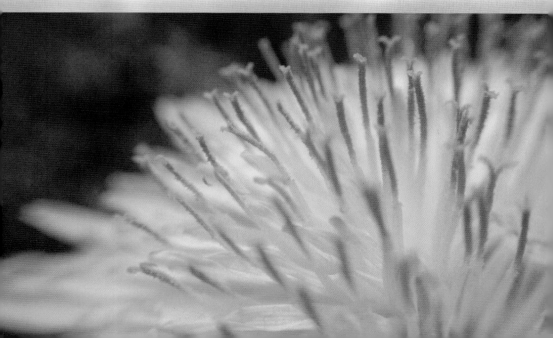

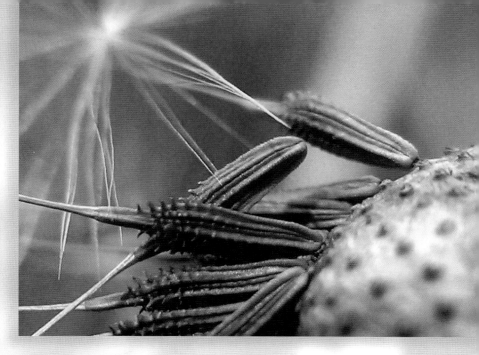

Plate 10. (above) *Taraxacum officinale,* Dandelion seed
(Photograph by Guido Masé)

Plate 11. (below) *Arctium lappa,* Burdock flower (Photograph by Guido Masé)

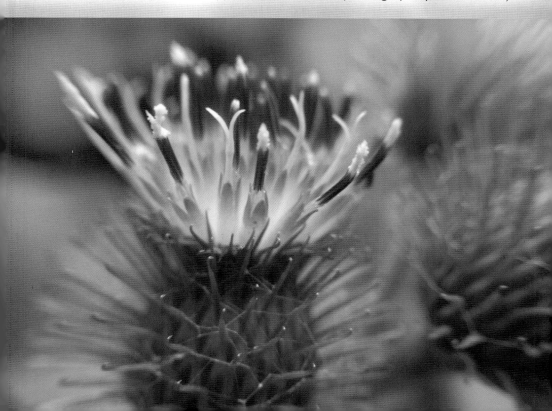

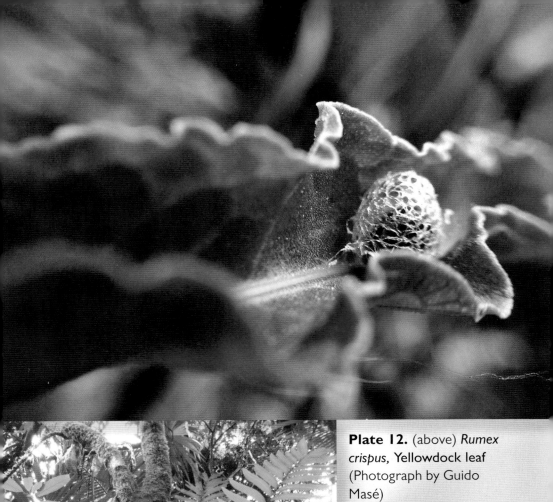

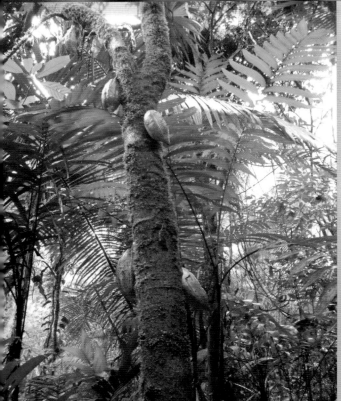

Plate 12. (above) *Rumex crispus,* Yellowdock leaf (Photograph by Guido Masé)

Plate 13. (left) *Theobroma cacao,* Chocolate pods (Photograph by Anne K. Dougherty)

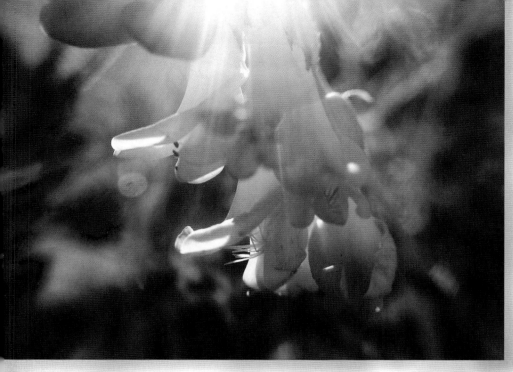

Plate 14. (above) *Astragalus membranaceus,* Astragalus flower (Photograph by Guido Masé)

Plate 15. (below) *Astragalus membranaceus,* Astragalus leaf (Photograph by Guido Masé)

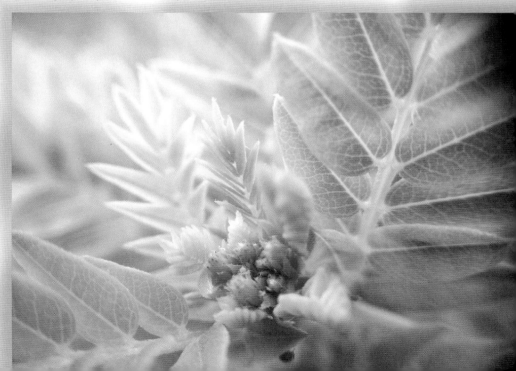

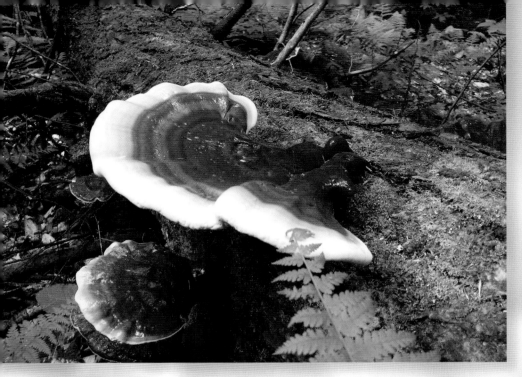

Plate 16. (above) *Ganoderma tsugae,* Red Reishi (Lingzhi)
(Photograph by Guido Masé)

Plate 17. (below) *Crataegus monogyna,* Hawthorn flower
(Photograph by Anne K. Dougherty)

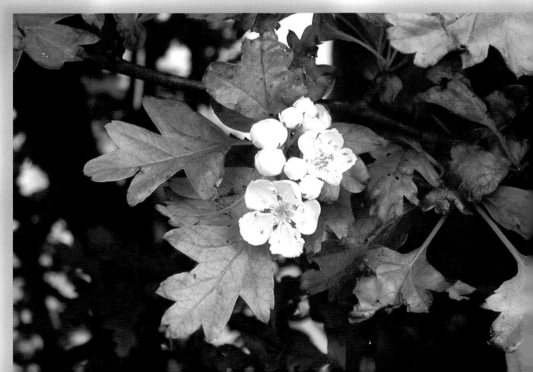

These were botanicals from the Apiaceae or parsley family, such as wild carrot root, parsley itself, anise, asafoetida, and opopanax; herbs from the Brassicaceae or mustard family, such as shepherd's purse; and roots from the Gentianaceae family, such as gentian and centaury.

Gentian (*Gentiana lutea*) is considered one of the bitterest plants we know.[4] Even small quantities of amarogentin, one of its constituents, elicit strong reactions on the tongue and throughout the digestive tract.[5] It is a beautiful plant, growing to four feet and featuring a riotous spike of yellow flowers, and Mithridates would have had to search for it at higher elevations, in the sunny meadows above the tree line, during his wanderings in the mountains of Pontus. Its flavor is actually very similar to that of the true poisons—deadly nightshade (*Atropa belladonna*), for instance—and, being experienced in trying these poisons, Mithridates could not have helped but notice the similarity in taste. Gentian, however, is completely nontoxic, and herein lay the king's genius. He thought that the regular consumption of a plant that tastes like poison might somehow fortify him against the occasional ingestion of a truly toxic herb like belladonna. As we shall see, this strategy worked quite well—too well, in the end—and relied on a couple of important ideas. First of all, our physiology appreciates a good challenge. And second, historically we have lived in an environment full of a wide diversity of botanical chemistry that provided that challenge.

THE XENOBIOME: IS THERE AN OPTIMAL OPERATING ENVIRONMENT?

Any living system exists in the context of its surroundings. Fields respond to the quality of the soil, the water that flows through them, and the weather they experience. Mice living in the field respond to the grass seed that ripens every fall and to the predators flying above the open expanse or hiding in the hollows. Bacteria living on and in the mice respond to their hosts' feeding patterns, their living situations, their social interactions. Even the inner milieu of the bacteria is responsive to the environment of the mice and field, altering the chemistry it expresses.[6] This reflects a profound degree of interconnection, where one piece of the web of life affects many other pieces in turn, at many different levels.

If we agree that ecological interconnection is indeed a reality, and organisms evolved in the context of their environments,[7] then it is not unreasonable to ask what environmental parameters, or ecological components, might be able to best provide the organism with what it needs to function well. In other words, are there any identifiable elements in the world around us that are crucial for health and, specifically for our discussion, crucial for our ability to consistently process and eliminate substances that might otherwise be toxic, irritating, and poisonous?

We know that food and water are necessary for survival. We also have a pretty good idea about some chemical constituents whose absence causes illness: vitamin C and scurvy, folic acid and neural tube defects in the fetus, and vitamin B_{12} and anemia,[8] to name just a few. Notice that these are nutrients we have identified by the immediate results of their deficiencies. Remove B_{12} from a person's diet, and within months she will develop very noticeable symptoms of fatigue and pallor, she will stop menstruating, and depression may ensue. We know these nutrients are important because it is easy to trace a direct cause-and-effect relationship between deficiencies and disease. But could there be other nutrients whose absence causes more subtle issues? It's possible that these issues would not even be evident on an individual basis, requiring instead a large population and long periods of observation. As we shall see, our species seems to be in the middle of just such an experiment, and the results are quite telling. But, for now, let's stay focused on the individual's physiology and its ability to process the daily barrage of chemicals to which it is exposed.

If we are talking about processing chemicals, we have to talk about the liver. While many tissues in the body have the ability to produce enzymes and antioxidants that help to neutralize toxins, none compare to the four-pound sponge located on our right upper abdomen, halfway hidden behind the rib cage. It is a tireless metabolic workhorse—but, curiously enough, if left alone it does very little. Isolated liver tissue and isolated liver cells do not seem to do much of anything, neither synthesizing bile nor producing high levels of metabolic enzymes. Researchers attempting to study how liver cells behave have learned that, in order to better replicate the conditions found in living beings, the cells have to be bathed not only in nutrients, but also in a cocktail of chemicals. It is only then that they begin to act like their true selves. This makes sense: any participant in the web of life becomes lost, sad, and confused when removed from its native environment. Cells taken out of the liver and cultured appear to be quite literally depressed—until you give them something to do.*

The cocktail of chemicals researchers apply to isolated liver cells varies depending on the experiment. Its precise composition comes from observing how cells metabolize "test" substances (such as aceclofenac, a pain reliever) and comparing it to how an animal's liver breaks down those same substances. If the cells work in the same way and at the same rate as in the living organ, then the chemical cocktail must be right (or at least close enough).[9] This technique is useful for creating experimental models of drug metabolism but doesn't tell us much about the true ecological context necessary for a complex, living organ, such as the liver, to work at its best—other than the fact that some type of context is absolutely essential.

We can perhaps begin to discover an answer by thinking about what types of foods humans have eaten historically. Our diets, as we shall see, have shifted over the course of recent history. Before we began cultivating vegetables and grains, some ten thousand to fifteen

---

*Although, interestingly, cells from other human organs, such as nerve or muscle cells, don't need much more than sugar and a few growth factors to respond to calcium and other electrolytes, much as they would in a living being. This implies that liver cells are more tied to the xenobiome—the comprehensive chemical environment in which it evolved—than other tissues are. This makes sense, given their role.

thousand years ago, we mostly consumed meat and wild plants.[10] Toxins came from bacteria (spoiled meat or contaminated water), the bites of venomous insects or animals, or directly from poisonous roots, barks, leaves, seeds, and berries. On this canvas we can begin to paint the picture of the xenobiome, the comprehensive chemical environment in which the liver evolved[11] and without which it might feel like a fish out of water.

Standing in the middle an East African landscape, you take a moment to experience the silence. It is hot and sunny. Where you can see into the distance, a slight haze lingers from the night. There is a tall, wide tree far off—a massive baobab that served as shelter, whose fruits you pounded into a meal that also seemed to reduce the aches from your days of running. Your gaze returns to your feet, red with the fine dust that is the soil here, out of which grows the endless sea of grass.

You hear a snap like the crack of thunder, then a series of them, and though they seem far away, they are clear and ring brightly across the savannah. The elephants are tearing down whole trees, wrenching massive limbs to get at the leaves, prying what sustenance they can from the dry landscape. It's good to know they are there. You haven't found many animals yet, and resources are scarce. Perhaps the elephants have discovered something interesting.

As you begin to move again, you notice a sickle bush (*Dichrostachys*) and a tamarind tree beyond some taller golden grass. The roots from the first are starchy, bitter but nourishing, and the beanlike fruits of the second will make a great, bitter-sour complement (depending on how ripe they are). You collect a good supply of both to save for the evening meal.

To people who lived (or are still living) in this world, plants provided the bulk of the chemistry that their livers experienced on a daily basis. Meat may have been abundant and was certainly crucial in nourishing the species, but it isn't a source of much chemical diversity. Aside from iron, other minerals, and important nutrients like B vitamins, animal flesh is primarily a source of macronutrients, such as protein and fat. Even more crucially, most of the chemistry meat does provide isn't at all challenging to liver metabolism. Protein from the breakdown of the meat we eat is used by the liver to make our tissues, our enzymes, our plasma proteins. We would never dream of chemically destroying such a precious resource. So, in the end, though they may not always have represented the bulk of the calories and macronutrients, plants were certainly responsible for providing both the greatest sheer number of different individual chemicals to the liver and also its greatest metabolic challenge.

Plants are hardly harmless when ingested. Sure, many are poisonous, but we generally avoid these and don't tend to think of carrots as toxic (which, of course, they aren't). The reason we tolerate them so well, however, is based on millions of years of coevolutionary history. Starting with insects, plants have been producing chemicals that act as deterrents to browsing and feeding, and animals have been finding novel ways to neutralize these compounds.[12] This is a crucial adaptive strategy for insects and herbivores whose diets rely exclusively on the local flora, but it's important for carnivores, too. It is definitely important for omnivores (like humans) who count on a decent measure of plants as part of their diets. Without these adaptations, carrots *would* be harmful to our health.*

In sum, humans living on the East African savannah have access to macronutrients from starchy plants and meats but are also exposed to a wide range of chemicals from the botanicals they consume. Many of these chemicals are produced for protection and thus contain a certain element of toxicity—at least, until the animals eating them evolve methods of neutralizing them. We cope with potentially harmful plant chemicals by breaking them down into safer forms in our livers and intestinal tissue, and, as a result, experience no ill effects from

---

*If only from the apigenin, a potentially toxic flavonoid, as seen in Tsuji and Walle's "Cytotoxic Effects." Apigenin is still toxic to cancer cells, as noted in Cárdenas et al.'s "Antitumor Activity of Some Natural Flavonoids."

them today (with some exceptions, of course). Finally, our detoxification organs seem to require exposure to some of those plant chemicals to even be active at all.[13] The xenobiome therefore mostly comprises plants—they are largely responsible for the makeup and behavior of our chemical processing centers.[14]

You may wonder how a chemical might prevent a browsing insect or animal from consuming its plant. After all, if it's simply toxic, you could eat your fill, saunter off, and experience problems later on. This is hardly helpful to the plant, which might have been destroyed before your demise. What's required is a signal, a way to tell a hungry animal that it may not want to overdo the grazing. And this makes a lot of sense from the animal's perspective, too: it seems advantageous to get a feeling as to the toxicity of the food you consume before you eat a whole lot of it and end up in trouble.

So, to be of deterrent value, plant chemicals need to be able to communicate their toxic presence to the animals that might consider eating them. This, as you can imagine, is accomplished through the sense of taste, which is there to give us an idea of the possible chemical content of what we are eating.* Sweet things, highly desired, mean there are a lot of nutritious, carbohydrate-based calories on the way. Salty things imply a rich mineral content, which is also very important. Sour flavors are elicited by acids (think vinegar) and are a result of mild chemical irritation. Pungent, spicy impressions are generated by aromatic volatile oils and their associated compounds (again, as a result of mild irritation), and we can usually smell pungency before we taste it. There is a flavor called umami, or "deliciousness" in Japanese, which is linked with certain amino acids found in meats and other savory foods, as well as with MSG (monosodium glutamate). Finally, there is the bitter taste.

It is harder to define a single type of chemical responsible for the bitter flavor. With the exception of meat and the umami flavor, there usually is an underlying hint of bitterness riding on the palate together

---

*For an overview of taste/chemical detection, see Kinnamon and Cummings's "Chemosensory Transduction Mechanisms in Taste."

with any of the above tastes: whole, unprocessed grains contain the bitter bran, salty seaweeds may have a bitter opening bite (as does actual salt in crude, unprocessed form), lemon and grapefruit juice always mix bitter with sour, and aromatic plants taste bitter when eaten whole. The only common thread in the bitter flavor realm is that it is present in virtually all plants. While some are more bitter than others, on balance, both an apple and a carrot have more bitter flavor in them than a piece of beef (try the peel if you doubt me on this). We find the bitter flavor so often because it is linked to a wide range of chemicals that are very common in the plant world: chicoric, chlorogenic, cinnamic, and rosmarinic acids; flavonoids and other polyphenolics; coumarins and furanocoumarins; iridoids; lactones; cyanogenic glycosides; other saponins; and more. All of these were once toxic to insects and animals.[15] Some still are. So the bitter flavor seems to be the signal from the plant world to watch out—eat less—and activate your detoxification mechanisms. (As it turns out, when you feed animals extracts containing high percentages of these bitter compounds, such as rosmarinic acid, you end up with enhanced liver detoxification.)[16] Animals that tied their perception of bitter to enhanced liver metabolism fared better than their competition.

There is one more important class of plant chemical that has, in almost all cases, an extremely bitter flavor: the alkaloids. These molecules often have powerful effects on animals that consume them and, from caffeine to quinine, taste pretty revolting. Poisonous alkaloids, such as atropine, strychnine, and aconitine, are intensely bitter, and you would have a hard time consuming appreciable quantities of them. But I guess that's the point: the plant makes the chemical to keep the animal away, and the animal develops a broadly sensitive taste receptor to warn it about the chemical's presence. That warning comes to us as "bitterness."* A little bit, coming from the ubiquitous molecules

—————————

*There is widespread consensus that our ability to perceive bitterness is an evolutionary adaptation to the presence of potential toxins in the diet. See, for instance, Lindemann's "Chemoreception," as well as Scott and Verhagen's "Taste as a Factor in the Management of Nutrition."

whose toxicity we've learned to disable, keeps our livers functioning well. Too much might mean we've ingested something overly toxic. In either case, the perception of bitter implies a challenge to our physiology and especially to our molecular metabolism.

We are beginning to get a better picture of the xenobiome: it is a set of chemicals, mostly derived from plants, that either once were or still are toxic to a certain degree and possess a generally bitter flavor. Most of what we think of as bitter is no longer toxic to us (though it may still be to the insects that have not developed the same detoxification machinery we have).[17] But it certainly awakens the same defenses that it always has: we have retained the perception of the flavor and the responses that go with it. And here we are starting to see why adding bitter roots and leaves to the aromatic Egyptian kyphi might have been an especially good idea for the toxin-obsessed Mithridates. The ongoing exposure to a rich and potent xenobiome kept his liver on its toes, gave it a daily challenge much as a daily run challenges the cardiovascular system and keeps it in "good shape." Such a xenobiome, we will see, might be just as important as physical exercise itself. Challenge leads to resiliency.

AN INTERLUDE WITH GOLDILOCKS

Now, as any runner knows, excessive challenge can quickly lead to damage and set off a downward spiral of injury, stagnation, weakness, and further injury. But no challenge at all brings on weakness and stagnation even more quickly. The optimal path, it seems, lies in the middle. Intuitively, we know this to be true, but in recent years research is beginning to uncover how important this middle path is in the healthy functioning of our physiology.

Take, for instance, social and emotional development. Dr. Mark Seery, a psychologist and researcher at the University of Buffalo, has spent the last decade analyzing the effects of challenge on human beings, particularly in the realms of psychology, mental/emotional health, and cardiovascular fitness. By studying what happens to us when we are placed in situations where environmental challenge either meets or exceeds our ability to cope, he has helped articulate what researchers are calling the "Goldilocks principle" of stress: not too much, not too little, but just the right amount.

As you might recall from the children's fairy tale, Goldilocks is the somewhat-brazen little girl who wanders into a cottage inhabited by three bears and proceeds to eat their breakfasts, wreck their furniture, and sleep in their beds. During each of her acts of trespassing, she tries three different options in turn: the first is too much, the second too little, and the third just right. What Dr. Seery and his colleagues discovered is that, when it comes to stress, we fare best not when we experience the least amount; rather, children who have the greatest degree of psychological resiliency and mental health are those who experienced a moderate level of stress during development. Those who experienced very low levels of stress fare worse than their highly traumatized counterparts.[18]

This is a fairly common phenomenon: not only in exercise and in childhood development, but also in eating, sleeping, communicating, even gardening (ever noticed what happens if you don't "harden off" your seedlings?). Living systems do best when they engage moderately with their environments, accept some measure of challenge, and get stronger in the process. We have numerous cultural and philosophical aphorisms that ensconce this principle firmly in the realm of "common sense": what doesn't kill you makes you stronger; adversity builds character; necessity is the mother of invention; no pain, no gain. Even the Buddha is said to have recommended the middle path, between the extremes of total self-indulgence and total self-denial, as the optimal road to travel. In the end, like Goldilocks, we should avoid the challenges that overwhelm us (this porridge is too hot!), but seek out those that help us grow and adapt. Without challenge, we become less resilient. But with a little, we turn out just right.

Might this principle also apply to the chemical makeup of our xenobiome? We have already seen that plants have come up with molecular challenges to the organisms that eat them and that the process of adapting to those challenges has helped create the liver and metabolic tissues that we have today. Obviously we can overdo the consumption of botanical toxins, and this (as Mithridates knew all too well) can still lead to death. But the ongoing exposure to low levels of similar substances might actually be important in maintaining our overall resiliency (Mithridates was counting on this). Toxins, or former toxins, activate our metabolic machinery. Could it also be possible, as in so many other cases, that removing these challenging chemicals from the xenobiome makes us weaker and less resilient? Could there really be a "middle path" to tasting poison?

THE BITTER TASTE RECEPTOR: FEEL THE CHALLENGE

Before we can see what happens when we remove formerly toxic, bitter-tasting molecules from the xenobiome, let's take a moment to examine the "detector" our physiology uses to assess the degree of metabolic challenge that our food contains. The bitter taste receptor is part of a family of proteins known as TRs (taste receptors). There seem to be six different types of TRs and some degree of variation within each different type. For example, the receptor for sweet flavor is one type of protein, coded for by three genes, and able to detect sugars.[19] The receptor for umami is similarly simple and detects amino acids (protein).[20] Sour taste is mediated through two different receptor subtypes, able to detect hydrogen ions (responsible for acidity).[21] We have a receptor for fats and another for salt (sodium).[22] Each of the above receptors is manufactured from the information stored in three to five genes, consists of one to three different subtypes, and binds to a small range of substances—some, like the salty and sour receptors, only to one specific substance.

But the bitter taste receptor family, known as the T2R receptor family, is made of over twenty different subtypes, coded for by some thirty-four genes, and able to detect over one hundred often completely unrelated chemical compounds.[23] The diversity and complexity of human bitter taste receptors directly mirrors the diversity of a plant-based xenobiome and contains the physical record of our interactions with a series of botanical toxins over the millennia. This is proof positive that we use the bitter flavor as a signal for potential trouble from the vegetable kingdom. Only those substances that served as botanical defense mechanisms, and that were once toxic to our ancestors, stimulate the T2Rs.[24]

Low concentrations of bitterness are noticeable but not necessarily unpleasant. Highly bitter substances can be so distressing as to cause vomiting (and a good thing, too—stomach pumping free of charge, courtesy of the highly poisonous plants). Stimulating T2Rs has profound implications throughout the digestive system and in the liver, as we shall see when we review the pharmacology of bitter-tasting molecules. For now, suffice it to say that getting the signal of bitterness on the tongue increases antioxidant enzyme and bile secretion in the liver through the combined action of hormones, such as cholecystokinin, and nerves, such as the vagus nerve.[25] This combination of effects prepares us to interact successfully with the bitter botanical chemistry we have experienced throughout our evolutionary history. It is a cascade of reactions that keep us well protected, a carefully orchestrated series of steps in our dance with the xenobiome.

Interestingly, T2R receptors are found in many other tissues of the body, indicating that their chemosensory ability is not limited to the tongue. First and foremost, they are present in the throat, stomach, small intestine, and pancreatic duct,[26] where they reinforce the hormonal and neural signals first elicited on the tongue. Liver and gallbladder tissue also have T2Rs.[27] Researchers have discovered these bitter taste receptors in the airways of the lungs (where, if stimulated, they induce relaxation and opening), and even in brain cells.[28] Neurons might be sensitive to bitter stimuli, the scientists speculated, as part of an appetite-regulation pathway in the nervous system because, in fact, reduced food consumption and lower blood sugar levels are another profound consequence of the bitter taste.

Our physiology evolved the ability to perceive bitterness in order to protect itself from orally ingested plant toxins. The logical next step after receiving the "warning sign" such flavors represent might be reduced oral food intake, meaning that it makes good sense to eat less if you're detecting the potential for lots of toxicity. If true, this could be part of the reason eating more vegetables leads to less caloric consumption.[29] Filling your belly with indigestible plant fiber certainly plays a part, but the relatively bitter taste of most vegetables and salad greens might be involved as well. Regardless, it would be fantastic if we could help control appetite by stimulating T2R receptors. This might be another reason for the presence of bitter chemicals in our xenobiome.

As it turns out, this is precisely what bitter-tasting foods appear to do.[30] Perhaps through nerve-based interactions, perhaps through the initiation of hormonal cues, people who stimulate their bitter taste receptors empty their bellies more slowly[31] and feel more full. Interestingly, when infusing bitter-tasting substances directly into the GI tract, researchers found no such effects[32]—meaning that, although T2Rs are found in the stomach, intestines, and beyond, there is something important about the conscious perception of the bitter taste. We eat less, and food remains in the stomach and duodenum (the main "digestive" parts of the digestive tract) longer. These effects represent useful adaptations in our model of the xenobiome: eat fewer potentially harmful substances and process them more completely.

We will explore the hormonal connection to bitters when we explore their pharmacology, but, for now, it is worth mentioning an interesting 36-amino-acid protein known as polypeptide YY. It is secreted by cells in the small intestine in response to bitter-tasting molecules and also protein-based meals, and it appears to be involved in controlling appetite in humans. When both obese and lean subjects have higher levels of polypeptide YY circulating in their bloodstream, their intake of food decreases by 30 percent. The fact that bitter plant constituents stimulate the secretion of this hormone may be part of how they control our feeding behavior.

As we shall see, other hormones are also secreted in response to T2R stimulation and reinforce the signal to consume less food while also modulating physiological processes (largely in the liver) that keep our blood sugar levels under control. Blood sugar, or blood glucose, is an important fuel for every cell in the body, but chronically elevated levels are quite harmful and are the hallmark of a common metabolic dysfunction, type 2 diabetes mellitus. Perhaps T2R receptor signaling is involved in maintaining healthy blood glucose levels, as research from the laboratory of C. Shawn Dotson seems to suggest.

Dr. Dotson, working at the University of Florida, is very curious about how our tastes affect our eating. He has studied and documented a specific connection between T2R receptor stimulation and average blood glucose, finding that the greater the signal coming from the bitter taste receptors, the lower the glucose levels.[33] T2Rs influence numerous hormones and, in Dotson's opinion, present "potential targets for treatment of Type 2 diabetes mellitus."[34] His research, coupled with studies showing that specific bitter molecules from plants keep blood glucose low,[35] suggests a significant role for the bitter taste receptor in the management of diabetes.

So it seems that our xenobiome, the cocktail of chemicals we experience, is loaded with a variety of substances that, at one point, were toxic to animal and insect life. We have evolved ways, through the liver and digestive tract, of handily dispatching (most of) these substances. Naturally, the more of them we consume, the more active the liver's detoxification pathways are and the more engaged our body's molecular processing streams become. Additionally, it seems that these same substances have an effect on our appetite, making us eat less and keeping our blood sugar under control. Aside from macronutrients, our xenobiome is quite bitter, a context that provides (or, perhaps more accurately, provided) a daily challenge to our systems, mediated through the T2R receptor—a challenge that relies on age-old memories of poison encoded in our bitter taste receptors, and a challenge that keeps our metabolism fit.

Most animals can feel this challenge, and humans are no exception. Experiencing the bitter flavor induces a series of changes that include not only improved liver and digestive function but also reduced caloric consumption and blood glucose. And while these changes are happening on a case-by-case basis, what effects become evident in a larger population? What we need is a big group of people. We need to alter its xenobiome by dramatically reducing the presence of plants and their bitter secondary metabolites. And we need to watch what happens over a few generations, say, one hundred years or more. Based on what we've just learned, it might be reasonable to expect that, on average, the people in our group would eat more, gain weight, experience more type 2 diabetes and higher rates of digestive complaints and inflammation. But where might we find such a group?

THE "WESTERN" DIET: A GRAND EXPERIMENT IN XENOBIOME ALTERATION

Consider sugars and carbohydrates, the source of another important taste: sweet. Carbohydrates historically occupied a much smaller role in our diets than they do today. When analyzing traditional indigenous diets from around the planet, carbohydrate content is low compared to that of animal protein.[36] As human populations reach more northern latitudes, starchy vegetables and plants in general become a smaller and smaller fraction of daily calories, replaced largely by seafood.[37] Interestingly, plants—from berries to seaweeds—still feature prominently in the human diet and are specifically sought out as health-promoting foods, even at the higher latitudes, such as in native Inuit populations.[38] In these same populations, people are consuming fewer plants than average and carbohydrate intake is also extremely low. Levels of diabetes, inflammatory heart disease, and fatty infiltration in the liver (often a sign of toxic damage) are comparable to those of other indigenous groups.[39] So perhaps we should refine the picture of the xenobiome a little: rich in bitter plants, it also has a relatively low level of sugars and carbohydrates.

Not that low sugar consumption is anyone's choice; it is much more a matter of availability and circumstance. While bitter plants are virtually everywhere, sweet starches, gums, and other substances, such as honey, are fairly uncommon. Just as with bitter, we have evolved a powerful set of behaviors associated with sweet: we seek it out and are intensely gratified by consuming it. It is a taste associated with deep and profound nourishment, and it makes us feel loved, safe, and rewarded, much as a drug would.* Of course, there is an excellent evolutionary reason for this: energy-dense nutrition is vital in a competitive world. If we had our way, if we could give in to our taste-driven desires, we would get rid of bitter completely and eat all the sweet food we could possibly find.

Such a dream was impossible for the majority of human history. We may have complained about it, but aside from the diets of northern latitudes, our food was largely plants and meat with the occasional sweet treat. And in the frozen tundra of the north, forget about it—not even complex starches were available, dried blueberries being the best you could hope for. Even after the advent of agriculture and the domestication of grains, truly sweet food was still rare, with rice, bread, or other carbohydrates being quite coarse and often as bitter as they were starchy. Milling soft, refined flours was an intensely laborious and expensive proposition, which is why cakes and pastries prepared with them were largely a luxury of the aristocracy. The general population's resentment of their rulers' ability to gorge on sweet (and reap its druglike rewards) was still evident at the end of the eighteenth century: the

---

*For a comprehensive review of the druglike effects of sugars and our hardwired response to the sweet flavor, see Kessler's *The End of Overeating*—an excellent read by a former FDA commissioner.

apocryphal "Let them eat cake" was used to mock an overfed, out-of-touch elite and its cavalier attitude toward the peasants' hunger.

Interestingly, the aristocracy didn't just have the exclusive luxury of being able to fully indulge its desire for sweet. It also had a lock on illnesses like gout, cardiovascular disease, and type 2 diabetes.* But, to the rest of us, this wasn't the issue. The rich could avoid physical labor and get anything their hearts desired, including lots of sweet food. Understandably, we were jealous. We wanted to stop working our bodies to the bone every day, and we wanted sweet cake to eat every night.

As they say, be careful what you wish for. With the advent of large-scale industrialized agriculture and milling in food production (typically a Western phenomenon of the nineteenth century), all of a sudden large portions of the population had access to softer, whiter bread. Novel chemical techniques were used to make the flour whiter still—literally by bleaching it. When sugarcane processing and sugar production were mechanized and coupled to steam power at about the same time, Europe's largest import skyrocketed in availability and popularity. Now everyone could entertain the notion of dessert at every meal and contend less with the rough and somewhat bitter flavor of coarsely milled bread.

Industrialization arose part and parcel with urbanization, and as people moved to cities to support the new factories, much in their lives began to change along with the new landscape. First, people moved their bodies less. Factory work consisted of long, brutally intensive hours—but was often not as physically demanding as farm work had been. Second, the proportion of sweets and refined carbohydrates in the average diet began to rise. I feel that sugar found its role as an opiate during this time, a respite from the exploitation of industrial labor, a literal piece of the "pie in the sky" promised to so many workers. That role is one that it still holds today for many of us.

But crucially for our discussion, the diversity of plants in the aver-

---

*My favorite example of these maladies is Henry VIII, king of England during the first half of the sixteenth century.

age person's diet began to drop. This change was slow at first, with many folks still connected to the country and the wild, bitter botanicals such a life offered. Inevitably, after a few generations, however, families picked fewer dandelion greens in the spring, relying less on foraging for supplementing their meals. Instead, for most people, the supplement became an extra helping of carbohydrate. And while we blame so much of our modern public health concerns on the rise of sweet in the Western diet, we can't forget that at the same time we handily eliminated much of what was bitter and wild in our food. This is quite natural: it's exactly what a child would do if given the choice. But, as we saw when examining the xenobiome, it is a choice that deprives the metabolism of vital chemistry, key to keeping it challenged, awake, and alive.

During the twentieth century, this trend continued. Petrochemical fertilization ushered in a "green revolution" that, in certain parts of the world, allowed for a fivefold increase in grain production. The American Midwest, once a patchwork of family farms, is becoming a vast corn, wheat, and soybean desert, a display of order and dominance unequaled on the planet. Huge water, fertilizer, pesticide, and herbicide supplies are now needed to maintain this carbohydrate glut, all to provide a diet that is more and more devoid of the incredible biodiversity human beings had historically consumed. What has happened to us as a result? Because, as you have probably figured out, we are the guinea pigs in this experiment. We had no idea what might occur by upending the chemistry of the xenobiome, by thrusting a relatively rare flavor (sweet) to the forefront of caloric consumption and eliminating a ubiquitous one (bitter) almost completely, but that's exactly what we've been doing for almost two hundred years. In the developed world, we have decided that our diet should be free of uncomfortable foods, foods that are wild, bitter, fibrous, weedy, or otherwise challenging. For the last fifty years we've pursued this plan with fervent zeal. What do we have to show for it?

Let's begin by reflecting on the infrastructure that is devoted to satisfying our desire for carbohydrates. The largest impacts are agricultural. In sections of the upper Midwest, where corn dominates and average farm size (by state) is three hundred acres or more, industrialized agriculture focused on the intensive production of carbohydrates rules the ecology. Of particular interest are the chemical additives to the ecosystem. In all corn-producing states, ranging from New York through Iowa, Nebraska, and Wisconsin, over 11 billion pounds of nitrogen, and almost 4 billion pounds each of phosphorous and potassium, are added to the soil each year. Synthetic fertilizers are one thing, but of even greater concern are the herbicides applied to the same acreage to control unwanted, wild plants. Corn farmers applied 57 million pounds of glyphosate (Roundup), more than 51 million pounds of atrazine, and some 20 million pounds of other herbicides in 2010.* By comparison, all the herbicide applied to potatoes amounted to about 4 million pounds, of which more than half was actually fungicide.

Atrazine is an interesting chemical. It's fairly cheap, and it kills a broad range of weeds from lamb's quarters to couchgrass. It seems to persist in the environment, especially in the groundwater, for a long time. This fact, coupled with the increased risk in humans of hormone disruption and birth defects from low levels of exposure, led the European Union to ban it from use in 2004. In Italy, in the 1980s, fertile lands around the Po River were under intensive cultivation, and atrazine was a major herbicide used at that time. Media reports of contamination and subsequent ill effects were alarmingly frequent, and the use of bottled water became the norm. In the United States, U.S. Geological Survey (USGS) maps of herbicide use show heavy application rates (more than thirty-two pounds per square mile) in almost all of Indiana, Ohio, Illinois, and Iowa—the heart of corn country.

The effects of atrazine on plants are dramatic. This chemical attaches to a piece of the molecular machinery that is essential for converting light to energy, and, as a result, photosynthesis is disrupted

---

*From the National Agricultural and Statistics service, a branch of the U.S. Dept. of Agriculture, "Agriculture and Chemical Use Program statistics for 2010."

and the harmful effects of solar radiation are amplified. Weeds quickly wither and die. In animals, it winds its way into the metabolism of sex hormones, affecting fertility, growth, and development, with documented ill effects on amphibians, birds, and, more recently, humans. Though we've long known about the endocrine-disrupting effects of pesticides like DDT, we are only starting to understand how weed-killing herbicides affect our hormones, and it doesn't look too good. Ironically, some of the weeds, from kudzu to red clover, dandelion to wild carrot, might actually buffer the deleterious effects of agrichemicals. We are using massive amounts of toxins on our farmland to kill the plants that might be our best protection against the toxins themselves.

Fertilizer runoff can affect open bodies of water, which are delicately balanced ecosystems. Lake Champlain, running almost the length of Vermont's western border with New York, routinely experiences blooms of toxic algae. These cyanobacteria thrive in the high-phosphate environment created as streams traversing farms run into rivers and finally into the lake. Herbicide and pesticide use is becoming more of a concern for human beings who drink water both from lakes and from underground aquifers. The petroleum required to produce the fertilizers and toxins, harvest the grain, ship, process, and ship it again makes the whole operation fairly inefficient (and perhaps unsustainable). Finally, it is worth remembering that more fossil fuels are burned to turn some of that carbohydrate into beef, chicken, and pork. We've put our livestock on a high-sugar, low-biodiversity regimen, too—and that affects the meat we eat, and not in a good way, I'm afraid.

As is true in any living system, you cannot remove a challenge, a stressor, an adaptive pressure from one part of the web without affecting other parts in turn. In large areas of the developed world, we have conquered the short-term challenge of the bitter flavor and the medium-term challenge of hunger. But the longer-term danger of chronic disease, including diabetes, obesity, and heart disease, is a different matter. And we have shifted a huge part of the challenge to our environment—to our prairies, our rivers, our lakes. It's not too difficult to trace a link between a glass of soda, its corn syrup content, and a little more atrazine in the water. And in the end, water supply affects us all.

Place a graph of diabetes rates in the United States next to a graph of farm acreage devoted to corn. They both follow a disturbingly similar curve, rising slowly since the 1970s and much more sharply beginning in 1995. Granted, this is a simplistic analysis: many other factors, such as the production of corn for fuel (in the form of ethanol), complicate this simple correlation. But our taste for sweet has consequences both in the world around us and in the world inside us. It is interesting how much the one reflects the other. Our fields have lost biodiversity, are devoted largely to carbohydrates, and are fed by a fluid (through irrigation) that is both overabundant in nutrition and laced with toxins. Similarly, the products of our fields have created a xenobiome for our liver and digestion that is at once less wild and challenging, and at the same time hypersweet. The lack of challenge affects our ability to process poison, so in the end we, too, are fed by a fluid (through our bloodstream) that is both overabundant in nutrition and laced with toxins.

This can impact health in many ways. Generally, you start to see issues with digestive function first. The sweet flavor does very little to activate the gut, being mostly about rewarding the brain. It lacks most of the stimulating effects elicited by the T2R bitter taste receptors. This was not a problem in the past, since anything sweet usually came from whole plants loaded with bitter, metabolism-activating chemicals. But now, sweet starchy foods flow like ghosts through our stomach and intestines, moving along but hardly making a mark. The body still recognizes them as sources of sugar and sends out signals to control the inevitable rise in blood glucose levels. But without bitters as a companion, the starches pass quickly into the small intestine and are met by a sluggish digestive enzyme response. Pieces of carbohydrate begin to ferment, acted on by bacteria instead of by our digestive fluids, and the gas that results may cause bloating, spasming, and even nausea. After some time of not experiencing the bitter flavor, the valves between compartments of our digestive tract grow slack, losing their tone. Food slips through even more easily. This may lead to heartburn, worsened by overeating, by lying down right after a meal, or both. The lack of bitter stimulus may also be connected to sluggish bowel function, with occasional periods of constipation.

The unchallenged digestion eventually has a harder time handling proteins, too. If they are inadequately broken down, proteins, such as gluten (from wheat) and casein (from milk), can be somewhat irritating, stimulating a mild (and sometimes not so mild) immune reaction. And inflammation in the belly may be a source of considerable distress, making digestive issues worse in a vicious cycle and also relaying an impression of this distress to the central nervous system via the vagus nerve. If aromatic plants help relax and rebalance the signals coming to the brain from the gut, a diet lacking bitters does the exact opposite: our mood has to contend with a daily background level of irritation and tension coming from the belly.

The speed with which blandly sweet meals move through the gut may complicate matters once the simple sugars they contain begin to enter the bloodstream. In nature, even the sweetest of substances, like honey, are wrapped up in a great deal of fiber. This fiber, which consists of indigestible starches, literally "traps" the sugars present in food and slows their rate of absorption. This is largely what our digestion expects—table sugar is an unknown food, in the evolutionary time line—and it reacts to glucose entering the bloodstream with the assumption that it's coming from a whole-plant context. But what is the difference between a whole-plant ideal and a refined-carbohydrate reality?

To understand the difference, let's examine the chemistry of the two. A whole-grain meal contains some digestible starches (which end up getting broken down to glucose), along with some soluble and insoluble fiber. A refined-grain meal simply contains the digestible starches—the refining process has removed everything else. Now, let's assume that both meals have the same amount of digestible carbohydrates in them, say, fifty grams. We know that those fifty grams of refined carbs will travel more quickly through the gut and enter the bloodstream more quickly because they're not trapped in a fiber matrix.* But our pancreas, a major organ involved in blood sugar control, doesn't know this. It simply assumes that all carbohydrates we eat are bound to indigestible fiber, because that's all that it has ever known.

So the fifty grams of carbohydrates from the whole-grain meal enter the bloodstream at a given rate, a rate that the pancreas is used to, and as blood sugar levels slowly rise, the pancreas secretes insulin in response. But when the fifty grams of sugars from the refined meal enter the bloodstream, they do so at a much more rapid pace. You can actually approximate this same rapid rise in blood glucose with a whole-grain meal; you just have to consume one hundred grams of carbohydrates instead of fifty. And, since it knows no better, the pancreas assumes this is exactly what you've done. So it secretes more insulin, preparing the bloodstream for a flood of sugar that isn't coming! And a few hours later, the result is low blood sugar, or hypoglycemia. The pancreas overshot its target, glucose levels drop, and the brain starts to crave—you guessed it—more sugar, the sweeter the better. We're riding the sugar roller coaster.

We are now beginning to see the results of our experiment in xenobiome alteration. We have removed the bitter flavor from our diets, both by reducing the amount of wild, weedy foods we consume and by refining and overdosing on starchy staples. This has been a natural response driven by deep-seated instincts: bitter makes us think of poison and makes us want to eat less, while sweet rewards our pleasure

---

*For more on this, consider the concept of the "glycemic index," which pegs the speed at which different foods enter the bloodstream as glucose. Table sugar, as a baseline reference point, has a glycemic index set at 100.

centers and makes us want to eat more. The consequences have been a series of imbalances in the human physiology: digestion has become sluggish and ineffective because the xenobiome is no longer stimulating, and blood sugar levels have begun to seesaw in dangerous ways that eventually increase resistance to insulin and promote the rise of type 2 diabetes.

Since you cannot alter one component of a system without affecting the whole, we are finding that our environment has suffered, too. We have shifted short-term challenges we used to experience in the endless search for nutrition onto different pieces of our ecological web. The global rise in carbohydrate consumption has prompted the development of industrialized agriculture, increasing environmental pollution dramatically, especially pollution of our water resources. After years of planting grains to feed our hunger, a "sugar-industrial complex" may now be determining what we eat. Either that, or there's some powerful graminaceous magic afoot.

Several ideas have been advanced about how to correct the symptoms associated with our newly altered xenobiome. Eliminating carbohydrates, and especially processed carbohydrates that have been separated from their fiber, seems like an obvious solution. Many people end up doing just that when they remove wheat products from their diet, as wheat accounts for up to 90 percent of the refined grain consumed in the United States (not including sugar). Others simply cut out carbohydrates completely and train their bodies to use lipids as energy by approximating a "Paleolithic" diet rich in meat protein and fat (and this may make them less reliant on bitter plants as a result— remember the Inuit). These approaches certainly can help to manage digestive complaints, obesity, and diabetes. They are intuitive ideas, and any plan should rely at least in some measure on moderating sugar intake.

Another approach is to supplement the digestive juices with enzymes taken orally. These are catalysts that break down the major classes of macronutrients we need: proteins, fats, and carbohydrates.

They are usually produced in abundance by cells in the mouth, stomach, pancreas, and small intestine—but only in response to adequate stimulation of bitter T2R receptors. If such a stimulus is absent, one certainly could add in enzymes from the outside world, though this seems like bailing water from a leaky boat. Better to find the hole and plug it. There is also preliminary evidence that long-term digestive enzyme supplementation might make gut juices even weaker, in essence adding to an already addictive pattern: first the sugar, then the enzyme.

We know that the problem exists. Our guts are weaker and more hypersensitive; our carbohydrate intake has contributed to epidemic rates of obesity, diabetes, and cardiovascular disease; and our environment is being saturated with poisons whose effects we can't escape. We also know that our xenobiome has been dramatically altered, made less diverse and less wild. Might part of the solution come from this less visible angle, rather than simply carbohydrate reduction or a pill?

Might part of the solution be hiding in the unwanted plants, the bitter, weedy roots and greens that intrude on our fields and gain footholds in waste places? They have been perennial companion species. Often in the past they were used as sources of food (in many places they still are). They are rich in bitter constituents, especially their roots—which we might have favored for nutrition as they also contain many digestible (and indigestible) starches. By activating our bitter taste receptors, they reawaken an ancient reflex, our birthright really, that makes us able to engage with a diverse botanical environment and the chemistry that comes with it. It is a challenge we were born to take and, furthermore, it seems to be a challenge without which we suffer and stagnate. Bitter plants, long sources of potential toxins, may at this point be so entwined in our metabolic machinery that we cannot live without them. Herein lies the heart of the mithridate, the bitter antidote to all poisons, an elixir of life.

THE TRADITIONAL APPROACH

If we think bitters might be a viable solution to the gastrointestinal and metabolic disturbances of modern life, there should be evidence in traditional herbal medicine that these plants improve liver and digestive function, and possibly correct the effects of diabetes. Of course, it is hard to separate the bitter flavor from the general context of an indigenous cuisine, where most meals contain a good measure of bitter vegetables. Nevertheless, historically, certain bitter herbal preparations have been viewed as more "medicinal" and have been used as a supplement to all diets for a range of complaints. You can still get tonic water at any grocery store—featuring the bitter taste of quinine (and lots of corn syrup, too). Let's examine these types of formulae and see what virtues they were thought to hold.

One of the first ever documented, at least in the European/ Middle Eastern context, must certainly be the mithridate. The herbalist Crataeus and his king put together a blend that was rich in both aromatic and bitter constituents, and though some had very intense flavors, all lacked any toxicity. This basic formula has remained unchanged ever since—which is why I think Mithridates made the first high-test digestive bitters. In all likelihood, the herbs were finely ground in a mortar and pestle and comminuted one with the other until a powdery mix remained. This could have been sprinkled on food, rolled into a large pill, or mixed into wine as the Egyptian priests who supplied some of the ingredients had always done. But the addition of so many local bitter plants to the aromatic cocktail was a new one. At the very least, their use was brought to the level of a fine art at the royal seat in Sinope.

The main use for this preparation was as an antitoxin, to allay the king's paranoid obsession with protecting himself from those who might wish to poison him. This application makes a lot of sense, given what we know about the effects of bitter T2R receptor stimulation and the importance of wild, bitter plants as part of the xenobiome. The net result must have included an increase in detoxification activity by the liver. But the mithridate also became prized for its action in response to a variety of other common issues, mostly arising from wounds and trauma, but also from digestive complaints, stiffness, weakness, old age, and debility. It was thought to decrease overall vulnerability (from *vulnus,* Latin for "wound"), and eventually the legend of Mithridates, his epic victories in battle, his old age and ruthlessness, and his secret remedy became conflated into a myth that the remedy itself conferred nearly complete invulnerability.

By blunting the effects of poisons and also apparently decreasing inflammation through the entire physiology, the mithridate secured its place in history. Physicians and pharmacists, beginning with the followers of Galen more than two hundred years later, tried to copy and amend the formula, prescribing it for many similar complaints. Galen was aware of the mithridate, noting its use against poison and for digestive disorders, calling it "an incomparable antidote for all internal indispositions of the body."[40] He renamed his variant on the recipe *theriac,* meaning "antidote." It is interesting to note that this word literally means "from the wild" in ancient Indo-European tongues— a nod to the importance of ingesting a little wildness to counteract toxicity. Now Galen was a good physician, but he tended to prefer conjecture over empiricism. Often his idea of how the theory of medicine should pan out trumped his actual observations of illness and recovery. Unfortunately, in European medicine for the next fifteen hundred years, this trend continued.

The original mithridate, and its derivatives such as the Galenic theriac, became adulterated with a variety of substances, such as animal bile, snake flesh, and more. These additions were perhaps the result of a theoretical notion that if a snake could survive with all that poison inside it, there must be something magical about its very nature that can be transferred to those who eat it. Of course, this is a false concept—but it sounded good in theory, so medicine ran with it, as usual. Eventually, another misguided notion took over: that if poison tasted bitter, the antidotes must taste sweet. So by the eighteenth century, even the word *theriac* had been bastardized into *treacle,* which was a sickly sweet mixture of sugar water and ineffective vestigial quantities of aromatic and bitter plants. Needless to say, it was not very useful stuff.

Fortunately, as the original bitter remedy was being diluted to ineffectiveness by the "authorities" in the medical field, folks living in the country were still harvesting the same wild plants and blending them together using the same basic structure: some aromatics to rebalance tension, some bitters to stimulate digestion and liver function, and no actual poisons. These remedies were seen primarily as bitter digestive aids and taken around mealtimes. Despite being largely ignored by mainstream medicine, they have persisted throughout history for one simple reason: they work. Numerous such remedies can be found in the marketplace today. But some of the other benefits ascribed to the mithridate (such as less inflammation and more youthful vigor) were part of the virtues associated with these blends, too.

The Italian *amaro,* or "bitter," is an alcoholic mix very much along these lines. It contains special (and often closely guarded) combinations of bitter roots and leaves, from plants such as gentian and artichoke, blended with aromatics, such as citrus peel, ginger, clove, and more. Some, like Fernet Branca, are quite bitter. Others, including Averna, have sugar added to make them more palatable. More commercial preparations, such as the cherry-red Campari, are a bit less bitter, but are still cut from the same mold. Cynar, definitely an acquired taste, is an artichoke-based liqueur that I remember being fairly ubiquitous, "enjoyed" by young and old alike before or after meals.

The *amari* are still used primarily to enhance digestion, though their aromatic qualities also make them useful for relaxing into convivial conversation after sharing food. They are recommended for symptoms ranging from heartburn and indigestion to gas and bloating, irregular bowel function, and, more generally, any issue relating to the belly. But one often hears, especially from old-timers, that taking a daily shot of a good *amaro* keeps away infection, reduces inflammation, and helps to encourage resilience and strength. These folks, noticing a slight decrease in digestive strength that comes with advanced age, tend to love their bitters even more. The improvement in liver metabolism that accompanies the bitter taste may have positive systemic effects, too. Regardless, people in traditional cultures don't turn to digestive enzyme or hydrochloric acid pills when they feel an issue in their bellies. They turn to bitters.

Throughout Europe, this cultural tradition is well established. Swedish bitters, a somewhat laxative blend containing senna, may have come from a Paracelsian formula dating back to the sixteenth century. Absinthe, not exactly a classic bitter but still used in much the same way (and possessing a similar flavor), was popularized in France and throughout the world, starting in the late eighteenth century. "New World" preparations, featuring new bitters like quinine but also more classic roots, such as gentian, became popular around the same time (Angostura and Peychaud's are two of the more famous brands). In the United States myriad bitter tonics were marketed during the nineteenth and early twentieth centuries for nearly every ailment. But two main points stand out in the more recent history of these formulae. First, they are just the tip of a cultural iceberg that includes a range of homegrown remedies that never made the history books. And second, all of them are considered digestive and liver remedies first and foremost. This is no surprise, given what we know about the stimulation of bitter taste receptors in humans. So, from a cultural perspective, the bitter flavor is an important conscious addition to food and has traditionally been associated with a healthy, happy belly.

What about herbal medicine? Do bitters have a distinct therapeutic focus, and how are they thought to work from a traditional perspective? If the answers to these questions reinforce the idea that they figure prominently in maintaining the correct xenobiome for liver and digestive function, we will have further evidence that bitter plants have a crucial role to play in bringing us closer to a state of overall wellness.

Generally speaking, bitters are used in herbal medicine in much the same way as they are used in a broader cultural context. Herbalist David Hoffmann is of Welsh extraction and training but has lived in the United States in the recent past and served as president of the American Herbalists Guild. He groups the basic actions of bitters into three functions: they stimulate the release of digestive juices, aid in liver detoxification, and help regulate blood sugar. Additionally, Hoffmann mentions that bitters can be used to stimulate a weak appetite and reduce inflammation in the gut wall.

Christopher Hobbs, an acupuncturist and American herbalist, has commented at length about the value of bitter herbs. He cites improvement in digestive function, though he also notes metabolic effects, commenting that symptoms such as fatigue and inflammation may be related to poor chemical processing by the liver. He also repeats the general formulation principle for bitters first recorded by Mithridates: some bitter, nontoxic herbs; some aromatics; and a little sweetness to blend it all together.

Rosemary Gladstar, who lives in the mountains of Vermont but spent long periods in California, recognizes the crucial role bitters have to play in balancing liver function. She emphasizes how a healthy liver improves physiological function across the board, particularly the metabolism of reproductive hormones. Thus, Gladstar recommends bitters for balancing a range of women's complaints that may be linked to hormone imbalances. For instance, her "bitterroot blend" calls for dandelion and yellowdock roots, Oregon grape root, wild yam rhizome, and a little Vitex berry. She recommends simmering it in tea—quite bitter, I'm afraid—and, handing you the cup, remarks, "I've seen many tenacious cases of reproductive problems respond well to liver tonic herbs."[41]

Deb Soule, a folk herbalist and amazing gardener living on the Maine coast, recommends a classic liver blend made of gentian, thistle, burdock, ginger, and licorice (again, a somewhat simplified but classic

Mithridates-like formula—intensely bitter roots and leaves, some aromatics, and a little sweet licorice to tie it all together). She emphasizes that "herbalists believe that health and vitality begin in the digestive tract"[42]—and by now we should see why this is so.

In Chinese herbal medicine, bitter herbs are highly valued. All effective herbal remedies are thought to contain at least some element of the bitter flavor. The applications focus on conditions that are "damp and hot," characterized by chronic inflammation and perhaps swelling—an immediate recognition of the importance of bitters beyond just good digestive function. Regulating excess that might accumulate in the physiology due to overeating and especially overindulgence in sweets is a crucial virtue ascribed to them. Finally, they are thought to improve the ability to store vitality from the food we consume—simply put, to digest and absorb nutrition more effectively.

In Ayurveda, the medical art of the Indian subcontinent, the bitter flavor is also held in high regard. The *Charaka Samhita,* compiled by the physician Charaka one to two hundred years before the time that Crataeus was studying in Pergamon (perhaps 200–300 BCE), is an extensive treatise on a very old medical art. In it we find bitters used as purifying agents, to improve digestion, to regulate bowel function, and as remedies for poison and worms. An interesting quote states that "though itself is nonrelishing," the bitter taste "destroys nonrelish."[43] I take this to mean that, though bitters taste bad, they were thought to help with a poor appetite and perhaps even nausea.

It would seem that traditional herbal medicine uses bitters for all the functions connected to T2R receptor stimulation. They improve all aspects of digestion, from poor appetite to overeating to everything in between. Liver metabolism is always mentioned. And blood sugar balance comes up frequently as well. Most references talk about a dose of herbal bitters that ranges between one-quarter and one-half teaspoon of a liquid preparation, though doses of some traditional liqueurs, such as *amari,* can be ten times that. Because of their value in modulating digestive function and the metabolic changes associated with eating, they are usually taken around mealtime. And most herbalists you talk to would say that it is vitally important to taste the bitter flavor on the tongue while you consume these herbs. Of course, if you are, in essence, harnessing a poison detection system, you'd better engage it fully right at the front door!

But after ringing that front doorbell, bitters go on to stimulate more activity inside the house. All botanical medical systems ascribe deeper virtues to these plants, linking them to reduced inflammation and irritability throughout the entire physiology, from nerves to skin, and also to increased activity of tissues in general. How might this happen? We will explore some biochemical mechanisms that are at work when we discuss the pharmacology of bitters, but traditional herbal medicine has some good ideas to offer, too.

English phytotherapist Simon Mills proposes an interesting model. He contends that bitters have broad systemic effects, in part by stimulating neurological and immunological tissue present in the gut. Nerves, including the vagus nerve and also smaller fibers and bundles (known as ganglia), like those that make up the solar plexus, relay a lot of information about the state of the gastrointestinal tract to other areas of the body. Immune cells sample the belly's contents constantly, adjusting the type and quantity of chemicals they secrete and thereby affecting inflammation throughout the physiology. Mills contends that, just as needles (or fingers or cones of burning mugwort) can stimulate distant areas of the body in practices such as acupuncture, herbal chemistry can interface with the wide absorptive area of the digestive tract. Each molecule acts like a small "needle," balancing the release of hormones, the impulses of nerves, and the activity of the immune system through a mechanism he dubs *acupharmacology*.

When you consider that the inner lining of our guts is about the size of a football field, you can begin to appreciate the vast sensory apparatus we carry inside us. It truly is a complete and highly sensitive interface with the world. We spread out everything we put into our mouths across this vast field, chemically altering and absorbing some of it, and interacting with all of it. Bacteria teem in this environment, complicating the picture further and helping us remember that, on a microscopic level, our digestive tracts are distinct and balanced ecosystems. In this context, the food we eat and the chemistry it contains create what could be called patterns of "weather" for this ecosystem—with daily, even yearly, cycles of activity. I wonder if bacterial colonies comment, in their own ways, on these changes: "Feels like it's gonna be a sweet one again today, friends" or "We were all doing fine until the great bitter glut, and now the Bifidobacteria have overrun the neighborhood . . ." But, all joking aside, the idea of acupharmacology presupposes an awareness that a xenobiome exists, is vitally important, and can end up affecting the whole human being (for good or ill) if it is altered. In this context, bitters are like a lightning storm: dramatic and eye-catching, and providing crucial rain.

While the articulation of acupharmacology is quite new, there is also an old concept, still much in vogue at the turn of the twentieth century, known as "dirty blood." Of course, there is no actual "dirt" in the blood, and if there were a poison or pathogen coursing through our veins, we would likely need more help than what herbal bitters could provide. The concept here is that our internal environment might turn a little more "pro-inflammatory" on occasion. The chemistry bathing our tissues can get a little bit off and the result is more allergies, breakouts and rashes, irritation, heart disease, even anger. Sound familiar? It reminds me a little of the herbicide-laden fluid we use to bathe corn country. Through stimulating liver metabolism (a major filter of the bloodstream, after all), bitters help correct this condition by "cleaning" the blood. If we allowed bitter weeds to grow in cornfields, we might clean our aquifers, too—and help with pest control as well. But that's a tale for another day.

While the idea of dirty blood has been exploited for many an herbal "detox" program, and used to market a variety of interesting (though potentially dangerous if they contain harsh, habit-forming laxative herbs, as many do) supplement products, it nevertheless still holds a kernel of truth. After all, the liver does indeed metabolize harmful substances, and this function is enhanced if the xenobiome is rich in bitter-tasting molecules. And perhaps the altered xenobiome we have created for ourselves has engendered a deficiency problem rather than a toxin-pollution problem—we are not necessarily polluted and dirty; we may just be missing bitter plants.

The often-touted oxidative hypothesis of aging and inflammation—stating in very warlike terms that our tissues suffer at the hand of free radicals that need to be "quenched," or vanquished, with antioxidant chemicals—might be only part of the truth. We need to consider the idea that the problems we are experiencing could be due to a xenobiome that is missing some key elements, elements without which proper function is lost. Their deficiency is not as visible as deficiency of the major vitamins and takes much longer to become apparent, requiring maybe a few human generations to be fully evident. If our blood is dirtied by anything, it might be sugar. More likely, our internal environment is just missing its familiar, diverse botanical influences.

Traditional perspectives teach us that bitters are important parts of our internal ecology, creating the right environment within. They literally touch every part of the gut, wherever T2R receptors are found, and send signals through nerves and hormones to the whole body. Their chemistry, though wildly diverse, is something we should seek out and embrace because of its safe and broadly beneficial effects. We should worry less about "bad" foods, toxicity, and fear-based reactions to what we eat and more about providing the essential ingredients for optimal gut function. These are easily found in bitters.

It seems that human beings have always used bitter herbs for medicine, mostly to help with digestive and liver health, but also to balance blood sugar and control some more subtle changes related to inflammation, environmental sensitivity, and age. The challenge bitters embody was always viewed as an integral part of life—though, as is remembered in the Passover seder, it can be a difficult part. One can overdo it, as did Mithridates, who filled every moment and every meal with bitterness, aggression, and revenge. Failing to embrace it, however, leads to a worse outcome in the end: a slow degeneration in the glut of sweet, monotonous luxury. The traditional emphasis on bitters shows us an effective way to bring back the flavors our guts were born to taste, without necessarily needing to radically alter our diet: just a spoonful of bitter medicine can help all that sugar go down.

THE PHARMACOLOGICAL APPROACH

Our explorations of the bitter taste and the indications for bitters in traditional herbal medicine have framed a clear picture for the uses of these important plants in remedying digestive symptoms, bolstering liver health, and reestablishing blood sugar balance. We have also seen bitters employed to counter toxins, control allergies and asthma, improve the skin, and alleviate other chronic inflammatory diseases. They might be useful in a culture where gastrointestinal complaints, obesity, and diabetes are widespread. In fact, according to the xenobiome hypothesis, we may be experiencing these diseases at massive rates in large part *because* we are no longer using bitters. What does the science have to say?

A major mechanism of action for bitter tastants stems from the activity of the T2R receptors. As we saw earlier, these receptors (present all over the body, but especially in the gut, pancreas, liver, and gallbladder) induce physiological changes that lead to greater secretions from the gut, reduced movement and closing of the valves between gut compartments, and less caloric consumption. T2R receptors mediate the connection between the bitter herbs and our bodies. But what exactly is going on after they are stimulated?

Research geared at answering this question has largely proceeded on two fronts: the transduction (or relaying) of signals from T2R receptors can involve either nerves that connect to the brain or hormones released into the bloodstream (often both transduction pathways are active). The nerve responsible for relaying messages from the mouth and gut back up to central processing is, of course, the vagus nerve—that thick bundle of neural fibers that both listens to and controls the heart, lungs, and digestive organs (and more, like the muscular fibers of the iris). The vagus nerve is clearly awakened when T2R receptors are stimulated, and the nerve kicks into action. It sends information up to the brain, where it is processed and integrated with other sensory input, and then it carries signals back to the gut musculature and secretory glands to slow movement and increase secretions. This is just what we might expect, given the traditional uses of bitter plants.

The role of the vagus nerve in digestion, food intake, gut motility, high blood sugar, and obesity was reviewed extensively by Hans-Rudolf Berthoud at Louisiana State University in Baton Rouge, in his study "The Vagus Nerve, Food Intake and Obesity." He examines how taste begins the process of vagal signaling (a phenomenon familiar to anyone who has noticed increased saliva production when tasting something bitter). He ends up linking increased vagal tone to less food consumption and describes how this affects obesity. He goes on to show how different foods activate vagus nerve fibers all the way down the gastrointestinal tract and notes that T2R receptor stimulation activates the same hormonal secretions that are stimulated by high-protein, high-fat meals. Carbohydrates, on the other hand, barely affect the vagus at all (though they may awaken some serotonin pathways). In summary, it is clear that the nervous system, through the vagus nerve, plays a very important role in coordinating muscular contraction (which is generally reduced), digestive enzyme secretion (which is increased), and hormonal secretion (also increased) throughout the digestive tract. It is also involved in liver function, primarily stimulating the uptake and storage of sugar from the bloodstream. Animals whose vagus nerve has been severed eat more and have higher average blood sugar levels after eating sugar.[44] This, of course, is not surprising.

Understanding that the nervous system can carry the signal for bitter through the entire digestive tract, liver, and pancreas helps us see that a simple taste can have wide-ranging effects. These effects are reinforced by a few important hormones that increase the "reach" of the vagus nerve and have profound repercussions in the physiology. Those hormones are cholecystokinin (CCK), peptide YY (PYY), and glucagon-like-protein 1 (GLP-1). Keep in mind that these hormones have received research attention. It is very likely that we are barely scratching the surface here, and much more is yet to be discovered about the signaling and functioning of digestive and metabolic feedback loops. That, however, hasn't stopped the older Italian gentleman from sitting at a bar in the late-afternoon light, sipping his *amaro,* and cursing at the soccer scores. I am grateful for that.

Cholecystokinin (CCK), released by cells in the lining of the small intestine, was first named because of its ability to stimulate the contraction of the gallbladder (also known as the *chole cyst,* or bile sack). We now know that it is a hormone crucial to connecting the brain and gut, with effects that stretch far beyond increasing the flow of bile. Taken as a functional unit, these effects coordinate the activity of digestive tissues and synchronize them with the motility of the gut. This ensures that food moves through at a rate that precisely matches our ability to digest it. In practice, this means slowing down muscular contractions, increasing enzyme and bile secretion, and providing a feeling of fullness[45]—precisely reinforcing the vagus nerve.

We first release CCK into the bloodstream when the T2R bitter taste receptors are stimulated on the tongue.[46] This is a big part of why, though bitters may awaken the appetite in the short term, they actually reduce caloric consumption in the end. It is also why bitters are often taken before meals. But if we remember that the T2R signal is there to warn us about toxicity, it is interesting to note that high doses of CCK also have a strong effect on the emotion centers of the brain, prompting outright panic. In fact, CCK is injected into subjects (at levels far, far above those achievable by T2R stimulation) in order to generate anxiety so researchers can test new anti-anxiety drugs.[47] Fear. Challenge. Poison.

As we continue down the gastrointestinal tract, there are more

T2R receptors, as well as detectors for fat and protein. All of these, when activated, stimulate the release of more CCK.[48] The liver synthesizes more bile, the gallbladder contracts, more enzymes are released from the pancreas, and the valves between the esophagus and the stomach, and between the stomach and the small intestine, close. Muscle contraction slows. Food is more likely to be thoroughly digested. Additionally, if there are any carbohydrates in the gastrointestinal tract, their absorption is slowed and blood glucose levels don't rise as much.[49] This pattern is beginning to sound familiar.

By the time we reach the end of the small intestine and the beginning of the colon, activated T2R receptors begin to stimulate the secretion of two additional hormones—polypeptide YY (PYY) and glucagon-like-peptide 1 (GLP-1).[50] In short, the first serves to strongly suppress appetite. The second encourages the release of insulin and enhances the body's insulin sensitivity. As a result, we feel more satiated and our blood sugar levels are lower. As we saw when we were examining T2R receptors, PYY, if administered before a meal, reduces consumption in both healthy and obese individuals by almost a third.[51] GLP-1 is so good at boosting the body's insulin response that analogues are being researched as antidiabetes drugs.[52] That is an admirable endeavor, but I offer the idea that we might already have an even better option.

When used habitually and perhaps before eating, bitters not only slow down the entry of sugar into the bloodstream, they also make us eat less and sensitize us to insulin. This is the perfect prescription for an epidemic of insulin resistance, diabetes, and obesity. This is not some kind of mysterious coincidence, nor an accident of design. The epidemics are there because the bitters are not, and, as a result, our built-in sugar buffering mechanisms are slowly atrophying. We are seeing it on an individual level, meal by meal. We are seeing it on a cultural level, diagnosis by diagnosis. And we are seeing it in our environment, acre by acre.

Research has examined the use of bitter plants in humans in the same conditions for which they've always been famous: regulation of digestive function, improvement of liver function, regulation of blood glucose, and improvement in hypersensitivity diseases, such as allergies and asthma.

Gentian root, an old standby, was administered to a group of 205 patients with a range of dyspeptic, or "bad-belly," symptoms, including nausea and vomiting, heartburn, gas and bloating, spasmodic pain, and constipation. All were quickly and effectively relieved.[53] Liquids containing both gentian and wormwood (another classic bitter) stimulated gastric and pancreatic enzyme secretions, as well as bile release from the liver.[54] Even the humble (but bitter) dandelion was lauded for its effects on incomplete digestion, gas, and bloating.[55]

Bitter preparations rich in flavo-lignans from milk thistle are now world-renowned liver protectants. They are the best (and only) antidote to poisoning from the deathcap mushroom, *Amanita phalloides,* which kills by liquefying the liver over the course of forty-eight hours (Mithridates would be proud—of both). They are also quite useful in the management of cirrhosis, a slower kind of poisoning that is usually brought on by alcohol.[56] But even simple preparations featuring only bitter artichoke leaves still exert an action that is both liver-protective and digestion-enhancing in humans.[57] Extensive pharmacological research underpins the use of classic bitter herbs, such as dandelion,[58] in supporting liver health and improving its ability to detoxify poison.

Certain plants, such as bitter melon (*Momordica*), are exceptional antidiabetic agents, comparable to conventional medication (though milder).[59] Even relatively abundant bitter constituents, such as chlorogenic acid (found in everything from chicory root to garden lettuce), reduce blood glucose after eating sugar, exerting their effects in part through the liver.[60] And we have seen clear evidence that stimulating T2R receptors has a profound influence on hormones that govern insulin sensitivity in human beings. Bitters may be milder than conventional drugs in managing diabetes but, if taken habitually, they still have therapeutic applicability.[61] They certainly appear to be excellent preventive agents. They have these powers by virtue of a positive rearrangement of the xenobiome, providing needed cues for balanced metabolic activity.

Finally, there has been some interesting human research lately that is exploring the ability of bitters to manage inflammation and irritation beyond the gut. Plants such as milk thistle, gentian, burdock, and yellowdock are featured in discussions of allergies, sinusitis, asthma, and generalized inflammation.[62] This all makes sense from the analysis of the key components of our metabolism and the crucial role bitters seem to play in the health of the liver and digestive tract. When these organs are happy, processing what we ingest with vigor and efficiency, we are generally happier. But perhaps more important, there is less inflammation in all our tissues, and we suffer fewer effects from toxins and irritants. How crucial this is in today's world! Like a strong fire that burns hot and clean, we want our metabolism to process food with a sense of purpose and an almost passionate engagement. We can get there by rising to the challenge the bitter flavor offers.

WHY BITTERS?

We are in the middle of a cultural experiment. The hypothesis is simple: challenge yourself less, and you will have a happier, healthier life. We have observed the ill effects of forced, excess labor for millennia. We have struggled against malnutrition, sometimes making do on wild plants alone, for millennia. If given the opportunity to rest and eat, who would refuse it?

The hypothesis is also dead wrong. Human beings are not like vintage automobiles, meant to be rested and admired. We are meant to move. We are meant to struggle, occasionally. And we are meant to eat tough and bitter foods, ones that we might rather avoid if we had the choice. Just because excessive challenge has beaten us down (some would say forged us in fire), over the course of evolutionary history, doesn't mean we should now reject it outright just because we can. There is a middle road to follow, and it may be time for us to walk it. Unless we do so, our slow cultural degeneration into earlier and earlier sugar poisoning will inevitably continue, and our slow and steady pollution of the environment will only become more acute.

We have recognized the crucial role of exercise. No one contends that a sedentary life is healthier than an active one. But what about food? Concepts in nutrition are identifying important pieces here and there, but nutrition has yet to give us a broad and clear vision of how and what to eat. Unfortunately, it never will—we cannot piece together an "intellectual" cuisine by identifying all the key chemicals of the xenobiome and ascribing recommended daily requirements to each one. Nor can we bypass cuisine itself by just supplementing our physiology with elements they would have produced in the context of a traditional meal—elements such as digestive enzymes, hydrochloric acid, or even glucagon-like-peptide 1.

Such elements have to be a natural expression of a living, vibrant human being in order to be effective. How can we stimulate this expression? Through bitter, wild plants. They hold a chemical diversity that is often unfathomable to our analytic machines. When we do uncover a specific layer of its complexity, we only reveal a deeper one. And at every turn, its richness interfaces with ours so completely that it is as if we were one large organism—plant and person evolving together, coherently coupled. Many are starting to recognize that wilderness is crucial to our health—the experience of nature itself, the presence of wild bacteria and parasites inside us, even the (relatively) tame garden soil under our fingernails.[63] So, too, we have to add the wild back into our food. This will build our resilience, to be sure. But I will guarantee you this: any human who tastes the wild and weedy plants and feels a benefit will never look at a sterile cornfield the same way again.

We must celebrate some of the most vulgar (literally meaning "of the people") plants because they are the most bitter. It is the bitter flavor that holds the key to identifying wildness in herbs. It is the bitter flavor that activates our digestion and metabolism. It is the bitter flavor that gives us the signal that our food is challenging and worth waking up for. We don't need to live off these plants, or to consume them in more than modest quantities. Excessive bitterness can overtake our life. But walking the middle path in the land of poisons ensures a healthy, stimulating xenobiome and this is what will correct the deficiencies in the Western diet.

So we return to Mithridates, the poison king. He tasted bitterness early, when he was still a child and his mother killed his father. But this challenge made him strong. He rose, and took revenge, and took the kingdom back. In the process, he had to kill his mother, but this, too, gave him strength and with it he fought Rome's eastward advance. All the while, he was tasting poison and blending antidotes, consuming daily doses of bitter herbs from the wild lands of his kingdom and beyond. As his strength grew, so did his anger and bitterness, in a vicious cycle that, though it made him exceedingly powerful, consumed him as well. In the end, we find him almost all alone, with one last faithful guard beside him, having killed his eldest son and been wholly betrayed by his youngest. The bodies of his family members, who died poisoned by his own hand, lie strewn around him. As the enemy closes in to capture and torture him, he takes a deep draft of his most potent poison to end a vengeful, angry life. But, as the story goes, it has no effect on him. That is the most bitter irony of all: his daily use of wild plants had made him invulnerable to the toxicity of his own poison. He pleads with his guard to run him through with a sword—and gets his final wish.

We must not follow his path too far. We need not fill our lives with so much of the bitter flavor that we lose the appreciation for its sweet rewards. It is dangerous to walk too far into the poison realm: the confidence that comes from overcoming challenge can quickly become a hateful, resentful arrogance. But that is not our way. We can appreciate a measure of bitter on our palate and experience its benefits without letting ourselves be overtaken by a choleric humor. We can thereby release the addictive hold that sugary sweetness has on our psyches, acknowledging that often there is difficulty in life and embracing the opportunity to meet it head-on. In so doing, we return to an ancient stream that flows through the lives of plants and people. Within it runs water that is nourishing but also challenging, clean like the crisp bite of gentian root. Though not exactly good, its bitter flavor is real. As you taste it, I watch your eyes brighten, your brow furrow, your back straighten. You are ready. *Per aspera, ad astra.* Through challenge, to the stars.

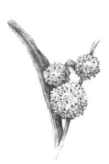

WORMWOOD

ARTEMISIA ABSINTHIUM

Circling around the North Star is the constellation many know as the Big Dipper. In the Indo-European mythology, which holds the roots of Greek and Roman legends, these stars were part of a larger grouping known as Ursa Major, or the Big Bear. Because of its constant presence in the night sky of the Northern Hemisphere, as well as its special location, it was always regarded with respect. So it is not surprising that it is named after an animal that, almost universally, is considered a powerful spirit-guide, a shamanic healer, keeper of the secrets of nature.

In the Greek pantheon, the cult of the bear evolved, some say, into the cult of nature and the hunt. The animal was replaced by an equally powerful goddess: Artemis, often pictured with a bow and a stag, lady of the growing moon, and, like the bear, queen of all healers. She was swift and effective in all her pursuits, but also challenging and often intensely harsh—transmuting rival hunters into animals and chasing them down, if not killing them outright. She had a taste for revenge, and many both on Olympus and off tasted her bitter anger.

I have always felt that the genus of plants to which she lends her name, the *Artemisias,* are very aptly named. They are all powerful, wild plants. The undersides of their leaves almost always have a silvery quality that reminds me of moonlight and makes them stand out on moonlit walks in the garden. They all have a history of use that includes ceremony, from the sagebrush of the American West to the cosmopolitan mugwort, found in almost every city sidewalk crevice and country ditch. And they are all intensely bitter herbs.

GROWING AND HARVESTING
WORMWOOD

It is easy to grow wormwood, but remember that it has little tolerance for other garden plants. Perhaps contributing to its dark reputation, the plant secretes substances from its roots that inhibit the growth of other species (a trick known as "allelopathy"). It sprouts readily from its numerous, small seeds and grows into a strong and woody perennial—meaning that every winter it leaves behind a hard and twisted stalk, which sprouts with new silvery growth when spring returns. Unless it's cut back regularly, this growth can get a bit rangy, straggly, and unkempt—but with regular harvest (for distillates and other fancy preparations), the shrub is kept in check and is actually fairly well behaved.

I like it planted in the corner of a bed, where it has room to grow without impeding others, and also where there is a good chance of brushing up against it: its odor, which is unique but contains hints of cedar, clove, and camphor, is not unpleasant and its foliage delicate, lacy, and silvery. If you have the luxury of space, consider devoting a whole bed to wormwood, or at least one very large container: that way it won't bother other plants, and you will have an amazing garden feature, especially if you like to visit your herbs on nights with a full moon. Wormwood does well in a wide, terra-cotta planter embedded in the center of a stone patio, not requiring much fertilizer or watering (think of its relatives, equally at home in the desert or a city sidewalk). When it flowers, clusters of small yellow buttons appear on a long spray—tiny flowers with almost insignificant silver-green petals. It can be harvested at this point, and hung in bundles from the rafters for aroma and also to dispel pests. But for medicine, the month of June is probably ideal: before the flowers arrive, when the leaves are still a little juicy and highly aromatic, wormwood yields its virtues to the skillful herbalist.

USING WORMWOOD

Of the *Artemisias,* wormwood is the most bitter by far. Its intensity is the reason for its name: so strong that even worms are expelled when you consume it. But beyond this use, it is also a classic bitter herb that possesses a lot of aromatic qualities—an incredible combination for digestive health in general. In fact, its essential oil profile, rich in substances like thujone, gives it a rich and somewhat notorious reputation among bitters: it is the secret ingredient of true "absinthe," a distilled preparation with a rich and checkered history. So Artemis returns: challenging, yes—but also dream-inducing, stimulating, erotic: the virgin huntress all men desire but can never have.

Warning

Of all the plants in this book, this one is perhaps the most difficult to work with. It is expressly forbidden for pregnant women, and those nursing small children would do well to avoid it, too. Part of its challenge comes from the intense bitterness, but the volatile oils present in wormwood are also quite strong and not for the faint of heart. The combination, however, is what makes this herb distinctive—so, if you are neither with child nor planning to conceive, consider its use in moderation. Quickly effective and somewhat magical, it's worth having in your home apothecary (if only for that little bottle of artisanal absinthe to show your friends).

There is no way I would ever recommend an infusion of wormwood. Even a cupful of its tea would turn the stoutest stomach. For general medicinal use, or to add as a bitter in drinks or cocktails, the most common preparation is the tincture. This allows for a little taste, all-important when using bitter plants, but doesn't overwhelm with a mouthful of fluid.

Wormwood Tincture

Fresh or dried wormwood
100–150 proof vodka

To make the tincture, the fresh herb (or dried, too) is steeped in at least 100 proof vodka or ideally some stronger spirits—something closer to 150 proof. Some would say that the best tinctures are made with wormwood harvested the night of a full moon—but regardless of your timing, chop the leaves finely and loosely pack them in a mason jar. Cover them with your spirits, and, shaking occasionally, allow them to steep for at least two weeks, though four weeks is ideal.

After this time, the tincture should be strained, the leftover leaves pressed to remove all the juices, and stored in a dark place.

Remedy Recommendation

Five drops of this preparation is adequate as a digestive tonic for upset stomach, gas and bloating, irregular bowel habits, or gastro-intestinal inflammation. Some might require up to thirty drops. For intestinal worms, twice that dose two or three times a day is the usual recommendation (but please consult a qualified herbalist before starting any antiparasite regimen yourself).

 ## Absinthe (Wormwood Spirit)

Wormwood tincture (made from the fresh herb)
Home distillation apparatus (see box on pages 88–89)

While the tincture is useful, the true magic of wormwood reveals itself once the tincture is distilled. For this purpose, as recommended by the alchemist-poet Dale Pendell (with whom I wholeheartedly agree), a tincture made from the fresh herb is the only choice that is truly effective.

You take the strained, pressed, fresh wormwood tincture and run it through the distillation apparatus described in the section on peppermint. Placing the tincture in the sealed distiller in a simmering water bath will yield a clear spirit, between 150 and 190 proof, depending on how long you let it go, which is the basic foundation of absinthe.

It can be taken as is, mixed in roughly equal parts with water, or you can reinfuse the distillate with other herbs of your choice: anise, ginger, and a little peppermint are all traditional choices. But the heart of the absinthe itself is the distilled wormwood spirit, which is easy enough to make.

Now, absinthe has an interesting reputation. The Parisian bohemians of the nineteenth century ascribed magical, inspiring qualities to this preparation. Poets, philosophers, artists, and madmen have all reveled in the mystery of *la fée verte*, or the "green fairy" (so-called because of the emerald-green color of the spirit—add fennel seeds and a little peppermint to your wormwood distillate and you will see what I mean). Many of the effects are thought to be linked to thujone, a potent chemical that is part of the volatiles found in many *Artemisias*. It seems to have stimulating, and perhaps hallucinogenic, effects.

The dose of wormwood distillate required is about one-half ounce, and only preparations made from the fresh plant contain adequate quantities of the essential oil to be potent. All the commercial preparations available on the market today contain virtually no thujone—so while they are nice and green, there is very little of the magic present. The reason for this is that thujone is toxic when consumed at high doses, or for prolonged periods, and thus is outlawed at effective concentrations. That is all the warning I will give.

Wormwood Candies

> 1 cup distilled wormwood remnants or simmered
> wormwood
> 2 cups white sugar
> 1 tablespoon butter
> $^2/_3$ cup honey
> Confectioner's sugar

While the absinthe carries off all the aromatic qualities of the plant, what's to be done with the leftover material in the distiller? It is a dark, thick, intensely bitter substance one drop of which activates all the recoil mechanisms our digestion possesses. I generally use it for making one of my favorite bitter preparations, incredibly useful for eliminating sugar cravings, and based on a recipe passed down to me by my Austrian uncle Harald (an herbalist and master pastry chef, whose go-to tonic is the elderflower tisane).

You can use the remnants of the distillation process or you can simply simmer a lot of wormwood in water for fifteen minutes or so (this removes all the volatile components and concentrates the bitter ones). You will want about a cup of intensely bitter wormwood fluid, obtained through either method.

Gather your cup of wormwood brew, two cups of white sugar, a tablespoon of butter, and two-thirds cup of honey. Also, get yourself a candy thermometer and either a cookie sheet or a nice slab of marble (which is what my uncle recommended—its cool temperature allows for better hardening of the candy). Dust the marble with confectioner's sugar. Mix the brew, white sugar, and honey together, and slowly heat it to a boil.

When the thermometer reads 275°F, add the butter and stir well. Let the mixture reach a temperature of about 305°F (hard crack stage), then pour it slowly over the marble slab. This should be left to cool until it's not tacky anymore, then cut into one-inch squares and left to cool completely. My uncle would finish it off by dusting everything with another generous measure of confectioner's sugar and individually wrapping the candies in small pieces of wax paper, but this last step is optional.

Keep these on hand for children, or anyone else with a sweet tooth. They quell the craving with a minimum of calories and, over time, a sort of aversion to sweetness begins to develop (try it and you'll see why). But my uncle recommended these for everything from digestive complaints, nausea, and irregular bowel habits to skin complaints, sore throat, and lung congestion.

Perhaps by harnessing some of the systemic effects of bitter plants, these intense wormwood candies are actually broadly medicinal. And what I've always liked is that, by distilling a tincture, you divide its aromatic, inspiring, ethereal fraction from its bitter, digestive, grounding components—a little of both sides of Artemis.

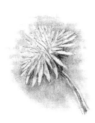

DANDELION

TARAXACUM OFFICINALE

There is a yellow flag on your lawn. In fact, there are many. It is April, and the dandelions are flowering (though the exact timing may vary, depending on location). If you don't do something about it, the flowers will become gray puffballs, and the seed will disperse on the wind. And then there will be more. Once, upon returning from a trip abroad, I found my garden full of bare, skinny dandelion stalks, their seeds long gone into the fertile open soil I had been nourishing and protecting for the sake of my vegetable and medicinal herb starts. For a moment, I felt the horror of the suburban weekend warrior. It was a good horror—in the same instant, I had to acknowledge that the entire situation was now out of my control. That's a good thing to do sometimes.

There is perhaps no other plant that is as iconic as the dandelion in the modern battle for the perfect green lawn. It features prominently on the front of many brands of synthetic herbicide. It has a long, fragile, persistent taproot that is difficult to eliminate, so we have resorted to chemicals in an attempt to eradicate it from our lives. It alters the homogeneity of the turf. It is a sign that we are not perfect in our devoted service to the *Poaceae*—the grasses that control our lives, to whom we sacrifice huge swaths of forest land, agricultural field, and living space. "Human slaves," they seem to whisper, "you are neglecting your duties. You cannot allow even one rebel to survive—or we shall withhold our sugar from you."

But like all good rebels, the dandelions are irrepressible. Mow them down, and they simply flower closer to the ground. Pave them over, and they will find and expand any cracks. Poison them and, in the end, you only succeed in poisoning your own children, for the dandelions adapt, resist, and continue to spread. But just as you can't keep a good rebel in chains, you can't keep a good idea down, either. They are like that thought that nags at the back of your conscience, the one you keep dismissing because it is too challenging, too risky, too ugly to entertain. It keeps waving its little flag for a reason: it is the best medicine for you right now. And so I feel it is with the dandelion: the weed we love to hate is perhaps the best catalyst to deliver us from the bondage of perpetual, hypnotic, addictive sweetness. So, back in my garden, I did the only thing an herbalist could do: I knelt down in the soil, found a new dandelion, and ate the whole thing—root and all. It made me feel a whole lot better.

GROWING AND HARVESTING DANDELION

If you have any difficulty finding or growing dandelion, you either live in the tundra or in the desert. This plant with the characteristic toothed leaf is cosmopolitan and generally very easy to find. You can seek it out in any lawn or park, provided that you know there aren't any synthetic fertilizers, herbicides, or pesticides being used. This is certainly how I collect the greens in springtime, a habit I picked up from my family in Italy. A few weeks after the snows melted in the lower Alpine valleys and the stronger sun began to warm the soil, we would head out for short walks with a sharp knife and a wicker basket. The best dandelion "crowns" were small, tight, lime-green in color and had no flower buds on them yet. We would slice the whole crown off at ground level, put it in the basket, and move on. Back home, after a little cleanup rinse, they would receive a quick chop and a generous dousing of olive oil, vinegar, and salt. Often this was dinner, maybe with just a little cheese and prosciutto. Other times they were the centerpiece of a bigger salad. I remember them being bitter, crunchy, salty, and delicious.

The true bitter quality of the dandelion is found in its root. It is not as intense as some of the other bitters, such as gentian or artichoke, but it is nevertheless very effective. There is a fine line to walk if you want to harvest it for medicine: the wild roots are very difficult to extract from the soil and are often quite spindly. On the other hand, if you grow dandelion in your garden, the roots get nice and fat and are a whole lot easier to dig up. The downside of cultivated dandelion is that it becomes much starchier and, therefore, less bitter than its wild counterparts. This is because, as is the case with most roots, the bitter principles are found in the outer cortex and the nutritive, sweet starches are in the inner flesh. While both are important medicinally, it is the bitter we seek: so my compromise is to allow more and more dandelions to grow in the perennial beds that are going fallow—areas where the soil is still loose, but where I haven't added compost for a couple of seasons. For example, after I harvest echinacea root from a garden bed, I simply leave the soil open and won't fertilize or plant anything for a year or two. Weeds inevitably spring up, and among the lamb's quarters, amaranth, purslane, and sorrel you're bound to find a good crop of dandelions. Not too fat, not too skinny, not too easy, not too hard: Goldilocks shows us the middle way in the garden, too.

So rather than striving to eliminate this weed from our lives, we should be harvesting it and using it daily. It is a gentle bitter, not overly challenging yet still amazingly effective. Its safety is legendary. And it seems to work so hard at making its presence known: one of the first flowers in spring, one of the most attractive seedheads to children, one of the most common weeds in cities and empty lots. It isn't too pushy, but nevertheless it's relentless: no wonder many herbalists choose it as their icon, repurposing a symbol that, to many in this culture, still has so many negative connotations. Herbal medicine works slowly, seemingly in the shadows, and yet cannot be eradicated: so, too, the dandelion, pushing up through concrete, reminds us that nature still wants to connect with us. Dandelion root tincture was the first tincture I ever made. It can help catalyze so much good change—if only we heed the signal of its yellow flag.

USING DANDELION

The dandelion leaf gets more and more bitter as the season progresses. This does not mean it should be avoided—on the contrary, its medicinal effects become more and more pronounced. While herbalists regard this leaf as a mineral-rich botanical to be infused for kidney and urinary health (and with a strong diuretic action), it is also useful as a bitter tonic when added to salads. It enlivens our unchallenging iceberg, romaine, and baby spinach concoctions with its wild touch. Eaten regularly, it has all the benefits of the bitter herbs: it helps control overeating, primes digestive function for fewer postmeal symptoms, and improves the liver's metabolic effects. If only we found dandelion leaf more often in our restaurant salads!

 ## Roasted Dandelion Root (A Coffee Substitute)

Freshly harvested dandelion taproots

A classic liver tonic made from dandelion roots is actually a decent substitute for coffee. These roots, along with chicory roots, are still prepared this way and brewed as a morning beverage throughout both Europe and the American South.

Take your freshly harvested taproots and mince them until they are about the consistency of coffee grounds. Then, in a cast-iron skillet and on low heat, roast them until they are dry and a toasty, nutty aroma begins to waft up from the pan. Just as with coffee, you can opt for a darker or lighter roast. Then simply take the skillet off the heat, allow everything to cool, and store the roasted roots in an airtight container.

These can be used in a French press or even a drip-style automatic coffeemaker, either straight or mixed in with a little coffee or chocolate. It makes a delicious, bitter morning beverage that goes great with cream and is very good at waking up an appetite for a nice, nourishing breakfast.

Regular consumption of this coffee substitute will bring all the benefits of bitters to your physiology: fewer digestive complaints first and foremost, but also a reduced level of systemic inflammation due to improved liver function. The positive effects of this humble weed on all manner of gut troubles have been known for centuries, and its yellow flower has always signaled to herbalists that it is specifically useful for the liver and gallbladder, sources of yellow bile.

A century ago Guthrie Rankin, a Scottish country doctor who became a member of the Royal College of Physicians in London, gave a lecture on digestive and gallbladder "colic" (painful, recurrent cramps and spasms), in which he extolled the virtues of the dandelion. I can only imagine how this went over in those rarefied circles (though it couldn't have gone too badly, as his lecture made it into the *British Medical Journal*).

 ## Dandelion Root Tincture

> Fresh dandelion roots
> 100 proof alcohol

For quicker access to its medicinal powers, I suggest preparing a dandelion root tincture. The roots can be harvested either in the spring or the fall: earlier in the season, they are more bitter and stimulating. Later on, they store up a reserve of starches for the winter and are more nourishing. These fall roots are not at all inferior: the starches are actually quite useful for the beneficial bacteria that live in our intestines. In practice, you can harvest the roots and make a tincture anytime you have the opportunity to do so.

Fill a mason jar with finely chopped fresh roots, and cover them with 100 proof spirits. Allow the jar to rest in a cool, dark place for at least four weeks, then strain and preserve the liquid.

Taking between one-quarter and one full teaspoon of this tincture around mealtime, either straight or mixed with just a little bit of water (or other bitter herbs of your choice), will give you a quick and convenient way to avail yourself of dandelion's power. Your belly and liver will be grateful.

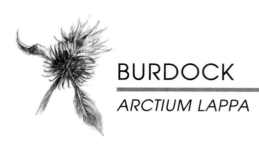

BURDOCK

ARCTIUM LAPPA

Like so many weeds, burdock is much maligned despite its virtues. In Japan, where it is still used as a staple food, there is a story of three roots getting into a hot bath: first the burdock gets in and then quickly jumps back out because the water is too hot. Next the carrot tries, and it likes the bath so much that it stays in too long and turns red. Finally the daikon radish enters, washes itself quickly, and emerges white and clean. The implication is that darker skin is dirty and undesirable, but I feel the opposite is true: the dark, fuzzy, bearlike skin of burdock is the most beautiful of the three and also has the best flavor. It is wild, nutty, and gently bitter. And it is by far the most nourishing. Again, what seems most undesirable might be the best medicine.

HARVESTING BURDOCK

Every year in the fall we get out our digging forks and head to a wild patch of weeds by the elder grove, close to the edge of the wood. Here the burdock has been thriving in the rich soil, opening its wide leaves in May and growing larger and larger over the course of the summer. The foliage is huge now and lends an almost tropical feel to this unkempt corner of the garden. Rising out of this mass of silver-green are thick stalks, some over five feet tall, covered in golf ball–sized burrs that are green or brown, depending on their stage of maturity. But we seek out the plants with no stalks, the ones that have reached the end of their first season of growth—for once burdock sends up its flower and sets its seed, the whole plant dies and its root is worthless. These first-year plants, however, hold a delicacy that is both edible and medicinal. I like to watch folks harvest it: easing out the long, straight taproot is a test of patience.

The trick is getting the whole thing out of the ground in one piece. I have routinely seen wild burdock roots that are two feet long, though they can surpass even this length, given the right soil. They seek deep mineral nutrition from the subsoil and carry these nutrients up into the plant and, by extension, into those who consume it. Using a digging fork and long digging sticks made of smooth, well-worn hickory, we loosen the soil where the leaves meet the crown of the root and begin to work our way down into the earth. Every once in a while a gentle tug reveals that there's still a long way to go. Sometimes, you will hear a muffled "pop," followed by a sigh of disappointment coming from the more impatient diggers (the taproot has broken off). But the patient ones emerge from the foliage with a thick, dark-brown, fuzzy root that tapers to a point and reveals, like a geological core sample, the structure of the soil: a foot of brownish topsoil is followed by a layer of gray Vermont clay and finally a pebbly, rocky mix that still clings to the end.

USING BURDOCK

Cooking with burdock root is the traditional way to consume this bitter herb. Its flavor is quite mild, and in Asia it is a regular addition to soups and stir-fried vegetable dishes. It used to be popular in Europe, too, added to soups mostly, but it has fallen out of favor over the last few hundred years, like so many of the more traditional foods. This is a shame, because its regular consumption is quite beneficial and it is much more nutritious than the carrot, which is the standard cooking root these days. Fortunately, there has been a resurgent interest in burdock over the past few years, and I am starting to see more and more of it in the produce departments of natural foods stores. It's a whole lot easier to bring it into your life if you can find it next to the leeks in a supermarket cooler, but the trade-off (as with dandelion) is that these cultivated roots are less bitter than their wild counterparts (and you don't get a chance to test your patience when you harvest them). Still, it is better to eat a store-bought burdock than none at all. And when consumed regularly, its benefits will still be evident. Before you cook with your roots, clean them gently with a cloth or potato brush. Don't scrub too hard—you want to preserve a good amount of the bitter peel. You can use burdock just as you would a carrot. It can be sautéed, cut on a bias and stir-fried with other vegetables, or diced and mixed with celery and onions as the base for soup and stock.

One of the major reasons burdock is good for the belly is the bitterness of the outer peel. But the complex of starches in the root itself has some highly valuable properties, too: some of the carbohydrates are digestible by humans, but many others contribute to a cocktail of soluble fiber that helps regulate colon function in a couple of ways. First, it can soften a hard stool and add a little bulk and firmness to a softer one. Second, the soluble fiber is rich in "prebiotic"* starches, food for the beneficial bacteria that inhabit the lower part of our digestive tract. These bugs are important for maintaining a healthy colon, and they help control levels of inflammation there by keeping pathogens at bay. We are learning more and more about our colon's ecology and how to promote digestive health by adding different strains of lactobacilli and other bacteria. This seems like a decent approach, but burdock and its prebiotic soluble fiber can help, too, by making sure that the right food is present for the good bugs to eat. Given the right environment, so the argument goes, the right ecology will thrive.

Herbalists value burdock for its bitter digestive qualities. But as we've seen, improving digestive function and liver metabolism can have important implications elsewhere as well. This is particularly evident with this weedy root: its softening starches, coupled with its general bitter effects and power to rebalance the colon's ecology, combine to make it an excellent anti-inflammatory for the digestive tract. As we saw in Simon Mills's concept of acupharmacology,

---

*Prebiotic is starch that probiotic bacteria consume preferentially.

reducing inflammation in one mucous membrane can bring down irritation in other tissues, too. Burdock is perhaps the best example of this effect. It has been used traditionally for all manner of skin complaints, from simple rashes to eczema and psoriasis, as well as acne in both children and adults. It is so safe and gentle that it can be simmered into tea and used in any situation. Even pets, especially dogs, who sometimes have irritation or "hot spots" on their skin that can lead to a persistent itch-scratch cycle, find relief with this simple remedy. American physicians of the nineteenth century called it "alterative," meaning it has the power to alter a stubborn, unresponsive condition. For this purpose it must be consumed regularly, as part of meals or as a cupful of suppertime tea. If given the chance, it acts patiently and persistently to address chronic skin and digestive issues—helping to get at the root of the problem, just like a patient and persistent herbalist digging for burdock in the thick Vermont clay.

Burdock and Seaweed Appetizer

Thinly sliced burdock root
Equal parts vinegar and water
Seaweed
Oil, salt, and pepper to taste

One of my favorite recipes doesn't even involve cooking: simply slice the burdock into thin matchsticks and soak these in an equal-parts mixture of vinegar and water for about ten minutes. Drain, then mix with a little seaweed (arame is great, but shredded nori works, too), sesame seeds, minced garlic, and grated ginger. Add a little oil, salt, and pepper to taste.

This crunchy, savory, and spicy preparation makes an amazing appetizer that, because of its medicinal bitter quality, also primes digestive function and prepares the palate for the meal to come.

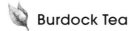 **Burdock Tea**

> A few tablespoons fresh, diced burdock root
> 1 cup water

For more medicinal preparations, take fresh roots and dice them. Dry them in the oven at the lowest possible temperature or on a screen in the sun. Then take a few tablespoons of the roots per cup of water and simmer them for a few minutes.

The tea that results is a mild bitter preparation, excellent for the digestion, especially if you are feeling debilitated, worn out from a long illness (or from food poisoning), or suffering from deficient appetite.

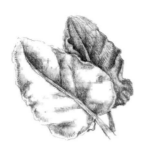

YELLOWDOCK

RUMEX CRISPUS

If your heart is full, and you need release, turn to the curly dock—or so the legend goes. Alternatively known as garden patience, sour dock, or yellowdock after the color of its roots, old herbalists who know of such things say that this plant can help us let go of the influences that are blocking our progress, impeding our understanding, or simply weighing us down. While this may indeed be the case figuratively, it has literal truth as well: there is no safer or gentler bitter when it comes to ensuring regular bowel function. But isn't it interesting that in traditional medicine a remedy for constipation can also help with stuck, stagnant emotion? The folkloric record is full of such correspondences.

GROWING AND HARVESTING YELLOWDOCK

This herb has another "signature" that connects it back to the heart as an organ of feeling. Herbalists speak of these signatures—images, signs, or shapes found in the physical form of plants that echo their medicinal uses—when picking out remedies from the forest and field. So it is with yellowdock that, as its seed matures in July, you begin to see a pink three-winged, papery calyx that holds inside two or three seeds shaped precisely like little brown hearts. These seeds twine themselves in spiral fashion up the green stalk, often three or four feet in height. By August, the entire plant turns brown and the seeds are borne off on the backs of animals or on the water beside which this plant loves to grow. They release the small hearts into the streams of the world so that new life may be born.

In the early spring, the first tender leaves of this plant can be harvested as food. They are tangy and tender, making a great addition to soup or omelets. One note of caution: their sour taste is linked to a high oxalic acid content, which can be dangerous for those with a history of kidney disease (same as with rhubarb or sheep's sorrel). But, otherwise, the diuretic effect they offer continues to reinforce the general idea of release and movement: the leaves can help with water retention, edema, bloating, and fluid stagnation in the body. Additionally, in the spring there is a sticky mucilage that forms right where the plant emerges from the soil: because of this, the crowns were traditionally collected and mixed with animal fat to make dock-leaf ointment, a remedy for all kinds of cuts and skin irritation. For our purposes, the bitter yellow root is used. It spirals down into the earth much as the seeds spiral up the stalk, and it's rugged and dark with a bright yellow core.

In the wild, yellowdock prefers open soils and a good bit of moisture. It is often found where human activity has disturbed the topsoil and left a place for the seed to germinate. This, however, means that you see it at construction sites or on roadsides—not good places to harvest roots. So I actually cultivate the root in the shadier spots of the garden, where there is a little moisture, without adding any fertilizer. You can purchase or collect the seed and just scatter it where there is open soil. This is best done in the fall, so that when spring arrives vigorous plants will emerge, mature, and (if conditions are good) set more seed. Though it can be an invasive plant, it is simple to control in the garden: the young plants can be easily pulled up and they don't take over quickly.

After a full season or two of growth, the roots will be ready for harvest. Yellowdock is a perennial, so you can wait longer if you wish— the roots will get bigger. Since they can branch considerably under the soil, consider using a digging fork or a small shovel to help. The best time to do this is after the whole plant has turned a rusty brown: this both ensures that the root is completely mature and that there will be a good amount of seed to scatter after harvest. After they are freed from the soil, cut the tops just under the crown, taking time to notice the beautiful golden cross section, rich in brown rays. Wash and clean the roots with a gentle scrubbing, as there is often a good amount of clay in the crevices. I recommend chopping them at this point, while they are still fresh, regardless of your plans for processing: it is much easier than trying to slice them when they are dry.

USING YELLOWDOCK

Yellowdock root is a classic "blood cleanser," favored by Europeans and also by Native Americans who quickly discovered the powers of this herb when it began to spread, following the arrival of the first colonists. It was used for everything from recurrent infection, anemia, and rheumatic disease to boils and tumors. Considering its bitter qualities, this range of applications sounds familiar—but the chemistry of this plant sets it apart from some of the other bitters. It contains small quantities of a substance called emodin, found in several species from aloe to rhubarb, which has a mild stimulant effect on the colon and also underlies yellowdock's anticancer activity.

Sometimes I run into folks who have been habitually using over-the-counter laxatives for months, maybe even years. Their bowels have lost the ability to move without this external stimulus. A slow transition to a higher-fiber diet, rich in bitter greens and herbs, can help considerably—but often, at least in the initial stages, some yellowdock tincture is necessary while the laxative dose is being reduced. With a little patience, you can retrain the colon to respond to the stretching of its wall as it fills with stool, and the dependence on artificial sources of stimulation can be successfully broken. When this happens, there is marked relief: not only are irregular bowel habits uncomfortable, but laxatives can often cause cramping and make life even less pleasant. This simple remedy is both safe and effective, and should be in pharmacies next to the stimulant and bulking remedies.

But perhaps more important, it is extremely rich in iron and other minerals, making it a key bitter used in pregnancy and debilitated conditions. Again we see a signature in the living plant for these traditional uses: its "rusty" quality, evident in the dry stalk but also in the reddish splotches found on the fresh leaves, is considered a sign that it is rich in iron. Obviously, it isn't the iron content that causes these features—but it has always been fascinating to me how these patterns come together sometimes.

That a remedy for constipation contains large quantities of bio-available iron is a bit of a paradox: usually, iron pills have the opposite effect and lead to sluggish colon function. This is another case in which the whole package provided by medicinal plants ends up being more well crafted than any combination humans might have engineered. And despite its effectiveness for ensuring regularity, its use as a source of easily absorbable iron is highly valued in the herbal world. If a person has anemia associated with an iron deficiency (such as might result from an inadequate diet or from excessive blood loss), yellowdock really shines. To this end, we usually prepare a syrup. It preserves well, tastes good, and corrects iron deficiency quickly and effectively.

Though this may be its greatest virtue, the systemic effects of having regular digestion are not to be underestimated. Far from simply alleviating discomfort, yellowdock (and most all bitter remedies) can help resolve long-term "stuck" conditions. As a result, there is often less anger and irritability, more comfort in daily life, and a greater willingness to be open to the love of others. I know this seems like a stretch for a weedy, simple plant—but for the right person it can make all the difference. After all, since the days of Hippocrates, a backup of bile (known as *choler* in Greek) was linked to anger, tension, and headaches. By helping us release the old patterns we hold on to (and a little bile as well), bitters such as yellowdock can counter the choleric tendency in our modern culture.

Yellowdock Tincture

>Fresh yellowdock roots
>100 proof alcohol

Unlike some of the milder bitter roots, yellowdock makes a tea that is a little too strong to be palatable, even in small doses. So for medicine I usually employ a tincture made from the fresh roots. Cleaned and minced, they steep well in 100 proof spirits and, if put up for three to four weeks, produce a tincture that is my go-to remedy for mild constipation. Its applications are numerous: a sluggish bowel during pregnancy, or the irregularity that accompanies travel or unfamiliar situations—all yield to its gentle action.

It is not habit-forming, unlike other stronger plants (senna and cascara sagrada, for instance). It is even safe to give to children. For adults, I recommend half a teaspoon of the tincture taken before the evening meal, or twice a day, if necessary. For children, the dose depends on age. Best to avoid it for youngsters under eighteen months; fifteen to twenty drops until about age five; and thirty to forty-five drops until the teenage years, at which point adult doses are fine to use. Though it is safe for long-term supplementation, yellowdock is usually employed for periods of two to three weeks at most.

 Yelowdock Syrup

>8 ounces minced, dried yellowdock root
>1 quart spring water
>Raw honey

Take about eight ounces of minced, dried yellowdock root and simmer it in a quart of spring water, over low heat, until there is only about a pint of fluid left. Strain the liquid, which should be dark brown and rich-smelling, and mix it with an equal part by volume of raw honey (meaning, if you have two cups of fluid, mix it with two cups of honey).

That's it! The syrup will keep indefinitely if refrigerated, and for a few weeks if left out at room temperature.

Remedy Reccomendation

Take a couple of tablespoons of yellowdock syrup with meals, once or twice a day, to ensure good iron levels. Because of yellowdock's ability to regulate bowel function, this is a beloved tonic for pregnancy: it helps keep energy levels up and corrects any mild constipation.

4

Tonics

Nourish and Balance

> *We need the tonic of wildness.*
> HENRY DAVID THOREAU, 1854

In Neolithic times, Ireland was ruled by a series of tribes,[1] many of which left lasting monuments to their presence in the form of sacred wells, barrow mounds, and standing stones at special sites. During transitions between different ruling peoples, fierce battles raged that consumed many lives and forged a strong mythology populated by warriors, goddesses, and healers of divine power.

One such healer was Dian Cecht, a noble figure in the Tuatha De Daanan and cousin to the king, Nuada. His tribe of tall, beautiful, shining folk waged war against the Fir Bolg for dominion of Ireland, perhaps around five thousand years ago, though the true dates are lost in time. In their first battle on the western coast, Dian Cecht gained much renown for blessing and enchanting a deep well. It is said that, when the warriors of the Tuatha De Daanan were injured in any way, simply descending into the well and bathing in its waters would restore them to complete health. There was, however, an exception: any piece severed from the body could not be made whole again, meaning, by extension, that decapitation still meant death.

Dian Cecht, his son Miach, and daughter Airmid would sing incantations over the wounded soldier as he descended into the well. Dark and deep, with spiral staircases intertwining on the inner walls, it held cold and restorative water. The soldier would reemerge whole, energized, and ready to return to battle. Thanks to this ritual, in the end, the Tuatha De Daanan, children of the moon goddess, were able to overcome a race of nature worshippers whose temples were the fairy hills of Newgrange and Knowth.

But the Fir Bolg did not pass quietly into history: during the four-day-long battle, a great warrior among them was able to completely sever the hand of Nuada, the king. Despairing, the king ran to Dian Cecht to be restored, but the well could not help him. So the great healer fashioned a silver hand for his master and skillfully attached it to the arm. Both hoped that, thereby, Nuada could maintain rule of the tribe, for Brigid, the matriarch, had decreed that only one whose flesh was whole could lead the people.

Unfortunately, the silver hand, though fully functional and as alive as any flesh, was not good enough for Brigid. The Tuatha De Daanan fell into turmoil. During this confusion, Miach and Airmid, the great healer's children, returned to the battlefield and found the severed hand of Nuada. Over the course of nine days, and using a deep and healing magic, Miach restored the living hand to the king, and thereby, the king to his throne. Such an amazing act of surgery had never before been witnessed, nor has it ever since.

Now, though both may work quite well, there is a difference between a silver hand and one of living flesh, and Brigid clearly knew this. One is the product of technology—advanced, remarkable, effective, but still a construct, an approximation. The other is a product of life itself—our true substance, warm, sensitive, integrated into the whole. The first is our best patch. The second is true healing. So, whether it was out of amazement and disbelief, fear of incredible power, or simply jealousy, Dian Cecht had to challenge his son to a display of healing skills.

Three times the father took a sword to his son's head, each time lopping off a bigger and bigger portion. Time after time Miach healed himself, blood returning to the veins and brain, skull, and hair growing back as they were before. The third time was by far the hardest. And when the sword came down for the fourth time, the great healer found that he had completely severed his son's head—and from this wound there was no return. Miach had died, and with him a great deal of the magic of the healing well was also lost.

Dian Cecht and Airmid buried Miach close by, and while the father quickly left the grave, sister Airmid lingered for days, through foggy, damp mornings and sunny afternoons and rain clouds that, rolling low overhead, darkened the sky over the green, green hills. After a time, strong seedlings began to sprout from her brother's barrow: each one was unique, growing at its own pace and in its own manner. They grew taller, quickly. There were 365 in all, some say one for each bone, joint, and sinew in Miach's body, others say one for every day of the year. But Airmid recognized in each a virtue and power to heal the ailments and ills her people might encounter, and she began to speak and sing to the green plants, and they sang back, so that soon she knew their secret ways. Gathering them up into her cloak, she grouped and arranged them according to their strengths.

But her father returned to the grave before she could hide the magic plants. Seeing what she had done, Dian Cecht seized the cloak and scattered the herbs to the winds. Here I cannot help but think that jealousy was at work—jealousy that simple, humble herbs could accomplish what he might never be able to achieve, jealousy that nature in her own time could work healing that ten thousand men could not comprehend. Or perhaps he simply wanted to hide the knowledge from most people, leaving it to be passed on, as a precious gift, by a select few. Regardless of his intent, this is what he accomplished: Airmid remembered each of the plants that had sprung up from her brother's grave, and some say that, to this day, she heals the sick and wounded from her home in the hills of Connemara. It is a good thing for us that she did remember and in so doing kept alive an essential part of our cultural knowledge. We find today that, despite our technology, the basic nature of life and health remains elusive. Some of Airmid's most magical plants were her tonics. By following their tendrils as they intertwine with our physiology, we may learn something about that basic nature in the process.

A NOTE IN HARMONY

The word *tonic* has a range of meanings. In its simplest form, it refers to tone: the degree of tension, or activity, in a tissue. For example, a well-toned muscle can withstand the load of a heavy weight longer than a muscle with poor tone. In pharmacy, the word often has a more uncertain meaning. Generally, tonics are considered to be remedies that are safe and foodlike, and that enhance physiological function rather than directly treating disease. While this is a commonly accepted definition, "tonics" are also sometimes viewed with skepticism (and rightly so, considering some of the preparations marketed as tonics in the nineteenth century).

Because of these many layers of meaning, I prefer to use a metaphor to describe them. So consider the concept of *tonic* in music, and, more specifically, the concept of the tonic note. This is the frequency of sound upon which a musical scale is built. In a C-major scale, the tonic is the *C* note. It provides a sense of resolution when it is sounded, closing a measure in a satisfying manner and returning the listener to the fundamental element of the piece. The other characteristic of the tonic note is that it harmonizes with all the other notes in the scale. Regardless of whether we are playing in C-major, C-minor, or a pentatonic variant, any note used will sound fantastic when voiced alongside a *C*. Here's a great definition: in music, the tonic is the most basic summary of the whole piece, the root to which the song returns in the end, and the note that harmonizes with everything along the way.

So, too, herbal tonics act as an important foundation for the daily unfolding of the song that is our health and vitality. We already saw this idea expressed in the concept of the xenobiome, the chemical environment that our metabolic physiology needs for optimal function. Indeed, bitters are often considered tonic because they enhance and normalize the activity of the digestion and liver. But Airmid's remedies reach more deeply into more pervasive processes, and their action was always considered more precious. They may show effects on the liver and digestion, too—but their effects at all levels of the human system make them truly tonic.

Part of this has to do with absorption and distribution of the plant chemistry we eat. Some of the most bitter substances, such as iridoids from dandelion and gentian, generally aren't very well-absorbed. What does enter our system is metabolized by the liver and leaves through the bile without circulating in the bloodstream much at all.[2] This, of course, isn't an issue as most of the action of bitter plants is mediated by the T2R receptors that line the whole gut and provide plenty of places for iridoids to exert their influence.

But tonic plants, just like the tonic note of a song, interface and harmonize with every piece of our melody. Some, like bioflavonoids, are somewhat bitter and thus work on the digestion, but they continue by acting on the lining of the blood vessels, our livers, and the environment inside our cells. Others, like saponins, have digestive effects but also go deeper by interfacing with patches of immune tissue as they move through the belly. All of them bring into focus the idea of complex systems interacting: a cocktail of chemicals from plants blending seamlessly with the processes of the human physiological network. So we are going to need to extend the idea of the xenobiome beyond the sphere of digestive and metabolic activity.

Another word that is often seen in the context of plant medicine is *holistic*. And though it may be overused, it has a very specific meaning and describes the activity of tonics well. In essence, holism is simply the broad self-similarity of a network: every tiny piece holds within it the image of the whole, akin to what occurs in a piece of holographic film. If you cut it in half, you don't get half a picture: you still get the whole; it's just a little fuzzier. Similarly, in music, the tonic note holds within it the entire composition: it just lacks elaboration. The progression of notes in a simple melody is, at its core, an initial variation on the tonic note. And even though a song can get extremely complex and detailed, it always recalls the melody, and the melody holds the tonic note, returning to it to anchor the piece. Music is holistic.

Herbal tonics are remedies whose effects can reverberate through every aspect of our being. As such, they might be the most important, enriching elements of the xenobiome. They may seem like no more than simple food, but their chemistry and activity make them unique: the more we examine these herbs, the more we find that they act pervasively, and in remarkably coordinated fashion, to increase resilience. All traditional healers and visionaries knew this—they worked quietly and subtly in their communities, using this gentle rebalancing medicine. In so doing, they saw echoes of the divine in their gardens, in their remedies, and in the people who used them. Hildegard von Bingen, a mystic, healer, and composer who lived in twelfth-century Europe, wrote extensively about the tonic qualities of plants, trees, and places (found in *Hildegard von Bingen's Physica*). In *Heavenly Revelations,* she also composed intricate, tonic-driven chants that beautifully express her rapture with the holistic nature of the world. Listening to her *O viridissima virga* (O greenest branch) is like taking an herbal tonic. We return to the root, we experience reconnection, we are nourished at a very deep level. It is so gentle, so powerful, so much like coming home.

The tonic, in its most positive sense, is an expression of love from the plant world to our own. It is evidence of our coevolution. Everywhere we look, we find locks in our bodies that are opened by these botanical allies. Airmid, and many more wise women following in her lineage, knew this basic fact: go to the tonic herbs, nourish the human being, yield, sing, and watch the resonance.

TURNING GENES INTO HEALTHY HUMANS: EPIGENETICS AND IMMUNITY

To be perfectly honest, all the herbs I talk about in this book are at least a little bit tonic—in the sense that they are safe, gentle (though often quickly and deeply effective), and rebalancing over time. But, as we shall see, there is a difference between a distilled, aromatic, peppermint spirit and a tablespoon of cooked hawthorn berries; a difference between ten drops of bitter dandelion tincture and a boiled broth of reishi mushroom and *Astragalus* root. The berries, roots, and mushrooms are the tonics. Sure, there is a lot of overlap between the categories of plants (with some, like garlic, perhaps belonging to all three). But tonics are unique in that they are coupled with the process of genetic expression and the process of immunity. The science of epigenetics, which studies genetic expression, shows how tonics affect the balance of cancer-promoting and cancer-suppressing genes and the balance of cellular metabolism. An analysis of immunology will show us how tonics speak to the effector cells of the immune system and alter the immunological chemistry of our blood and lymph.

Tonics have the distinctive ability to modulate the function of these two essential processes, and to do so in coordinated, simultaneous fashion. Amazing pharmacological detail substantiates this claim. In addition, traditional herbalists have a strong record recommending classic tonics—like ginseng, wild blueberries, and red clover, among many others—for the worn-down, fatigued, and chronically inflamed. They unburden us or, more accurately, we slowly collect a growing burden when they are not in our lives. Eventually, this burden can manifest as heart disease, chronic pain, even cancer. But before we explore how tonic plants interface with our physiology, let's take a closer look at epigenetics and immunity.

EPIGENETICS

Imagine yourself on the border between Montana and Idaho, almost exactly on the Continental Divide that separates the waters that flow into the Atlantic from those that flow into the Pacific. At nine thousand feet, there are still clusters of old—but small—spruce and fir trees here and there in the meadow. The grasses are short and mixed with a range of wild plants. The slope is steep, and rising above you are the rocky tops of Mt. Jefferson and its ridges. Behind you is a brown and deeply fissured rock wall, crumbling into a pool of water and graced with goldenrod and purple chiming bells in this late summer season. From this pool a small stream tumbles down and into a steep valley, winding its way north as it prepares to hairpin around the mountain and flow east.

This is Brower's Spring, and its water will flow into what becomes the Missouri River, and from there on into the Mississippi and out, past New Orleans, into the Louisiana bayou. At first the flow is overwhelmingly governed by gravity, though long ago, before the mountains had their present shape and the valleys were cut into them, even the clear-cut path that spreads out before you was uncertain. Once, the water from the spring could have flowed west instead—early in the development of this landscape, so much could have been different. But now the course is clear and, as the river basin opens wider, more waters swell the stream so that once it reaches the broad prairie, the water flows in a channel that stretches five football fields across.

It would take a lot to push this flow around, both at the widest point and at the source. In both cases, canals and dams might make a difference but would require incredible energy and time. At our time-scales, the river's course looks pretty fixed (except, of course, when it floods). A water droplet from Brower's Spring is fairly certain to flow past Vicksburg, Mississippi, at some point (assuming it doesn't evaporate beforehand).

But once in the Mississippi Delta, this certainty changes somewhat.

Sure, the droplet will enter the sea somewhere along the Louisiana Coast—but where exactly is governed much more by a complex tangle of local factors. Wind, rain, runoff, fish, boats, plants, and even simple chance, as well as its interaction with other droplets along the way, will all play a role. Finally, somewhere out of the branching delta, the water will reach the Gulf of Mexico.

The story of water's journey to the sea is very much like the story of a new skin cell. Though once, long ago, before skin even existed, the ancestors of this cell could have chosen myriad different paths to travel, now it is locked into a course that has been well-worn by hundreds of generations of skin cells before it. When it grows, it won't become bone, muscle, nerve, or vessel: it will be skin. Once it reaches maturity, it will look a little different from its neighbors, depending on a complex tangle of local factors, ranging from inflammatory chemicals, to sun exposure, to elements from the diet of the human being on which it grows. It may switch back and forth between a few different states during the course of its month or so of life. Finally, as with all skin cells, it will die and be replaced, leaving a protective and waterproof layer of protein behind. Unless, of course, something unexpected alters this plan—unless a flood occurs and the river breaks its banks. The skin cell might then find a different course, forget its manners, and start dividing out of control or perhaps perish before its time.

During the first weeks of development, the human embryo is just a ball of cloned cells. Each of these cells is more akin to a drop of rain far above the Continental Divide, back on the border of Idaho and Montana: it hasn't committed itself to any path quite yet. It will hit the ground somewhere along the ridgeline just west of Mt. Jefferson, and percolate through the soil, or perhaps run off some stones, and join the underground plume of water that feeds Brower's Spring. But it could also become part of the Great Salt Lake, if it falls only a few more feet to the west. As it falls, its possibilities are diverse, but once it arrives on the ground, it soon becomes locked into a well-defined course.

Though all our cells (and there are over fifty trillion of them) have the exact same DNA—an identical genetic blueprint in their nuclei—they become very different during development. They choose a river to join then stick faithfully to its course, though still retaining the ability to make some final adjustments in the end. This analogy of a landscape was first developed by Conrad Waddington, a geneticist and evolutionary theorist who worked in the latter half of the twentieth century. He compared the fate of a cell as it differentiates from its embryonic state to marbles rolling down a furrowed slope: they pick valleys to follow and end up resting in the lowest points. Using energy, a marble can be pushed up and over a ridgeline, or back up a valley—but, in general, it will follow its course once it chooses it, just like our water droplet. The science that attempts to describe this landscape is the science of epigenetics—the study of how our genes become our bodies. The landscape is a series of chemical and environmental factors. These factors govern how the blueprint of life is expressed. They determine how and when specific cell types form and how they behave once they've settled on their path.[3]

Now, while this is pretty important stuff, how applicable is it to daily life? There are two answers. The first is that understanding epigenetic factors and how to modify them might help prevent, and possibly even treat, cancer—helping the river stay within its banks. The second is that epigenetic factors govern the cell's behavior during trauma, infection, and inflammation—the path the droplet takes once it reaches the delta. Though we can't turn back the clock to an undifferentiated embryonic state using plants, we might be able to have a positive impact on factors associated with cancer and chronic inflammation. In this sense, the science of epigenetics is extremely relevant.

Genetic material can be used for two main purposes, as far as we know today. It can either be used to create proteins for structure and catalysis of metabolic reactions (about 2 percent is used for this purpose), or it can be used to create chunks of RNA that end up affecting the genome in turn. These are known as retrotransposons, free-floating functional copies of pieces of DNA, often used to alter when and how genes are active. The instructions for their production account for over 40 percent of our DNA blueprint.[4] We're not sure about the rest. The transcription of DNA into mRNA (another type of functional DNA copy, used as a template for assembling proteins for enzymes, muscle tissue, or hair) and its translation into proteins has been well described;[5] what is more interesting are the feedback patterns that occur when proteins affect the DNA, in turn, "switching" particular genes on or off.

How is this "switching" accomplished? This is another way to frame epigenetics—as a collection of factors that turn genetic material on or off. After all, a skin cell contains all the information needed to become a nerve cell—it's just that the nerve cell genes are "off." The process of picking a streambed to follow to the sea is governed by which areas of the genome are active. Our cellular physiology does this by attaching different types of molecules to DNA and to the scaffolding that supports it.

Let's take a moment to visualize the more than six billion base pairs that make up our DNA. Of all that genetic material, very little is actually accessible at any given time. It's mostly packed away into chromosomes, unless the cell is dividing, in which case it's slowly being unraveled and copied. While it's packed away, the molecular machinery that "reads" the information can't get access to it. The packing is accomplished by wrapping the DNA around spherical proteins known as histones. This is the only way you can fit six feet of double helix into one-one-thousandth of an inch. But it also serves to protect the genetic material from radiation and harmful chemicals.

If you were floating in the intracellular fluid and could cross through one of the pores in the nuclear membrane (all the while watching thin ribbons of mRNA threading their way toward the protein-assembly stations that are the ribosomes), you would enter a soupy realm bustling with activity. Proteins and enzymes, along with pieces of RNA, would be flowing in and out of view, coming and going from a cluster of giant, dense scaffolding. This scaffolding is made of histones, arranged into chromosomes, gatekeepers of the genome. Around certain areas of the chromosomes, you could make out ghostlike loops of DNA suspended in the haze, drifting toward each other, with lots of molecular activity around them.[6] Steroid receptors, activated by their hormonal triggers, would be gliding along the loops. A variety of molecules from the outside world might be at work, too. In short, you would be observing a stew of molecular machinery, extremely complex but endowed with the typical "fuzzy" organization found in so many ecosystems.

The loops of genetic material that are unwrapped from their histone scaffolding are legible thanks, in part, to a structural change in the scaffolding itself—an epigenetic change. Some of the molecules in the stew are responsible for adding small hydrocarbon chunks, known as acetyl groups ($-C_2H_5$), to the histones.[7] This allows the histones to release their grip, and the DNA, unbound, begins to float freely inside the nucleus. Now it can be read, its instructions can be followed, the chain of events that leads to physical structure and function can begin. The instructions might include directions to unwrap other areas of the chromosomes or to attach other types of molecules to other histones, which, in turn, might lead the currently active genes to have different ultimate expressions in the organism. The web of interactions between genes, histones, and the molecules surrounding them defines a complex system, a network of organized complexity (to return to Warren Weaver's words).[8]

Some of the most interesting players in this network are proteins known as sirtuins, from a protein first discovered in yeast and called Sir2.[9] These proteins have since been well characterized in human beings,[10] and they generally remove acetyl groups, both from histones and from other molecules. The sum of their effects seems to increase a cell's resilience, reducing inflammation and increasing life span.[11] Their presence allows for the successful "packing up" of DNA, and their activity is stimulated by increased stress, DNA damage, increased energy usage, and the presence of harmful chemicals. All in all, recent evidence suggests that these molecules are the central regulators of such diverse yet all-important processes as the cell cycle, cellular self-destruction, cellular metabolism, and DNA repair.[12] If we could trace a link between tonic herbs and sirtuin activity, we might find clues as to their deep rebalancing power.

Another important epigenetic mechanism takes place on the DNA itself. Certain base pairs, the "rungs of the ladder" in the double helix, may have another type of small hydrocarbon chunk, this one called a methyl group ($-CH_3$), attached to them. This acts as a sort of "roadblock" for the protein machinery charged with reading the DNA. Even if the instructions are floating free from their histone scaffolding, they are literally illegible. And it seems as if the areas of highest methylation (where methyl groups are attached to the DNA) are those right before what's called a "promoter sequence"—a flag for the start of an active gene. Methylation thus keeps our cells from even starting to copy that gene into mRNA. So, if the acetylation of histones offers a flexible way to make large sections of the genome available, methylation of DNA hard-codes certain genes on or off.[13] And, as it happens, these codings can be acquired during our lifetime and passed on to our offspring. Epigenetic changes have been experimentally documented to extend over at least three generations.[14]

Dysfunction in methylation has been linked to cancer[15]—where normally dormant genes, silenced perhaps since those first weeks of embryonic development, lose the methyl groups on their promoter regions and become active again. But, in practice, this is a rare occurrence. Modification of DNA's scaffolding, the histone protein chains, is much more commonplace—and these modifications can change fairly radically, depending on the situation and the environment.[16] You might expect to find some degree of influence here from tonic plants. And, of course, you would be correct. Let's see why.

In the cellular nucleus, a complex balancing act is taking place. The instructions stored in the DNA, encoded in a giant organic library, are packed in dense stacks. But rather than being just simple storage shelves, these stacks have special abilities. They can find their way around the library all by themselves, lock and unlock bookshelves, and bring different volumes together to create a meaningful story. They are aided in this by a cloud of enzymes that place and remove chemical elements, such as acetyl and methyl groups, on the books and shelves and, in so doing, affect what is visible, legible, active. Only the active instructions participate in this dance. The rest of the genome sits quiet, tucked away, dark—until the miraculous event of cellular division literally turns the library inside out and duplicates it. Along the shelves are books that describe how to grow, how to rest, how to perpetuate inflammation, how to repair and renew tissue, how to respond to signals from other cells.[17] All this complex cloud of activity is set in motion at the moment of fertilization, when sperm meets egg (the raindrops above the ridge). As cells divide, each settles into a pattern (the river's course) but can also respond, within limits, to changes in its environment and thereby alter its expression (the many channels in the river's delta).

Many of these responses are modulated by proteins, such as sirtuins, which rearrange the stacks in the library of the genome and close up huge sections after they've been read. They also activate and deactivate a web of other enzymes (we will explore them more when we get deeper into the pharmacology of herbal tonics), which, in turn, open or close other parts. Sirtuins are the custodians of a very important set of genes and gene-activating enzymes:[18] they regulate how a cell responds to environmental stressors by increasing its resilience, longevity, and self-repair function or, if necessary, helping to drastically reduce cellular activity through a process called "autophagy," or "self-eating."[19] In other words, they increase life span and reduce the damage a cell might suffer during inflammation, while also ensuring that they don't become overextended, bloated, or wasteful.

If we are talking about wellness from a cellular perspective, our sirtuins seem to be crucial. Their activity is, however, tied to their environment: not only what genes are active, but also what the chemistry surrounding them looks like. The activity of sirtuins and, by extension, the activity of genes relating to cellular resilience, metabolism, and repair, are extremely sensitive to the xenobiome.[20]

Here we return to the tonic plants. It seems that certain molecules they contain, known as bioflavonoids (and other polyphenols, such as the curcuminoids, coumarins, and stilbenoids), are some of the most potent activators of sirtuins.[21] These molecules are found in many different plants but are highly concentrated in tonics, such as chocolate, hawthorn, blueberries and grapes, green tea, dong quai (*Angelica sinensis*), *Schisandra,* and more.[22] These are the molecular interfaces between the inner world of the nucleus and the environment all around us. Epidemiological research that looks at correlations between plant flavonoid intake and disease is extremely interesting, and well summarized in Jeffrey Blumberg's review.[23] Flavonoid consumption levels are linked to significantly lower rates of heart disease, stroke, and certain types of cancer. The lowest documented rate of flavonoid consumption globally is in the United States.[24] We will come back to what this means for us, and why these flavonoid molecules might be so important for keeping us vibrantly healthy and resilient. But for now, I want to leave you with one final thought. Yes, these compounds are essential for helping our cells respond to environmental stress and challenge, and they do this by modulating epigenetic activity through proteins, such as sirtuins.[25] Yes, they protect us from the most common diseases associated with old age. Yes, they come from plants. But what is their role in the botanical world?

It turns out that plants overproduce these molecules when they are under stress. Imagine that—when a hawthorn tree experiences drought or inclement weather, it generates more of the same molecules that our cells use for modulating protection, resilience, and longevity switches.[26] This makes sense—that's what the plant is using them for, too.[27] But the beauty of this whole system is that if we regularly consume the plants richest in flavonoids, we tap into a botanical-signaling system that is highly sensitive to the conditions in the air, water, and soil around us. This signaling system grabs our genome and directs its expression through epigenetic mechanisms that have evolved over millions of years of plant consumption.[28] We have allies in the wild, tonic, flavonoid-rich plants. They whisper to us at the deepest level of our beings, where our physical substance unfolds out of the genetic blueprint, and they direct this unfolding as a conductor does her orchestra.

IMMUNITY

Let's stay at roughly the same spot, deep inside the nuclei of our cells. Backing out a little, we pass into the thick fluid of the cell itself. Here a host of molecules, each participating in a complex dance of chemical reactions, keeps the cell active and in good repair. Eventually, we cross outside, beyond the fatty membrane that separates the cell from the fluid all around it. Studding this membrane are proteins and sugars that have an incredible diversity of roles: channels for transport of nutrients, receptors for signal molecules, docks for anchoring to other cells, markers for identification, and many more. It looks something like a very small planet, mostly covered in a greasy ocean, with occasional cholesterol islands and an array of different, gigantic trees growing out of (and into) its surface. This landscape is in flux, with the "trees" gliding along and even changing shape in a kind of hyperaccelerated tectonic drift.

A new type of cell appears in the periphery. First there is only one, but soon there are more. They are much, much smaller spheres, but they, too, have a whole range of different outgrowths on their surface: delicate bands of protein and sugar they can use to communicate, exchange genetic material, and interact with their environment. These are bacteria—*Staph* in this particular case—and they probably shouldn't be here. One of them brushes up against the outer surface of our cell.

Almost immediately a stream of proteins begins to form a cloud around the bacteria like a swarm of blackflies around a hiker's head.

They start to connect with the tendrils growing out of the invader's outer layer. Some are repelled, but others succeed in creating small openings in the bacteria's cell membranes, and a few of the pathogens fall away. If you were an immune cell, you could smell this activity, it would be attractive to you, and you would slowly make your way to the scene. Soon enough, one does: with surprising agility for something so large, a white blood cell appears, extends long fibrous arms around the bacteria, and eventually engulfs them all. Inside, they soon meet their demise, and the white blood cell places pieces of them on its outside surface: "Here's what I found!" it seems to say. As we shall see, it has some important friends who might be very interested in the discovery.

The above image is that of the innate immune system in action. This system is in part a collection of molecules, such as the defensins that swarmed the *Staph,* that help an organism withstand attempted colonization from harmful pathogens. In animals, this chemical activity is reinforced by cellular players like the white blood cell (a dendritic cell, also known as a macrophage, which lies in wait in our tissues). But the molecular component of the innate immune system is extremely ancient, being the primary immunity for insects and found throughout the plant world as well.[29] We share a "first line of defense" with plants and fungi in the age-old struggle of multicellular organisms attempting to stay alive in the face of an overwhelmingly viral and bacteriological world. Plant defensins, so similar to our own, repelled potential invaders for millions of years before the first animals ever swam the sea.[30]

The molecular components of innate immunity evolved in concert with the pathogens in the environment and still provide a remarkably effective barrier to infection. Coupled with dendritic cells and other white blood cells, including the "natural killer" cells, they protect us from simple cuts, bacteria, many viruses, and developing tumors. All the players in the innate immune system are highly sensitive to what pathogens produce, especially their surface markers. In fact, researchers use a substance called "bacterial lipopolysaccharide" to induce experimental inflammatory reactions.[31] They directly aggravate innate immunity by injecting a huge number of bacterial surface markers into skin or muscle tissue. Furthermore, not only is the innate immune system exquisitely sensitive to foreign molecules, it is also extremely specific and only mounts reactions to those molecules and not, say, to tissue in our joints, digestive tract, or upper respiratory passages.[32]

The innate immune system has a rapid response, too. Within minutes, defensins, complement proteins, and dendritic and natural killer cells are on the scene of a wound or viral incursion, helping to prevent infection. This defense mechanism is highly effective, and it's crucial that it function well. Those with genetic illnesses that affect the production of immune-active proteins experience debilitating, lifelong disease.[33] As we age, or experience frequent, recurrent immunological challenge, all aspects of immunity suffer somewhat.[34] Still, innate immunity continues to protect us extremely well from everything from the common cold to a *Staph* infection on the skin.

Vertebrates, however, lay claim to a special trick: our immune systems have the ability to remember. This memory is encoded in another type of molecule, the antibody, which is precisely tuned to one particular substance (known as an antigen, or "*anti*body *gen*erator"). When antibodies bind to antigens, they greatly facilitate the capture and destruction of whatever may be causing problems.[35] And once we can make antibodies to a particular substance (usually a snippet of DNA from the pathogen or a unique cell surface marker), we retain that ability and can muster it quickly during any future exposure. Far more often than not, the combination of innate immunity and antibodies neutralizes any potential threat from an organism that might want to colonize us.

Our capacity for making antibodies and thus remembering what we have encountered resides with the adaptive (also known as the acquired) immune system. It is a collection of white blood cells that, unlike the cells and proteins of innate immunity, can discriminate in its attacks. Its memories are stored in special white blood cells called "B" cells. This is where antibodies come from. But the true heart of the adaptive immune system is called a "T" cell. In short, T cells serve as direct killers, or, more often, coordinators of the overall immune response. They secrete chemicals that can stimulate the release of histamine (an inflammatory chemical notoriously involved in allergies) from the mast cells where it is stored. They can stimulate the activity of more dendritic cells and macrophages, speeding their cleanup of the affected area. They recruit and train B cells, and are thus essential for the production of antibodies. But crucially, they also act as the traffic directors of the immune response, helping to activate it when it's dormant or calm it when it becomes overactive.[36]

While there is broad overlap, there seem to be two general patterns of behavior for these "helper" T cells (also called regulatory T cells). These patterns are defined by the types of chemicals and cells involved. Very well described in animals,[37] our understanding of the patterns in human beings improved through the 1990s. Now, we know that there are many different types of helper T cells, sometimes specific ones designed to regulate our immune system's interaction with a single, specific pathogen.[38] Still, there seems to be a balance between two basic immune behaviors: a tendency to use antibodies (IgG) that bind up bacteria and viruses for capture and disposal, and a tendency to use antibodies (IgE) that stimulate histamine and other chemicals involved in inflammation.[39] In other words, T cells can help the cells of the innate immune system ingest and destroy unwanted material, or they can trigger a signal that stimulates a histamine reaction and causes redness, swelling, and pain. In practice, both patterns occur during inflammation: the first is the cleanup, the second is the gas pedal. Sometimes the immune system gets a lead foot, and though it's unclear why this happens, it can lead to conditions like allergies, asthma, and eczema.[40]

The link between innate immunity and helper T cells is the white blood cell that engulfed the *Staph* bacteria.[41] As you recall, it placed little pieces of what it found on its cell surface. It turns out that this is a message for a T cell. This signal will activate the helper cells, and they will coordinate the next phase of the immune response. If that white blood cell engulfs an allergen, like a piece of pollen, it displays it on its surface just like that piece of *Staph*. This would generally stimulate the "cleanup" behavior pattern in a helper T cell. But in some individuals, that T cell pushes the gas pedal and stimulates the release of more histamine instead. The inflammatory reaction gets more and more intense. In the end, the intensity of inflammation in all of us is linked to the interplay between both patterns of T cell activity. In fact, certain diseases where the immune system attacks healthy tissue (such as rheumatoid arthritis) are characterized by an opposite pattern, where the cellular "cleanup" processes get out of control and begin to destroy connective tissue. In the end, it seems most important that the two faces of adaptive immunity complement each other harmoniously.

If we could get a handle on this equilibrium—called the Th1/Th2 balance in reference to the first and second pattern of helper T cell (Th) behavior—we could have an impact on allergy, chronic inflammation, and hypersensitivity. This is yet another point of balance in the human physiology. It is a place in the network that is highly connected to other processes, affecting them profoundly. It is a place that is sensitive to fluctuations in the chemical environment, in the xenobiome. Every time we've located such a place so far, we've also found that plants have an essential, normalizing effect. As you might guess, we will discover that the immune system also pivots around such a botanical fulcrum.

Tonic plants are to the innate immune system what bitters are to digestion. Many of them possess starches, chains of various sugar molecules that look a lot like some of the sugar chains on the surface of a bacterium or virus. These chains, called polysaccharides, seem to wake up innate immunity, increasing the secretion of proteins like defensins and the activity of the phagocytic white blood cells.[42] That's not a huge surprise, if we remember that plants also use defensins to protect themselves. They help this immediate, quick-acting, ancient part of our immune system stay vigilant and effective. This is never a bad thing: innate immunity never overreacts unless told to by a helper T cell, nor can it ever attack our own tissue.[43]

Tonic plants go further, helping to regulate the Th1/Th2 balance and often shifting it more toward a Th1 response[44]—taking the foot off the gas pedal and restoring equilibrium. As we will see, this might be due to a similarity between chemicals, such as polysaccharides and bacterial surface markers. It is interesting to note that, over the past twenty years, an idea termed the *hygiene hypothesis*[45] has attempted to describe the rise in allergy, autoimmune disease, and even autism in terms of missing immunological challenge. Lacking actual pathogenic signals, helper T cells shift away from a cleanup pattern and begin to overreact to everything from pollen to gluten, even to our own tissues. Too much hygiene, so the argument goes, has confused the immune system.[46] Some have gone as far as purposefully infecting themselves with hookworms to successfully treat conditions like multiple sclerosis.*[47]

One association that has been extremely well characterized is that between asthma rates and rural farm life: it is an inverse association, meaning there is less asthma on the farm.[48] Researchers have been attempting to figure out why. Some say the bacteriological challenge from raw farm milk is the key; others say it's the milk's whey content.[49] Still others comment on the exposure to farm animals—children who sleep in the barn seem to have less asthma.[50] I suspect that a complex series of factors underlie this association, rather than one single magical element. Though it's seldom discussed, farm kids might be eating more wild plants, or at least doing more gardening.

Interestingly, "horticultural therapy," using small gardens for food and recreation, is considered a great addition to the conventional management of asthma in Japan[51] (not surprising, coming from a culture that also advocates immersion in the forest to relax and control

---

*For an engaging read on this topic and others relating to "rewilding" our bodies, see Dunn's *The Wild Life of Our Bodies*.

anxiety). So put it all together, and we come up with a picture that includes not only exposure to bacteria but perhaps also to a variety of diverse botanical influences—a rich xenobiome. Here we are getting very close to describing the biochemical basis for "nature deficit disorder"—a phrase coined by Richard Louv in *Last Child in the Woods* to both define a major problem in today's culture and at the same time offer a clear solution. Part of this biochemical basis might be a lack of direct ingestion of wild plants.

"The more high-tech we become, the more nature we need," Louv explains in *The Nature Principle*.[52] I feel this is a valuable insight, and not because nature is somehow always good and helpful. It's not. Simply put, elements from nature are crucial to our mental health (as Louv repeatedly shows), our metabolic health, and our immunological health. It is literally Thoreau's "tonic of wildness" that we should be seeking, and wild, unhybridized plants are a huge part of that. As we have seen, they seem to be such a huge part that, without them, our physiology suffers. The action of tonics includes the regulation of epigenetic factors that are vital for cellular survival and resiliency. We might also expect that some of their chemistry would impact diseases where immune function is disrupted, providing some of the same immune-active chemistry of pathogens, without any of the risks.

Of course, this is precisely the case. We will revisit how, and what it means for us, when we explore the pharmacology of tonic herbs. Suffice it to say that tonics like the medicinal mushrooms (*Coriolus, Ganoderma, Grifola, Lentinula,* and more) and sweet roots such as *Astragalus* have been found to reduce asthma, allergies, and symptoms of rheumatoid arthritis (where the immune system is attacking the tissue of the joints).[53] Additionally, they improve immune function and lessen infection, as seen, for example, in two types of patients with seriously challenged immunity: those undergoing chemotherapy for cancer and those experiencing nervous exhaustion.[54]

This dual action that is both balancing and enlivening comes up over and over again in our exploration of plants, and it's no coincidence:

we are built around these herbs. In exploring aromatic plants, we saw how they rebalance mood and help us engage with life, but this could have simply been a coincidence—useful, but not necessary. With bitters, though, we came to appreciate the role of wild plants in managing our ability to nourish ourselves—how we process food, handle sugar, and protect ourselves against poison—and we may have begun to feel that we are actually somewhat dependent on these plants for normal function. But tonics are the best examples of how the complex botanical world interacts with the complex human physiology: we are dance partners and need each other. The memory of tonic herbs is encoded as much in our genes and immune systems as it is in our myths and cuisines. Their memory holds the answer to Michael Pollan's challenge of how to "escape the worst elements of the Western diet and lifestyle without going back to the bush."[55] Incorporating just a little of the wild plants into our daily lives can make huge difference over time. And once it's reawakened, this memory leads us back to the barrow mound where, as visible examples of rebirth and renewal, the tonic herbs sprung up around Airmid. We, too, can gather them, yield to their gentle song, and watch our whole being resonate in harmony.

THE TRADITIONAL APPROACH

If tonic plants indeed have consistent effects on epigenetic regulation and immunological balance, we might expect to see them used in a traditional context for problems related to poor resiliency, overactive inflammation, weakness, and repeated infection. Let's take a look.

Perhaps the most famous and celebrated of all tonics is the root of *Panax ginseng,* a plant in the Araliaceae family that grows wild in rich, dense forests of northeast China and the Korean peninsula. It is commonly known as ginseng (though a few different species claim this name), and these days you can find it almost everywhere, especially in preparations purporting to boost energy levels. Though I approach these modern concoctions with skepticism, Chinese medicine does have a lot to say about herbal tonics and about ginseng root in particular. It is reported to have been used by the yellow emperor, Huang Di, as a tonic for longevity and well-being.[56] During the evolution of dynastic rule, ginseng became more and more prized, with wild roots (which can routinely exceed fifty years of age) being saved for the express use of the emperor. It was at this time, during the first few centuries of the Common Era, that this plant cemented its reputation as a life-enhancing medicine for a wide range of ailments.

One important use of ginseng, however, stands out and clearly illustrates how well this tonic works when it comes to increasing resiliency and literally "giving life." When the emperor was near death, and matters of succession required provincial leaders to assemble in the capital from the far-flung corners of the province, doctors would prescribe quantities of pure, old, wild ginseng roots for the ruler. This would keep him alive until everyone could arrive and settle the affairs of state. These types of anecdotes are recorded throughout Chinese history, a more recent one being the story of Wung-Wai Tso,[57] currently an honorary professor in the Biochemistry Department at the Chinese University of Hong Kong. An experience in his childhood must have profoundly affected him, because his work now centers on researching the medicinal activities of traditional Chinese tonic herbs.

When Dr. Tso was young, he often stayed with his grandfather while his dad was away. During one of his father's trips, his grandfather became weak and knew, as many people close to the end of life do, that his end was near. Consulting with local doctors, he was given a strong decoction made of ginseng roots. Thanks in part to this remedy, Dr. Tso's grandfather was kept alive for the two days needed for his father to return home. Ginseng's power, echoed over and over again in the traditional use record, is to enhance vitality, especially in the later years of life.[58]

Traditional Chinese tonics, such as *Astragalus* root, were also seen to have important effects on immune function. *Astragalus* was, and still is, used to enhance the *wei qi*, or "surface energy," thought to emanate from the rhythmic motion of the lungs and protect us from "evil influences" (in this case, that means the organisms responsible for respiratory infections).[59] The root is called *huang qi,* or "yellow leader," truly a noble appellation in a culture where yellow is the color of highest honor. It is often mixed with ginseng to increase vitality and resistance to infection. Other important immune-enhancing tonics in Chinese medicine are the medicinal mushrooms in general, and reishi (*Ganoderma lucidum, G. tsugae*) in particular. Reishi has various names that translate to "mushroom of immortality" and "mushroom of kings," and it is used for age-related problems, such as dementia, agitation, immune weakness, and fatigue.[60] Again, the traditional use record emphasizes tonics' role in promoting vitality and resilience, especially as we age, and in promoting good immune function. Often these tonics are seen as having a "sweet" flavor—nothing like sugar as we know it today, but quite satisfying nevertheless.

Chinese medicine has defined the category of herbal tonics. We will look at what types of plants the West identifies as tonics in its traditional herbal medicine, but before we do that I want to take a moment to review the modern take on old Chinese life remedies. Plants like ginseng, *Astragalus,* and the mushrooms, but also *Schisandra,* licorice, and jiaogulan (*Gymnostemma*) have received increased attention in modern times and are generally classed as "adaptogenic" herbs. *Adaptogenic* simply means that they are associated with an increased capacity to adapt to stress and challenge in daily life, whether that challenge stems from a mental, emotional, or physical source.[61]

This definition, perhaps originating from the work of Russian pharmacologist Nicolai Lazarev published in the late 1950s,[62] seeks to identify a class of medicinal plants that have safe, "nonspecific" effects on the physiology. These effects, depending on the person and circumstance, may include increased immunity, increased alertness, increased physical and mental performance, and, almost paradoxically, better sleep. As elaborated by Israel Brekhman (a student of Lazarev's) in the latter half of the twentieth century, all these effects boil down to one particular gift: adaptogenic plants increase the physiology's resilience in the face of stress. They simply make us more resistant.[63] This sounds exactly like what epigenetic and immune regulation may accomplish: we have seen that tonic plants may increase resiliency at the cellular level through epigenetic regulation. They also may decrease chronic inflammatory damage (one of the clearest signs that resistance is breaking down—just ask any runner during intensive training), while also increasing resistance to pathogens through immune regulation.

Thus, adaptogens don't simply enhance resistance at a cellular level, but they seem to be able to give the whole physiology greater endurance in the face of ongoing challenge. While any challenge to the human system may be stressful, it certainly doesn't have to be. As we saw when exploring aromatic herbs, it is our response to stressors that largely determines their impact. In other words, there are two ways to handle a difficult situation: either you lessen your perception of the problem, meaning you don't allow the stress to affect you (here aromatics shine); or you shore up your resilience, meaning you can endure the challenge longer (a traditional strength of tonics).

The idea that an organism eventually becomes overwhelmed when under prolonged stress has been well documented. We have seen that challenge is an important factor in promoting good health, but too much for too long can have adverse effects. Hans Selye, a physician who studied in Hungary during the 1920s but moved to Johns Hopkins in Baltimore and eventually to McGill in Montréal, Canada, described this phenomenon and its physiological basis in detail. His work earned him a nomination for a Nobel Prize in 1949. Selye recognized that human beings (and most animals, too) have a strong but limited capacity to handle disruptive influences. At first, there is a beneficial reaction—but, eventually, a state of exhaustion follows. As occurs with exhaustive exercise, this state includes increased inflammation, loss of function, and an inability to respond to any new challenges. In short, we have a finite capacity to deal with harmful stimuli, and when we reach that threshold, we can no longer adapt and respond.[64] Brekhman proposed that adaptogenic tonics raise that threshold. As we will see, others had already figured this out—and modern research has given us a good pharmacological understanding as to why tonics work in this way.

It is instructive to note that Brekhman's research on adaptogens started with the hypothesis that traditional tonic plants are adaptogenic. In order to research those plants directly, he traveled to the Primorski Krai (or "maritime province") of far eastern Russia. This province is bordered by the ocean to the east and China to the west—close to the home range of ginseng. It is heavily forested, mountainous, and untouched: the perfect place to stalk the wild, tonic herbs. Brekhman, urged by Lazarev to "search for the answer in nature,"[65] spent more than forty years here cataloging and researching the pharmacology of tonic plants, and in the process he thoroughly defined the concept of *adaptogen*. Poignantly, after working with astronauts, athletes, performers, chess masters, and more, he came to see these plants as possessing a "life-enhancing symphony of a formula to make people healthy, happy, to protect them from stress."[66] So it seems as if these herbs help sound a tonic note in all those who deeply explore their virtues.

In Western medicine, the historical herbal tonic had a somewhat different definition than the life-giving, resistance-promoting adaptogens featured in the Chinese medical system. Nevertheless, as we will see by exploring the idea of the tonic in European herbal medicine and in the practice of the Eclectic physicians, the ultimate effects are the same: it's just that in the West, tonics have been associated with a specific tissue or organ system. There are heart tonics, gut tonics, and lung tonics, for instance. This was true in Asia, too. The Chinese speak of yang, yin, blood, and *qi* tonics; of tonics for the spleen, the liver, and the kidneys. It seems that traditional herbal medicine has always recognized these herbs as enhancing function and improving resistance, and sometimes has tied their effects to particular pieces of the physiology.

Perhaps no other plant better embodies the European idea of a tonic than the hawthorn tree. The mythology surrounding this understory plant (which grows fifteen to twenty feet tall, much like an apple tree) is extensive. It is also called the whitethorn, and it's associated with the May Day feast. In warmer climes, it blooms white around this time and its fruits ripen over the course of the summer into red, juicy, bean-size berries that hide a hard seed. Dioscorides, whose compendium of herbal remedies dates to somewhere around 50 CE, references this tree. Galen mentions it. In more recent times, Nicholas Culpeper summarizes its uses as a general tonic and diuretic, emphasizing its importance in "dropsy" (now known as congestive heart failure). By the beginning of the twentieth century, its use in both folk and traditional medicine was well established, and its indications summarized by Maude Grieve: "used as a cardiac tonic in organic and functional heart troubles."[67] Modern Western herbalists all concur with Varro Tyler's more recent assessment that hawthorn has "a favorable effect on the heart itself which is especially noticeable in cases of heart damage."[68]

David Hoffmann makes an interesting point when discussing hawthorn, contrasting the use of this tree with that of remedies such as foxglove (*Digitalis*) and lily of the valley (*Convallaria*). The latter remedies are very strong, containing chemicals called cardioactive glycosides that are the sources of modern medicines used for heart failure—but if you overdose on them, these plants can be lethal. True heart tonics, like hawthorn, are different. As Hoffmann puts it, they "have an observably beneficial action on the heart and blood vessels. . . . How they work is either completely obscure or an area of major pharmacological debate, but flavones appear to be major contributors."[69] The hawthorn is about as toxic as an apple—meaning, not at all. And flavones, along with a variety of other flavonoids, are important parts of its medicinal activity. As we saw earlier, these chemicals work in part through their epigenetic effects—making cells in the heart and blood vessels experience less inflammation and more resiliency. Other flavonoid-rich berries, such as blueberry, bilberry, and even grapes, all have similar traditional uses for the heart and blood vessels. True tonics indeed.

Herbs that improve the function of other important organ systems also fall under the umbrella of tonics in Western herbal medicine. For instance, some of the aromatic herbs we explored earlier are considered "nervine" tonics, especially those in the mint family (the Lamiaceae). They are seen as enhancing the function of the nervous system—and we know why this is. Bitter herbs are often called bitter tonics, since they substantially improve the function of digestion and metabolism. Herbal bitters are perhaps some of the most well-respected tonics in European medicine, as we clearly saw when exploring these plants. This is what I mean when I say that all the plants in this book are somewhat tonic—they are safe, foodlike, and shore up the function of the organs they affect. But I have found it useful to separate the aromatic nervines and the bitter digestives from the more specific anti-inflammatory and immune-active tonics—both because of their chemistry and because of their clinical applications.

Other plants seen as tonic in Western herbalism include herbs such as red clover, melilot, cleavers, and sweet woodruff. These plants are generally used to reduce swelling, such as edema, in tissue (though they may also have some interesting immune-related activity). Then there are also some very astringent plants, such as oak, or even rose, that have similar uses. Here we see an application of the word *tonic* that is more akin to that of modern medicine: astringing, or "tightening up" tissues, literally improves their tone. The use of rosewater as a facial toner is a perfect example. I contend that these applications are a bit different from the classic idea of a "tonic" as an enhancer of physiological function. Nevertheless, all these species are also rich in flavonoids and tannins—astringent molecules all.

Immune-enhancing tonics are less clearly visible in Western tradition, certainly when we compare it to the Chinese record. Hildegard von Bingen does mention mushrooms, though she isn't too happy about their use. "One who has pain in his lungs," she writes in *Physica* in reference to a willow bracket fungus, "should cook this mushroom in wine and add a bit of cumin and lard."[70] One doesn't find lots of sweet roots like *Astragalus* in the list of tonics. It may have been that the right species were just missing, or perhaps that the focus in Europe was more on treating infection and securing heroic, battlefield cures, while in China, the concept of tonification was developed to a much greater extent. In Europe we often see a greater emphasis on bitters as a way to enhance liver activity and thereby stimulate resistance, from Galen's use of the mithridate to John Gerard's seventeenth-century recommendation of *Angelica* root as "an enemy to poisons."[71] This is a sound strategy, as we have seen—but it falls more under the aegis of bitters than of tonics.

So, in sum, much of the Western record looks to tonics as remedies that manage inflammation, improve physiological function, and enhance resistance, especially in the cardiovascular system. Almost everything else considered "tonic" would fall under the definition of an aromatic herb ("nervine tonics") or a bitter. Whereas the Chinese model looks to tonics as overall vitality enhancers that regulate immunity and often taste sweet, the European system considers tonics to be foodlike agents like hawthorn that soothe hot, inflammatory processes in the body and have a more sour flavor. The former often calls for nourishing vitality in the face of aging, stress, and damage, while the latter focuses on improving function and reducing inflammation. Both approaches are equally valid and useful in treating disease and maintaining health—and ultimately lead us to the same place.

Eclectic medicine was practiced for about one hundred years in North America, roughly from the 1850s to the 1930s. As a discipline, it made incredible contributions to the art and science of botanical medicine and to botany. Eclectic physicians cataloged over two thousand different plant remedies, three-quarters of which were new to the European colonists, since they came from species native to the Americas.[72] This was, at the time, a very unconventional approach to medicine. While both colonists and Native Americans knew about herbalism, "regular" physicians largely employed strong medicines such as alkaloids (for example, morphine) and minerals (like mercury, antimony, and tartaric acid). Bloodletting was still in vogue and embodied the general driving philosophy of technological medicine at the time. Illness was thought to be an expression of overactivity, of excess "heat," and therefore draining off some of that vitality (in the form of blood) was the solution. In the archetypal example of the fever, this approach seemed to work (though now we know that bloodletting simply weakened patients to the point where they were unable to mount a fever, without actually "curing" them at all).

In contrast to this idea that the vital reaction needed to be suppressed,[73] the Eclectics presented a vision much closer to that of Chinese medicine and Selye's stress response model. The physiology, they believed, is generally pretty good at resisting disruptive influences, whether splinters in the skin (pushed out by a strong inflammatory reaction) or ingested pathogens (eliminated, for instance, by coughing or vomiting). "But," wrote John Scudder, an Eclectic physician who worked in Cincinnati at the end of the nineteenth century, "if this resisting power be weakened, locally or generally, or if the exciting cause be too strong for it, then the cause acts, and disease begins."[74] Thus, it may be as important to strengthen Scudder's "resisting power" as it is to treat the disease directly. Going back to the example above, our approach changes if we see fever as part of the body's resistive response to a stressor like the influenza virus. In many cases, that response will lead to a successful elimination of the virus (in which case nothing needs to be done). Factors such as enhanced virulence or bacterial coinfections might alter the progression of disease and need to be addressed. But weakened resistance has an influence, too. This is painfully obvious in the immunocompromised patient, but may also be present in you and me if other sources of stress are taxing our limited capacity for an adaptive, resistive response.

Interestingly, the Eclectics noticed that, after prolonged debility or in hypersensitive cases, the body would increase secretions and inflammatory symptoms in tissue, and especially in the mucous membranes of the nose, throat, eyes, and lungs. This may be something like what we experience when we're very tired, when our eyes begin to feel as if they were burning and they tear up in response to the irritation. This certainly is a fair description of an allergic reaction, such as hay fever or the chemical sensitivities that may accompany chronic fatigue. Tonics were still considered the remedies of choice. Jones and Scudder say, almost with surprise, that "very peculiar, and apparently very dissimilar effects upon the secretory organs and tissues follow from the use of tonics, under different pathological conditions."[75] Meaning that, sometimes, chronic disease leads to a dysfunction in immunity that causes an ongoing, hot, hypersensitive, and hypersecretory condition, and tonics can bring this situation back into balance, too—seemingly decreasing activity instead of stimulating it. Sounds as if they were describing tonics' ability to regulate the Th1/Th2 balance of the adaptive immune system one hundred years before this balance was even identified.

The Eclectic view is, in the end, almost identical to Selye's and Brekhman's: we are great at adapting to change, it's what we're built to do, but there is a finite "pool" we can draw from to adapt. Once we drain that pool (either slowly over time, as with insomnia, or quickly, as with infection), collapse ensues. Tonic plants are used not to treat disease directly, but rather to raise the threshold of exhaustion—to improve adaptability, to enhance vitality, "to act directly upon the vital force of the entire system" as Scudder puts it.[76] Here, thus, we have a type of plant that was seen to act on every level of the physiology, to increase resistance to infectious threat, bolster resilience in the face of inflammation, and push back the fatigue and hypersensitivity that come from repeated stress. The traditional record is talking about modulating immunity and epigenetics, and identifies the plants that impact these areas as tonics. Once we account for aromatic nervines and bitters, it would seem that practitioners of botanical medicine figured out how to keep human immune function balanced and effective, and how to help human cells flow along their rivers of genetic expression with grace.

So we have the Chinese tonics, from ginseng, to *Astragalus,* to the medicinal mushrooms: sweet, nourishing, rich in polysaccharides and saponins that both stimulate innate immunity (nonspecific resistance) and balance acquired immunity (helping to coordinate resolution of inflammation). When we revisit their pharmacology, we will see that there is even more these plants can do to raise Selye's threshold of exhaustion. We have traditional European tonics, such as berries and other flavonoid-rich plants like nettle or goldenrod that tone tissue, strengthen the heart and blood vessels, and improve resilience in the face of inflammation. As we will see, the action of these plants extends to the immune system, too. But, crucially, we find a common thread through the traditional record: to truly achieve health, which is defined as being strong, vibrant, engaged, and resilient, we need to think about medicine that builds adaptability just as much as, if not more than, medicine that fights back against challenges. The latter strategy is being perfected by technological medicine. But the former has long been practiced by traditional herbal medicine. It relies on wild, tonic plants—because our physiology, at the level of the tissue, immune function, cellular function, and genetic expression, needs these botanicals as part of its xenobiome.

Our body has a complex cocktail of hormones that balance its internal functions. So, too, the ecology (of which we are a part) has chemical signals it uses to coordinate the function of its component organs. The flavonoids, phenolics, polysaccharides, and saponins found in tonic herbs may be tangible examples of such chemical signals, and evidence of the strong degree of coupling between plants and people. What is amazing to me is that you can actually see overlap between these two spheres, between the microcosm of human hormonal activity and the macrocosm of interspecies ecological signaling. The processes interlock. And it is here that I want to begin our discussion of the pharmacology of herbal tonics.

THE PHARMACOLOGICAL APPROACH

In the short term (meaning a matter of seconds and minutes), adrenaline (a.k.a. epinephrine) rules the stress response. It speeds the heart, opens the lungs, and gives us a rush of alertness to help us cope with the events at hand. Coming quickly on its heels is the hormone cortisol, secreted by the adrenal glands in response to cues from the brain (specifically from the limbic system and hypothalamus, areas we've encountered before). Both hormones are important, but while adrenaline is short-acting, focused, and extremely powerful, cortisol takes time, has more widespread effects, and isn't quite as dramatic. This is partly because it must enter the nucleus of the cell and interact with the molecules and enzymes that surround DNA in order to exert its effect, and this takes time. Cortisol's action centers on reducing inflammation, mobilizing blood sugar, and countering fatigue—the classic actions of a steroid, which is precisely what cortisol is. It has such dramatic effects that, when Edward Kendall isolated it from adrenal tissue in the late 1940s, it was hailed as a "miracle drug" that might eliminate chronic inflammatory diseases like rheumatoid arthritis.[77] Since then we have realized that this miracle is more problematic than we first thought,[78] but it is still a vitally important part of the adaptive stress response. For example, I couldn't run more than a mile or two without the cortisol my adrenal glands secrete: my ankles, knees, and hips would be in too much pain. This important hormone pushes back against both short- and long-term inflammation.

As you will recall, Selye's model of chronic stress exposure includes an eventual exhaustive phase. We likened the body's adaptive capacity to a "pool." Drain it, and collapse follows. That collapse is characterized both by an inability to tolerate further stress and by crippling fatigue and inflammation. You see it during endurance training. The human body can withstand remarkable abuse, but its resistance has to be built up slowly or exhaustion is inevitable. You see it in people who experience demanding workloads for long periods: even the strongest eventually succumb to chronic lack of sleep and repeated, daily stress. The pattern is always the same. During periods of overwork and elevated stress, human cortisol response is high, and more of the hormone circulates throughout the bloodstream.[79] This is also true in acute infection.[80] But in situations that bear the hallmarks of repeated, chronic stress and eventual exhaustion, cortisol levels are much lower than normal. We see this in post-traumatic stress disorder, chronic fatigue syndrome, and childhood stress (children often reach the point of depletion more quickly than adults do).[81]

In a fascinating piece of research coming out of Germany in 2002, Angelika Buske-Kirschbaum and her team explored the relationship between cortisol levels and chronic inflammatory hypersensitivity, specifically eczema-like skin inflammation.[82] The researchers discovered that patients with eczema had lower levels of cortisol, and that, perhaps to compensate, they secreted more adrenaline. This might be a useful strategy for managing an acute stressor, but long term it simply seems to lead right where we might expect: to less of an ability to handle inflammation and greater hypersensitivity. As the Eclectics and Selye predicted, we can quite literally deplete our "pool" of vital adaptive energy. Chronic, severe stress is linked to lower cortisol levels, and chronic hyperreactive inflammation inevitably follows.

What happens to cortisol once it leaves the adrenal glands? Unlike adrenaline, which is mostly gone in three or four minutes, it can take over two hours for cortisol levels to drop after a stressful stimulus.[83] Its levels are regulated, as is so much else in the human body, by a pair of enzymes that exert opposite effects: one inactivates cortisol by converting it into cortisone; the other reverses the reaction, changing cortisone back into active form.[84] As cortisol levels rise, the first enzyme kicks into gear in response—and hormone levels come back into line.

If there is a balance point in the human physiology somewhere, we should by now expect that plants have a role in that balance. It turns out that the metabolism of cortisol, a crucial stress hormone the levels of which drop in the exhaustive phase of the stress response, is quite sensitive to the chemistry of tonic plants, in particular to saponins. These molecules, a combination of a hydrocarbon "body" and a sugar "tail," have a soaplike effect: that is how they got their name. The body mixes well with fats and oils while the tail dissolves well in water. Plants like soapwort have been used for just this purpose—as gentle detergents, shampoos, and soaps.[85] Many saponins, like those in elecampane, are somewhat irritating when consumed (you try eating soap and tell me what you make of it) and can be used, in high doses, to induce vomiting or, more often, expectoration. Once in the digestive tract, saponins from plants like fenugreek and yucca have a well-documented ability to bind to and facilitate the elimination of cholesterol.[86]

It's important to recognize that the "body" of the saponin, which is most likely separated from the "tail" by intestinal microbes,[87] is absorbed into the bloodstream and has some interesting effects on cortisol metabolism. This mechanism may contribute to the activity of such saponin-rich tonics as ginseng, licorice, *Bupleurum,* alfalfa, and horse chestnut. In short, the leftover "body" of the saponin is absorbed from the small intestine and enters the bloodstream, where it first encounters the liver. Here, it either passes through or is combined with other molecules that increase its water solubility. It eventually leaves our system through the liver or through the kidneys. In both of these tissues, it encounters the enzymes that metabolize cortisol.[88]

This is the crux of the pharmacological activity of saponins as it relates to the hormone cortisol. The case of glycyrrhizin, the saponin found in licorice root, has been very well documented (and this molecule may have potential adverse effects, so approach licorice with caution, especially in cases of high blood pressure).[89] Its metabolic byproducts interact with the enzymes that change cortisol into its inactive form, inhibiting the breakdown of this important stress hormone.[90] So, in this illustrative case, we find that saponins, when ingested and altered by the gut and liver, can have effects that prolong the activity of cortisol. In the exhaustive phase of the stress response, they may therefore help reduce inflammation, fatigue, and depression. They potentiate the effects of our natural stress hormone, improving our ability to handle disruptive influences and sparing the adrenal glands, whose "pool" of stress hormones may be deficient already, from having to make more. No wonder tonics, including licorice, are traditionally used to address inflammation and fatigue.[91]

Saponins have other very interesting effects, mostly centered on the activation of innate immunity and the modulation of Th1/Th2 balance. Because of their soaplike quality, they create complexes with cholesterol (which is very fatlike) and also with the membranes of cells they encounter. They insert themselves into the membranes, leaving their sugar "tails" sticking out, and thereby start to look a lot like the surface markers of bacteria or viruses—a perfect stimulus for both the innate immune system and also the T cells that coordinate the acquired immune response.[92]

They make such a good stimulus that drug makers employ cocktails of plant saponins, cholesterol, and pieces of cell membrane to act as "adjuvants" to vaccines.[93] An adjuvant is a substance that wakes up the immune system so it can mount a strong reaction to the antigens present in the vaccine and thereby effectively train its adaptive arm to remember what it encountered. Researchers get pretty fancy in their adjuvant cocktails: depending on the types and ratios of saponins employed, you can shift the adaptive response toward a Th1 or a Th2 pattern.[94] In plants, you never find a single type of saponin; it's always a mixture. Ginseng, for instance, is thought to contain over twenty-five different saponins.[95] They certainly modulate cortisol metabolism, either raising or lowering hormone levels, depending on the context, but they also have both stimulating and suppressive effects on T cell function, depending on the saponin examined.[96]

In the end, it seems that saponins have the ability to speak to our immune system and, depending in part on the details of their structures and the context in which they are applied, either to increase or to decrease immune activity. They are always present in plants as cocktails—so in a weakened state, enhancement of function ensues, while in an overactive state, inflammatory responses are quieted. The pharmacology of saponins goes a long way toward explaining the rebalancing effects of tonic herbs.

But the story does not end here. Polysaccharides, which are long chains of sugars, are found in a variety of plant and mushroom species. With a few exceptions, such as celandine, *Arnica,* and perhaps juniper, all the species are traditionally considered tonics, especially in traditional Chinese medicine.* These species are plants such as *Astragalus,* ginseng, licorice, and *Bupleurum* that we have encountered before, but also tonics such as heal-all (*Prunella*), fenugreek, larch, oats, and *Perilla.* These species are mushrooms we have met already, such as reishi, shiitake, maitake, and turkey tails (*Trametes*). All in all, more than fifty-five well-characterized tonic species have rich quantities of these sugar chains, and all of them are recognized by the same receptors that white blood cells use to detect bacteria and viruses.[97] Polysaccharides form complexes with fat and cholesterol, much as saponins do, and in similar fashion serve to "prime" innate immune function, improving resistance to infection even in delicate situations—following surgery, stress-induced exhaustion, and the compromised immunity of advanced cancer.[98]

Polysaccharides go further. They help the physiology handle cancer directly by increasing immune surveillance, helping to detect and destroy malignancy before it grows out of control.[99] A patented polysaccharide formulation obtained from *Trametes versicolor* is known as Krestin in Japan,[100] where for more than thirty years it has been routinely prescribed in cancer therapy to strengthen immunity. It helps the patient withstand chemotherapeutic drugs while also having anticancer effects. Positive results are documented in the treatment of gastric, colon, breast, and lung cancer.[101] And while this preparation is usually administered by injection at cancer treatment centers, there is evidence that polysaccharides are active orally: they interface with the

---

*See Zhu's *Chinese Materia Medica,* pages 547–651, which covers the tonics.

immune system at sites along the digestive tract.[102] To this day I wonder why, given its track record, Krestin is not used in the United States for cancer and its associated complications.

Researchers are beginning to speculate as to why polysaccharides from plants and mushrooms have similar immune-activating effects as those on the surfaces of bacteria and viruses (without, of course, causing disease symptoms). It is becoming increasingly clear that these molecules are part of a very ancient signaling mechanism between single-celled organisms (such as pathogens) and multicellular organisms. Tonic plants have conserved similar elements found in very old common ancestors, and when we ingest them, their chemistry interfaces with our innate immune system, ensuring optimal function. Reviewing the research on the immune activity of these compounds across the animal, vegetable, and fungal kingdoms, Igor Schepetkin and Mark Quinn (biologists at Montana State University) remarked that "a common, evolutionarily conserved polysaccharide structural backbone may be shared between these diverse groups of organisms,"[103] and as a result multicellular beings capable of exploiting these signals from the plant and mushroom world always fared better in an ecology teeming with virulent bugs.

So we see a clear echo in the pharmacological exploration of tonic plants: saponins, their aglycones, and polysaccharides may account for a large portion of the immune-modulating activity traditionally assigned to these herbs. We have already seen how they can blunt overactive immune reactions, perhaps by balancing the Th1/Th2 response or potentiating the activity of cortisol, in diseases such as asthma, allergies, and rheumatoid arthritis. We've just examined the mechanisms behind their ability to address deficient immunity. Through hormone metabolism, innate immune activation, and the enhanced activity of white blood cells, tonic plants make a strong case for being an essential part of our xenobiome. Without them, we might expect to see a quicker progression to fatigue when under stress; a tendency to develop frequent, lingering infections; increased autoimmune reactions; and more cases of cancer. Look around. Chances are you know someone who is suffering from one or more of these complaints.

Again, we are finding that a plant deficiency in our xenobiome might be partially responsible for the unique illness patterns of the Western world. While a lack of bitters is linked to increased rates of diabetes, obesity, and digestive problems, a lack of tonics is linked to reduced vitality and tolerance of stress, disrupted immune function, and cancer. For instance, asthma rates in the United States have risen from about 3 percent of the population in 1980 to more than 7 percent in 2004.[104] Reidentifying the vitality- and resistance-enhancing qualities of tonics, so well known to the Chinese and the Eclectics, can point us toward viable solutions.

Enhancing immunity is important, but (as we saw in the physiology of cortisol) we have to remember that immunity and inflammation are linked. One requires the other, and a strong reaction to a stressor usually involves what herbalists call a "hot" response. During a *Staph* infection, this may be acceptable: the inflammation contributes to eventual resolution, and all returns to normal. But repeated stressors of a different kind, particularly noninfectious ones, can lead to the same type of "heat" without the same purpose, without closure. Our physiology has exquisitely sensitive mechanisms in place to help us handle both infectious and noninfectious disruptions. By increasing their resistance and longevity, cells can better weather the inflammatory storm. These are specific epigenetic mechanisms, as we have seen, controlled in large part by sirtuins. You will recall how this family of proteins is involved in the removal of acetyl groups from histones. They "close up" the stacks in the library of DNA, both protecting it from damage and regulating the expression of key genes involved in cellular growth, division, and inflammation. Polyphenolic chemicals found in tonic plants, especially the traditional European tonics, such as hawthorn, reliably stimulate sirtuin activity.[105]

Sirtuins exist at one of the hubs of the network of enzymes and transcription factors involved in epigenetics. This means that, if we can find a way to influence sirtuin activity, we can have widespread effects across the genome: we will be interfacing with a well-connected node in the system. Since polyphenols, and especially bioflavonoids, can do this, we might expect that these plant molecules would also have widespread effects across the genome. They can act as guides for the flow of genetic expression in the crucial "final mile" of the river, helping us to pick channels of greater longevity and resilience. Let's see how this might work.

Two transcription factors, activated by sirtuins and by the polyphenolic chemicals found in tonic plants, play a vital role in how a cell handles inflammation and how it resists challenge.[106] One, known as a forkhead protein, induces epigenetic changes that lead to increased life span, more efficient metabolism, and resistance to stressors.[107] Sirtuins activate this protein. The other, known as nuclear-factor-kappa-B (NF-κB for short), is responsible for turning on the genes needed for production of inflammatory compounds. In short, without NF-κB, cells and tissue simply can't get as inflamed in response to stress.[108] Sirtuins deactivate this protein. The net result of these actions, along with many others that sirtuins initiate in our cells, is prolonged life span, greater efficiency, fewer free radicals, less inflammation, and greater resistance. This is exactly what we see when organisms consume bioflavonoids and other polyphenols from tonic plants.[109] Their activity on sirtuins provides part of the explanation.

But what about cancer? If tonic plants and their flavonoids protect cells and increase their life span, we might wonder whether this could be detrimental in fighting tumors. Research shows that the converse is true: flavonoids inhibit cancer growth and lead tumor cells to commit suicide.[110] How is it possible that these plants and the chemicals they contain have opposite effects on healthy cells and cancer cells? The answer to this question frames the strengths of tonic plants very clearly: as we have seen over and over again, they help find a place of balance. Their effects depend on the context. And, in the end, through the modulation of epigenetics and immune function, they help bring the most basic processes of life to their most positive, healthful expression.

So while activating sirtuins is a big part of how flavonoids protect cells, their activity is not limited to this sphere. Take this example as a case in point. By stimulating sirtuins, tonics activate forkhead proteins, which, in turn, shut off self-destruct switches like the p53 enzyme system.[111] Conversely, part of what the self-destruct switches like p53 do is to inhibit sirtuins, reducing the ability of the cell to survive. You can see that we have a feedback system consisting of opposing, countervailing forces, a clear place of physiological balance deep in the most basic life processes of each and every cell. Sound familiar? Whenever we've run into such a balance point, tonic plants are there, too. This example is no exception. While flavonoids activate sirtuins, they also activate p53 and other self-destruct, anticancer genetic switches.[112] It is as if tonic plants are hedging their bets: by getting involved on both sides of a physiological balance, they can positively impact the system regardless of its state.

In a way this is similar to the progression of all chemical reactions. An overabundance on one side of the balance point makes it easier to transition to the other side. If a healthy cell is under threat from inflammation and is expressing more and more genes that will eventually lead it to self-destruct, the anti-inflammatory, prosurvival effects of flavonoids become much more pronounced. Alternatively, if a cancer cell is expressing more and more genes relating to growth and division, the effects of flavonoids on self-destruct switches will predominate. The tonics seem to say, "Well, if I can't attack this problem head-on, maybe I can stimulate the countervailing force and bring the situation back into balance." This is seen in heart disease, autoimmune disease and allergy, inflammation, dementia, and cancer—all areas where flavonoids and the tonic plants that contain them have positive impacts.[113] It is just as the Eclectics had hoped. It is also a physical embodiment of a very, very ancient concept: that at the moment of greatest darkness (or of greatest light), the seed of the opposite begins to sprout with vigor. At the winter solstice, when nights are cold and deep, the days start to get longer again. When a cell is threatened or compromised, the seeds of balance are already sown—but only if that cell is connected to nature, to its environment, to its xenobiome. If that is the case, it will experience what the Chinese recorded in the *Book of Changes:* "thunder within the earth: the image of the turning point"[114]—A journey back to balance.

WHY TONICS?

The modern world has its faults, certainly, but it has provided us with some amazing tools and technologies. This is clearly evident in the dramatic cures for infection and acute trauma achieved by medical science. The drugs and procedures used to combat these age-old scourges, which in the past decimated huge numbers of us, are remarkably, almost miraculously, effective. At the same time, however, we are struggling with new sources of morbidity and mortality. No longer is infection the leading cause of disease and death: now we have chronic inflammation, hypersensitivity, cancer, and heart disease staring us down in our later years. Tonic plants, with their complex cocktails of saponins, polysaccharides, and polyphenols, seem to offer a potential solution through their ability to modulate immune function and genetic expression.

I have returned to the word *modulate* throughout our exploration of tonic herbs for good reason. If we are to address the new diseases of the modern world, we will need to approach them with a slightly different mind-set. They don't respond well to the strong, direct treatments used for acute conditions. The lesson learned from flavonoids and their effects on cancerous cells as opposed to healthy ones should be applied to the prevention and treatment of chronic disease. Sometimes it's easier to balance a seesaw by standing close to the fulcrum and making small adjustments on both sides, rather than by jumping from one end to the other, throwing your weight around and attempting to control the inevitable repercussions.

Tonics come to us, unadulterated, from the ecosystem. They seem to be a necessary part of our xenobiome at very deep levels. They are used in conditions of weakness, deficient energy and immunity, dementia and exhaustion as much as conditions of cancer, inflammatory heart disease, allergies, and asthma. But they are much, much milder than technological drugs. Though they can lengthen the life span of healthy cells by "turning on" survival genes, they will never be able to increase cancer cell survival because the cancer cell has taken care of activating all those genetic switches already. Flavonoids are too gentle in their action to add to this effect.

Tonics are also complex medicines well suited to interacting with our complex physiology. It's impossible to overwhelm a chanting crowd by screaming your message by yourself, but get some friends to whisper an interesting thought to their neighbors, and the idea might spread, like a virus, from person to person until the chant changes. In the face of altered diets, increased stress, novel chemicals, and a much faster pace of life (as well as a longer life span), we would be foolish to think that a single drug targeting a single receptor site might be able to reverse the years of cultural and ecological effects on an individual human being. Medicine is beginning to realize this. Physicians are trying cocktails, "polypills," for cardiovascular disease in hopes that intervention at multiple levels might be more effective.[115] I would respectfully argue that nature has been handing us much more complex and multilayered polypills all along: they are the herbal tonics. Their effectiveness against the modern, chronic diseases is beyond dispute, especially when treatment is started early on. It is even possible that the chronic diseases exist, or are more widespread than they should be, because of an absence of these vital plants.

Dian Cecht was a miraculous healer. The silver hand he fashioned for his king, Nuada, was a technological marvel. It allowed the king to grasp his sword, to return to the fight, to wield his strength for the good of his people. But it did not make him whole again, and Brigid, the goddess-queen, could not let a man unwhole lead the people. Technology might make us work, but it can never make us well—it is impossible to be fully well, engaged, and alive through its gifts alone. True strength can only come from nature and our connection to the wild world that shaped our genes, our chemistry, our entire selves. Our technologies are certainly an expression of nature, but they cannot completely replace Henry David Thoreau's "tonic of wildness." We simply cannot remain whole that way.

Airmid and Miach, using deep, long-lost magic, made Nuada whole again. They did not try to replace the king's hand; rather, they reunited the king with what was missing. Their magic was mysterious, and its explanation beyond our ken. It also, as Airmid discovered, could not be crushed by skepticism, arrogance, or jealousy. The old magic simply transmuted, filling the healing herbs with its power. She recognized this right away, collected the plants, and kept their secrets safe.

Using medicine is like planting a seed. Both, to some degree, involve trust. We can try to control certain elements—enhancing the quality of the soil, timing the sowing in accordance with the season, even watching the weather for the most opportune moment. But, in the end, we must do just as did Airmid: sit, wait, watch, and hope. However, we have an advantage compared to the goddess of the healing plants. She has already paved the way, she has gathered the herbs and passed their knowledge on through generations. She remembers. If we can reawaken that memory, we can start to use tonics again for the ills that make our lives unwell. We can nourish people, as we would a garden. We can tend the growing seedlings, as did Airmid. Collecting them, we can use the plants as tonic medicine, yield, sing, and watch the resonance.

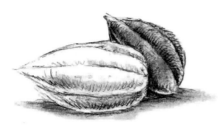

CHOCOLATE

THEOBROMA CACAO

The jungles of Central America and Mexico are a tangle of vines and hardwood canopy trees crisscrossed by a network of narrow trails. Warthogs and other foragers travel across this landscape and are stalked by the chief predator of this ecosystem—the jaguar. This mysterious nocturnal feline was always a totem animal for the cultures that inhabited these sacred lands. From these forests and hills radiates a power that ripples across the entire hemisphere, traveling down the *cordillera* of the Andes and up through the Southwest United States. This power still resonates from sites such as Palenque, perched on verdant hills where the jungle slopes rise up from the drier plains of the Yucatán Peninsula. Here, seated on a throne fashioned to resemble a two-headed jaguar, the lords of the Maya handed out justice, sacrificed the warrior-champions of enemy cities, and drank prodigious quantities of a magical, nourishing, enlivening liquid known as *kakaw,* cacao, chocolate.

The drink was, and still is, extremely nourishing in large part because of its substantial protein content. This is also why, when shaken or vigorously stirred, it forms an airy foam that is velvety and luxurious to consume (chocolate mousse is perhaps the epitome of this in modern times). To the Maya; their ancestors, the mysterious Olmec; and the Aztecs, who ruled the same lands following the demise of the Mayan culture, this foamy airiness was highly sought after. They employed elaborate rituals to prepare it for the royal family for whom the beverage was reserved. The basic trick consisted of pouring chocolate-infused water from great heights, sometimes over fifteen feet, into small cylindrical vessels over and over again. Servants, usually women, were employed for the express purpose of properly frothing the ruler's cacao. Spices and other special herbs were added to the preparation—and the result was complex, thick, foamy, and no doubt quite bitter. For even though it is one of the world's most excellent tonics, it is deeply bitter when unsweetened. This flavor transitions into an intoxicating and complex mixture of sour, floral, and uniquely *chocolate* notes. There truly is nothing like it. Its pharmacological effects warrant the blissful feeling with which it leaves you.

HARVESTING CHOCOLATE

Cacao pods appear in the jungle like ghosts, often creamy-white, about the size of small footballs, hanging directly off the trunk of their trees. They begin as greenish fruits, then mature into white, through yellow and orange, and finally to a reddish purple color so reminiscent of the final chocolate itself. But it is not this pod that produces the delicacy; rather, the seeds (known as "beans," as with coffee) are what hold the magic. At first, when the ripe pod is broken open, the beans are wrapped up in a whitish pulp. But after being fermented for a few days en masse, then laid out to dry, and finally carefully roasted at low temperatures, they achieve the complexity that is characteristic of the final product. In tropical environments, numerous species and varieties of cacao are grown on plantations. Low-end, commercial preparations are fermented and processed quickly, with little attention to detail. But the highest-quality beans are hand selected, carefully separated from their pulp, and freed of their papery skins without a single one being damaged. The result is more intense and complexly layered than the finest red wine—and may be a whole lot better for you, too. It is well worth the price.

You can often find cacao "nibs" at specialty and natural foods stores. These are broken-up pieces of the processed beans, rich in chocolate flavor but also creamy because of their high fat content. Cocoa butter, as cacao's fat is known, is semisolid at room temperature due to its high saturated fat content. Although this type of fat has received a lot of negative press over the past fifty years, cocoa butter is actually a very healthful product. It contains a high degree of antioxidants that prevent it from ever becoming rancid and contribute to the overall health benefits of chocolate. When you eat the nibs (or other low-sugar cacao preparations, such as 80 percent dark chocolate), you are partaking of a protein- and fat-rich food that is actually extremely healthful, provides nutrition essential for cellular function and repair, and tastes great. I grew up in a world where chocolate was maligned and called the "devil's food." This may, in part, be due to the intense pleasure derived from consuming it (hardly a reason for negative marks in my book). Rest assured that, when eaten close to its natural state, cacao has no demonic qualities. We might want to call it the "jaguar's food" instead. It is powerful, mysterious, nocturnal, and beautiful.

USING CHOCOLATE

The chemistry of the fermented and roasted chocolate bean is extremely complex. Right up front, its alkaloids set it apart from any of the other plants we've explored. Alkaloids are tremendously powerful molecules. From caffeine to morphine, humans have known about them for over three hundred years and have pursued their extraction with great zeal, as they have potent physiological effects. Cacao's chief alkaloids (technically, proto-alkaloids of the methylxanthine variety, closely related to caffeine) are called theobromine and theophylline—literally, "drink of the gods" and "love of the gods," respectively. Certainly not demonic. These molecules are not nearly as stimulating as those found in coffee or even black tea, yet they still have effects on the brain: a mild euphoria, a relaxed focus, an easier breath. In fact, theophylline in concentrated form is still used as a drug for asthma because it helps relax and open the airways. My favorite way to experience these alkaloids is by drinking large quantities of traditionally prepared cacao after a couple of days' fast. Because their effects are subtle, I feel them most strongly when I give my mind and body a chance to rest from the daily routine and stimulus that usually surrounds me. Taken this way, on a very empty stomach, cacao is one of the most pleasant intoxicants I have experienced. Its stimulating quality is offset by a relaxation and joy that is difficult to describe, but it suffuses me with deep and full contentment. It nourishes the belly, dispelling hunger and bringing satisfaction. Focus is clear, understanding is quick, and creativity is enhanced. It is no wonder the Mayan rulers favored it so.

But the intoxicating alkaloids are not the most powerful of cacao's chemicals. What intrigues me the most are its bioflavonoids. They are similar in structure to those found in green tea, though more diverse and present in abundant quantities. As we saw in our general exploration of tonic plants, these molecules have numerous health benefits, according to the modern research record. First, the flavonoids may have central nervous system effects, counterbalancing the alkaloids' stimulating quality with a gentle relaxing power. They also affect the cardiovascular system, where they can lower blood pressure, dilate blood vessels, and protect the heart. Coupled with cocoa butter, the flavonoids may lower elevated cholesterol, too (another example of whole-plant synergy in action). Put this all together and you have powerful medicine for the heart. Beyond this, there are the epigenetic effects that contribute to their anti-inflammatory, cancer-protective properties. All this seems pretty miraculous, but there is one catch: unlike pharmaceutical agents, cacao's chemistry needs to be experienced daily for a fairly long period to derive any benefits. I know, it's torture.

Cacao is easy to prepare and, if you begin with a high-quality powder, it's a highly nutritious, medicinal tonic unequaled in the world. The ritual of preparation, which can be simple or as elaborate as a Japanese tea ceremony, provides a focal point in the day that is subtly mind-altering and enlivening. It can be customized to suit individual tastes, timing, and preference (some love chocolate as a warm morning beverage). Its power flows from the jungles of the Western Hemisphere, from jaguar-guarded forests rich in dark, deep magic, into our hearts, through our bloodstream, and finally down into the hidden recesses of every cell. It is a gift with a joyful, euphoric touch. The Maya's tree of life, growing out of the richest hidden soils, was a cacao tree.

Mayan-style Cacao (Hot Chocolate)

1–2 teaspoons whole, raw cacao powder

A few spoonfuls milk, soy milk, or another liquid of your choice (including water)

1 teaspoon honey (optional)

1 tiny pinch cayenne or ginger powder, or a little vanilla or orange extract

The easiest and best way to get your chocolate fix daily is similar to the Mayan preparation. When you make it this way, you can also add other herbs and spices to suit your mood and tastes for the day. All in all, since there are so many excellent cacao products available today, the whole process is fairly easy and similar to brewing a cup of espresso.

Start with whole, raw cacao powder. This is crucial for a couple of reasons. Since we won't be growing or harvesting this medicine ourselves (unless you're lucky enough to be living on a Belizean plantation), choosing raw, organic cacao ensures that you have a potent variety that has been processed with care and attention and was not burned during roasting. Additionally, organic cacao is usually fairly traded, an important consideration when consuming a plant that has been linked to farmer exploitation and environmental degradation due to its global popularity. Finally, raw cacao contains all the fat of the original bean (unlike many standard cocoa powders). This helps to preserve the powder and also adds substantially to its nutritional value.

Take between one and two tablespoons of the powder and mix it with a few spoonfuls of milk, soy milk, or another liquid of your choice (including water). This helps to smooth out the powder a little, and makes the next steps a bit easier. Since cacao is so bitter, I like to add a teaspoon of honey, though this is not necessary.

Finally, put in a tiny pinch of cayenne, or ginger powder, or a little vanilla or orange extract. Pour hot water just off the boil over this mixture, stirring with a whisk or fork. If you're feeling inspired, you can make this cacao in the blender and add fruits like blueberries or strawberries for a special treat.

I usually have two mugs ready and will approximate the Mayan ritual by pouring the hot chocolate from one to the other. This has the effect of both cooling it down a bit and increasing its velvety frothiness. My favorite time for this drink is late afternoon, in the summer sun or after a snowy winter's walk.

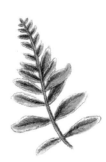

ASTRAGALUS

ASTRAGALUS MEMBRANACEUS

It may have been over five thousand years ago, in Central China where the Yellow River courses through rough and mountainous countryside before dropping into fertile lowlands, that the mythical Huang Di discussed matters of medicine with Shen Nong, the so-called divine plowman. Such accounts are largely mythological, and the timing is impossible to confirm; nevertheless, their work may have provided the spiritual basis for Chinese medicine in its most classical incarnation. Shen Nong, who was said to visibly radiate the qualities of the medicinal plants he consumed, cataloged hundreds of herbs while Huang Di, the yellow emperor, cemented the cultural and political foundations of the Middle Kingdom. Yet over two thousand years were to pass before the first compendium of plant medicine recounting Shen Nong's wisdom was to appear: *The Divine Plowman's Classic on Herbs,* as the text is known, details the effects and preparation techniques for some of the most important botanicals (most of which are still in use today).

Among these, the yellow leader, huang qi, also known as *Astragalus membranaceus,* stands out as a premier tonic. It is said to enliven the earth energy of human beings, while also helping to fortify the protective shield, which, like a sword, repels invaders attempting to assail our bodies. The herb is the root of a legume, cousin to the common field vetch so often found in farms across the world, rich and sweet and yellow and fragrant. I can imagine the two masters, walking in the wild countryside, examining and tasting the wild vetches and happening upon this particularly upright, bushy, and vigorous species with the cream-colored flowers. Shen Nong, the elder, was probably the first to try its root. Pulling it apart, he watched it peel like the membranes and fascia of our own tissue, and thought it might strengthen the vital force and resistance of those who consumed it. How right he was, and what a gift this plant has turned out to be for us all.

GROWING, HARVESTING, AND STORING *ASTRAGALUS*

The seeds of *Astragalus* are like small, black lentils. They are found in a small peapod, which, as the seed matures, inflates with pressurized air. This was quite a surprise to me the first time I saw it. When the seed is fully ready, it begins to rattle around in this fat, squishy pod, making a very pleasant sound. This may be the origin of the name *astragalus*: this Greek word refers to the small, cube-shaped ankle bones of animals, used in Hippocrates's time as dice. When thrown, they rattle across wooden floors and make a sound similar to the one made by this herb when, in October, all the seeds shake in the first cold autumn winds.

You can plant the seed, two or three per cell, in an early spring greenhouse and expect fairly consistent and vigorous germination. Thin the seedlings out so that there is a single one per cell and, once they are hardened off, plant them into deeply dug garden soil in full sun. It is best if the soil is not too heavy with a lot of clay, though *Astragalus* will handle a broad range of growing conditions. Just avoid excess moisture, as that may rot the precious roots. Then sit back and be prepared to watch the plant grow for at least four or five years, though ten-year-old roots are fantastic, strong medicine. Every fall, collect the rattling seedpods and plant more, if you'd like. In the fall of the fifth year's growth, loosen the soil around the crown, cut the stalks with a heavy-duty clipper (the crown will have expanded and sent up numerous shoots over the seasons), and pull up the long, branching, twining yellow root. Use clippers to cut off a small piece right away, clean it off, and taste it when it's fresh. Its full, soft, and sweet flavor is as nourishing to us humans as the fertile alluvial soils around the Yellow River are to plants.

The harvested roots are extremely difficult to slice in cross section, being very fibrous. So, traditionally, *Astragalus* was sliced lengthwise into long "tongue depressor" strips with a creamy white interior surrounded by a thin layer of rough brown root bark. This process also facilitates drying, which is important because the roots lack any antiseptic power and will quickly turn sour and get moldy if they are not processed with speed. The long slices are placed in the sun or in a hot, well-ventilated greenhouse and turned over periodically over the course of two or three days until they are bone-dry. Then they can be stored in tall mason jars for future use. Nowadays, you can find *Astragalus* in this form but also cut and sifted into small shards, or even powdered. All these preparations, if relatively fresh (less than a year old) are effective medicine.

USING *ASTRAGALUS*

The science behind *Astragalus* is remarkable. Modern research is validating the uses Shen Nong detailed for this plant. But though studies link it to improved immunity and reduced anemia when it comes to chronic infection, cancer, kidney disease, and more, its true nature is not difficult to discern. It is a nourishing tonic that builds our resistance to all manner of ills, including pathogens as well as chronic weakness. Therefore, recovery from protracted illness or long-term stress is another of its strengths. When appetite is poor, following a fever or a disease like mononucleosis, the root is simmered along with rice or another simple grain to enhance vitality and return strength to the convalescing patient. I have found this preparation, perhaps mixed with just a pinch of ginger powder, to be useful support for those undergoing the difficult courses of chemotherapy associated with cancer treatment.

Those who start taking plants like *Echinacea* in the fall should switch to *Astragalus* instead. It's a much more appropriate immune tonic and much more effective at keeping illness at bay. I find it especially useful for those who interact with the general public—teachers, retail workers, health care providers—and anyone with young children.

While its life-giving power is legendary in conditions of extreme depletion, such as cancer, compromised immunity, or recovery from prolonged infection, we don't have to wait until we are extremely weak to avail ourselves of this plant. In these viral times, when illness courses the globe in a matter of weeks (or even days), everyone would do well to get some *Astagalus* root every day once the summer season reaches its peak and the grain harvest begins.

Whether simmered into soup, stock, or grain, or rolled into tasty sweet treats, this herb directly enhances the life force. Its noble power, evidenced by the creamy-yellow color of the roots and flowers, is humbly hidden away in an unassuming (though very vigorously growing) plant. When cooking it in a big soup pot alongside onions, burdock roots, and garlic, think of Huang Di and Shen Nong in a cottage by the Yellow River, simmering their own pot, and sipping their *Astragalus* brew. The spirit of this plant unites us with those mythical leaders. The spirit of huang qi is a leader itself.

 ### *Astragalus* Broth

> 1 dozen 6-inch slices *Astragalus*
> 1 gallon water

This plant, like all tonics, is basically enhanced food. As such, it is usually cooked and not extracted. In Chinese medicine the "tongue depressors" are placed in cold spring water and then simmered for hours, or even days. More water is added as needed, and eventually a somewhat thick, creamy, and cloudy fluid can be strained out and consumed by the cupful.

For this simple decoction we usually start with a dozen slices, each about six inches long, per gallon of water. You get about two weeks' worth of medicine from this process, and it should be frozen to prevent spoilage as the liquid will only keep for three or four days in the fridge. Needless to say, this can be hard to do, especially if it represents an entire plant that you've tended for five years. So I supplement my garden's harvest with organically grown roots that I purchase. They are relatively cheap and easy to find.

Simple *Astragalus* broth is great, but this herb is most often added to stocks that are simmering on the stovetop anyway. Throw some slices into the cold water you add to your soup bases, or tie up about a cupful of shredded roots per gallon of water in a piece of muslin (for easy removal later) and simmer away. It is a fantastic addition to the soups and stews we make as the weather turns colder. And what perfect timing: one of the major virtues of this plant is to enhance the activity of both the innate and acquired immune systems, and as such it is perhaps the best preventive medicine for winter illness. Best to start consuming it while the leaves are still on the trees, though; it isn't useful once you get sick. But for those who get frequent colds, or whose respiratory tracts seem to be congested and weak all winter, this herb is just the ticket.

Astragalus Nut Treats

> Approximately 1 cup powdered, organic *Astragalus* root
> ¹/₂ cup nut butter
> ¹/₂ cup raw honey
> Shredded coconut (optional)

Some people find that it's difficult to simmer a soup stock, or maybe you don't care for soup. It is fairly easy to make a simple and tasty preparation that appeals to almost everyone, children included. This can be frozen and used as needed.

For this recipe, you will need recently powdered, organic *Astragalus* root (most likely purchased, since it is very difficult to powder the root yourself without appropriate tools). Mix together a half-cup of nut butter, such as peanut butter, almond butter, or even fresh tahini (sesame seed butter) and half a cup of raw honey. Then slowly add about a cup of *Astragalus* powder to the mix. You may need a few more tablespoons of the powder, depending on the consistency of your wet ingredients.

That's it! Roll the doughy mix into balls about an inch in diameter, and dust them with shredded coconut or more *Astragalus* powder. Then eat two or three of these every day to prevent upper respiratory tract infections, strengthen the lungs, and improve overall immunity.

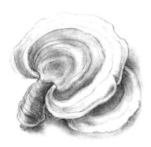

RED REISHI (LINGZHI)

GANODERMA TSUGAE

After crossing over an old rock wall, now half-buried under leaves, and fording a small stream, the path enters a section of the forest that is a little older and, in places, a little darker. There are fewer young hardwoods and more and more Eastern hemlock trees—evergreens with short, dark, flat needles on long branches overhanging the trail. There is less vegetation in the understory or on the forest floor, just a few ferns and the occasional patch of wintergreen or partridgeberry. In a spot up ahead are some small deciduous trees—a striped maple and a couple of very young ashes. They have taken advantage of a clearing in the canopy where an old hemlock died, most of its trunk severed from a craggy stump and lying across the ground.

There a prince of the forest has made his home. Five red fan-shaped polypore mushrooms are growing out of the stump, one almost two feet wide. They fan out on thick stems and all of them seem varnished in a shiny maroon lacquer reminiscent of antique furniture. In this stump dwells an amazing organism, and these visible parts are simply his reproductive organs. He takes up residence from time to time in certain hemlock trees after they become old and die, slowly digesting their wood and participating in the ecological web of the forest. Like the soil, the bugs, the birds, and the trees, we, too, can choose to meet this being that, despite usually only living three to five years, is nevertheless part of a very old lineage of forest dwellers. His skill consists of transmuting decay into life.

This mushroom is known as *reishi* in Japan and *lingzhi* in China. There are tropical species, such as *Ganoderma lucidum,* that prefer harder woods, and a species known as *Ganoderma tsugae* that thrives in our temperate forest and grows on hemlock trees. Regardless, as their name means in Chinese, they have been known as "divine mushrooms" and considered givers of immortality for at least two thousand years.

They are often found abundantly in their preferred places of growth, and herbalists have been harvesting them to extend and improve the lives of the members of their communities long before their specific uses were first recorded. Modern research is fascinated with these fungi: not only are they incredibly safe, they seem to have a profound balancing effect on immunity, stress hormones, heart and brain function, and genetic expression. They are the very definition of a tonic.

HARVESTING AND STORING RED REISHI

While many polypores (nongilled fungi that disseminate their spores from small pores, are nontoxic, and usually grow on trees) have long-lasting fruiting bodies, reishi does not. A few weeks after maturing, the shiny red fans will rot if they are not harvested and dried. So I always recommend harvesting them if you find some and they are mature, fully red and without their yellow-white outer ring. First, obtain a positive ID. Then visually inspect and touch the mushrooms. They should feel solid and strong, and give a satisfying "thump" when hit gently from above to release any remaining spores (and bugs). The undersides, though not boggy, should feel moist and firm. Using a very sharp knife, slice through the stem of the mushroom as close to the tree as possible. Carry the red reishi fan home in a soft basket to avoid excessive bruising.

It is much easier to slice this mushroom when it is fresh, so I usually do so once I get back from the forest. The whole fan may be hung in a warm, well-ventilated space and dried as is, but it will be much more difficult to process that way (though it stores longer when whole). Using a serrated knife, slice the fan into thin strips and string them together with needle and thread, leaving plenty of room between each slice. The chain may be hung anywhere there is good airflow, as the slices dry quickly. Once they fracture easily and there is no more trace of moisture, unstring them and store them in a tightly capped glass jar.

USING RED REISHI

The effects of reishi described in both the traditional and modern record are nothing short of legendary. Not only does it balance the mind, control elevated blood pressure, and aid in liver metabolism, but it also has a strong dual effect on immunity: it stimulates innate immunity, while also modulating the Th1/Th2 balance of the acquired immune system (and toning down the Th2 response, if necessary). The net result: fewer infections and less allergy and inflammation.

So while reishi is working deeply at strengthening and improving our immune system's response overall and perhaps also lengthening our life span, the major short-term effect I notice is that even small doses reduce allergy symptoms almost immediately. This is highly useful for controlling complaints such as hay fever, animal and pollen allergies, and especially chemical sensitivities. Be prepared for a range of side effects, though: more restful sleep, less anxiety and irritability, healthier blood pressure (for those with both high and low numbers), and a mysterious clearing up of rashes and skin issues.

It is very possible that mushrooms, like plants, are an essential part of our xenobiotic cocktails, and send important cues to our immune system without which we develop hypersensitivities and weakness. If this is the case, then the polypores like reishi deserve our special attention. After all, they have been injecting chemistry into the forest ecosystem for millions of years.

Reconnecting with these important medicinal species goes beyond the surprise of finding their beautiful forms, glistening red, in the dark of a deep forest. It gives us a chance to eat something that is neither plant nor animal, endowed with an often amazing intelligence. We can partake of the flesh of literal death-eaters, and in so doing may be able to also transmute destructive tendencies in our body and spirit into growing, life-giving expressions.

Red Reishi Stock

> 1 cup red reishi
> 1 gallon water
> Stock vegetables of your choice

The traditional method of preparing these polypores is to simmer them, usually for at least five or six hours, though it is not unheard of to cook the highest-quality wild red and purple reishi for up to two days. This longer-term process extracts the polysaccharide chains known as beta-glucans very well but also gets an appreciable quantity of the steroidal molecules (and their saponins), such as ganoderic acid, that don't dissolve in water very quickly. This makes a simmering soup stock an excellent extraction medium for reishi.

A cupful of slices may be added to a gallon of water and vegetables, cooked over low heat for two or three hours, then removed (reishi is very fibrous and not a tasty mushroom to eat). You might even be able to use the same mushrooms a couple of times before composting them.

Used this way, four or five days a week, reishi extends life, soothes a disturbed and restless spirit, and nourishes the heart and circulation.

Red Reishi Two-phase Extract

> Dried red reishi
> 100–150 proof alcohol
> Glycerin (made from vegetable fat)
> Water

Since simmering reishi slices for allergy and sensitivity is a bit too much to ask sometimes, I have used the following modified tincture recipe to good effect for extracting the full range of chemistry from this mushroom. In essence, we will need to combine two "fractions" of molecules into a final extract, but each one will need its own solvent and extraction process. The polysaccharides will dissolve quickly into a simmering water bath; the steroidal and triterpenoid molecules prefer a high percentage of alcohol. Unfortunately, the latter solvent can actually damage polysaccharides (think of 150 proof rum directly in your mouth) and weaken the final product. Thus the "two-phase" process. Once you've tried it a few times, it will seem less complex.

First, take your dried medicinal mushrooms, divide them into two equal parts and chop them well. Using the first part, prepare a tincture by covering the mushrooms with a solvent made of 75 percent alcohol (150 rum, perhaps), 15 percent glycerin, and 10 percent water. The glycerin, made from vegetable fat, is readily available at natural foods stores and helps maintain an emulsion when the next steps are taken. Set the tincture aside, and let it steep for four weeks, shaking it occasionally. Then strain it and measure its volume.

After you've strained the tincture, take the second part of the dried mushrooms and simmer them for at least one hour, preferably two or more, in twice as much water as you used for the total solvent volume. Keep adding water, if necessary.

At the end of the simmering, strain the mushrooms out and reduce the volume of fluid you have left by boiling it down so that it equals the volume of strained tincture. Take this off the heat and allow it to cool completely. Combine the simmered broth and strained tincture, mixing well with a whisk. Make sure you are adding the tincture to the broth and not vice versa to reduce the amount of concentrated alcohol the polysaccharides have to endure. The final product should be roughly 35 percent alcohol by volume.

This two-phase process is useful for extracting the chemistry of almost any medicinal mushroom. It produces a cloudy and thick remedy that can be used daily as an immune-modulating tonic (and for all the other benefits ascribed to this storied substance), but it can also be employed on an as-needed basis for allergy symptoms.

Remedy Recommendation

The doses range from about thirty drops once or twice a day (a good amount to start with for allergies and sensitivities) up to a full teaspoon two or three times daily (for severely disturbed spirit and heart, profound immune weakness or derangement, or recovery and convalescence). It keeps for years and is convenient to carry and administer. And the more you consume it, the less you'll need. If only all medicines worked this way!

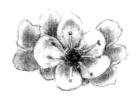

HAWTHORN
CRATAEGUS MONOGYNA

If you are brave and need some help in fulfilling your heart's desires, wise folk in the countryside might point you to a scraggly old tree in the middle of a pasture, its branches leaning eastward from years of flagging by the western wind, all covered in white blossoms. "Cut a piece from one of its stouter branches," they counsel in hushed tones. "But be advised: if you do not chant the sacred words, a wicked curse will follow you all the days of your life." Should you still feel courageous, you could wander up to the hawthorn tree, respectfully harvest a small piece of wood, and carve it into a talisman to wear close to your heart. The May, as this tree is also known, might then grant your secret wish and bring you the joy you desire.

In rural England and Ireland, folks still wait for the hawthorn to flower before tilling the fields or shearing the sheep. Its blossoms, which usually begin to appear on May Day, signal a time of fertility and growth and are considered a blessing from the goddess who watches over forest and field. But just as the branches carry thick and dangerous thorns, this tree is thought to have a dark side, too. Approach it with disrespect, or marry in the month of May, and she might hinder your progress, wither your crops, and spoil all your hopes. When it blooms, its flowers also remind us of the dual side of hawthorn: their smell can be both pleasant and a bit nauseating and has been described as the smell of arousal but also the smell of death. Its flowering boughs are brought to the maypole for fertility rituals, but it is also forbidden to carry them into the home, as this will surely bring death along.

Love and death, fertility and harvest—traditional herbalists revered the hawthorn tree. It seems to hold the threads of fate for those who live close to the land—and the modern research record assigns it an almost equal importance. It is one of the most-studied medicinal herbs, and the clinical results are always impressive, showing strong anti-inflammatory effects, especially in the blood vessels. But just as with the traditional uses, hawthorn shines at protecting the heart and enhancing its function. Not only that, but it has an impeccable safety record and can be confidently employed alongside conventional medication. All this is not surprising: its high flavonoid content makes it an incredible tonic. The lady of the May wraps herself deeply in our physiology, from our blood vessels to the double helix of our DNA. Like so many tonics, she may be more of a necessity than a luxury. No wonder such deep cultural rituals drive the use of hawthorn.

GROWING AND HARVESTING HAWTHORN

The Western Hemisphere has its native hawthorns, too, mostly found in the Pacific Northwest. In the East you can still find them by old farmhouses and in the forest next to stone foundations. Settlers brought trees with them and planted them close to home. Especially in New England, there are groves that have naturalized, tended by birds for whom the berry is a valuable food. Just like apples, these trees interbreed freely, making our local hawthorns very diverse and difficult to label with a standard species name, though all are of the genus *Crataegus*. Some of the leaves are heart-shaped and finely toothed; others so deeply lobed they resemble oak leaves. Some hawthorns flower early in the month of May; others a bit later. But all present the characteristic blossom of the *Rosaceae*—five-petaled, white, and shining. Their fragrance shifts as the flowers mature, just as the country folk say. And for making tea, the first flush of leaf and flower is the best part to harvest. It is definitely an astringent mix, but research shows that it contains a higher concentration and more diverse blend of flavonoids than even the fruit, which is extremely rich in these important molecules and also the part that is traditionally used. But the berries are difficult to infuse, unlike the leaf and flower—so I gather the blossoms in the month of May to save for tea, always with great respect and reverence.

Some hawthorn varietals set their berry early in the season, and by September it is already flushing red. Technically, the small red fruits are pomes, like apples, and contain two or sometimes up to four or five small hard seeds, surrounded by a firm and delicious yellow flesh. If you let them mature too far, the flesh becomes softer and quickly starts to spoil, so I usually err on the side of caution and harvest the berries just after they've turned bright red, while there are still some green fruits on the tree. The harvest is difficult to dry properly, so I usually process them right away. On my way home, I always make it a point to bury a little of my harvest here and there, in spots that might be spared the mower's blade. With luck, a few will sprout—though, as with appleseed, what you get is somewhat of a mystery. But all varietals of hawthorn are useful for medicine.

You can also sprout seedlings at home. To do this, harvest the overripe fruit, remove its seed, and dry it at room temperature. Next spring take your collection, soak it overnight, and plant two seeds per cell. Select the strongest sprout of the pair and, after a few weeks, transplant each into its own half-gallon pot. These baby trees can be kept sheltered for their first two winters, either mulched with straw outdoors or brought into the root cellar. But soon thereafter the little hawthorns can be planted out, either in the center of a circular garden bed or, as they do in Ireland, in a row as a hedge border where they function as a very effective (and thorny!) fence. If you want your hawthorns to produce well, or if you are trying to make a nice hedge, you will need to do some pruning in the early spring. This is actually a tricky process, and I encourage you to consult with an arborist to learn this ancient craft.

USING HAWTHORN

For medicine, hawthorn's tonic activity is all about the heart. Properly harvested and prepared, it has none of the darkness the lady of the May sometimes shows. It opens the circulation, reliably decreasing blood pressure, but it opens the heart in other ways, too. When used over time, even the posture changes, shoulders roll back, the forehead lifts, and one can almost see a radiance emanating from the solar plexus. Sure, this "energetic" effect is difficult to capture or assess objectively. But you might be surprised at how connected our emotional heart is to the physical muscle in our chest. Our autonomic nervous system and our heart are part of the same organ system, as we saw when exploring aromatic plants. So many times I've seen people, myself included, respond to hawthorn not only with lower blood pressure and a steadier heartbeat, but also with a softer, more tolerant, emotional connection to the world.

Safe, foodlike, highly effective when used habitually, often quite tasty—these red fruits embody all the qualities of a tonic. Though their effects are most pronounced on the heart, pharmacological research shows that they can substantially affect inflammatory balance and epigenetics as well (which may be part of why they are so helpful to the cardiovascular system). It continues to puzzle me why their use is not more widespread in the modern health care system. Perhaps it's become hard for us to trust that medicine might be found, already perfectly complete, hanging off a scraggly, thorny tree on the edge of a weedy farm field. Are we trying to say that there can be no good remedy without human tinkering? Or have we become afraid of whatever is unknown, unhybridized, uncontrolled?

Regardless, the hawthorn tree watches us from the edge of her field. She is like a lover, half-wild, passionate, full in her affection but vengeful in her anger. But she is also like a mother, older and wiser than her children, revealing the secrets necessary for a full and safe life. She holds the bookends of the most joyful season of the year, bringing in the May and celebrating the harvest with her great gifts. And if we embrace her, with affection and with respect, she opens our hearts and lets our feelings flow to their fullest. Don't underestimate her love, or deny her power. A true tonic she is, desiring little praise, but holding us safe in her gentle hand.

Hawthorn Tea

A few tablespoons hawthorn leaf and flower
Linden blossom (optional)
1 cup hot water

Because of this heart connection, I often combine the leaf and flower of this tree with the blossoms of the linden, to reinforce the aromatic effect on tension with the tonic, nourishing, and rebalancing effect hawthorn provides.

A few tablespoons of leaf and flower per cup of hot water is sufficient, or you can brew up to one-half gallon at a time using two cups of the herb. Strain it out after letting it steep for at least an hour, and store the tea in the fridge.

Remedy Recommendation

Usually a pint a day is sufficient and taken consistently over months noticeably brings down high blood pressure. It is delicious sweetened with a little raw honey or even maple syrup.

 ## Hawthorn Berry Jam

Fresh or rehydrated hawthorn berries (plain and simple!)
Vegetable mill

Hawthorn's cardiovascular effects are not limited to controlling blood pressure. In fact, the berry, in extract form, strengthens the contractions of an aging and failing heart. It reduces symptoms of chest pain, shortness of breath, and easy fatigability that come from a weak cardiovascular system or from poor circulation in people of all ages. And it does so extremely safely because, as with most tonics, it's basically just food. And while exotic fruits such as goji and acai are all the rage these days, I usually recommend that you save your money and focus on hawthorn and blueberries instead. They are as rich in flavonoids and as effective as any expensive tonic from far-flung corners of the globe.

The best way to prepare the berries as an ongoing heart tonic is to cook them into a thick, rich, unsweetened jam. I like to use the fresh berries, but if you have none, you can rehydrate dry ones by soaking them in barely enough water to cover them and leaving them overnight.

Take the berries and simply cook them in a steel pot, over low heat, stirring and mashing them in the process (a fork works fine for this). After an hour or so you will have a rich, reddish-orange mass interspersed with the hard seeds.

At this point, pass the pulp through a vegetable mill (the old kind with the hand-cranked handle that goes around in circles). This separates the seeds, which can be discarded. If you're familiar with canning, you can reheat the hawthorn pulp and preserve it that way. Alternatively, you can fill eight-ounce jars about three-quarters of the way and simply freeze your jam.

Remedy Recommendation

Take about two tablespoons of this medicinal treat daily—as is, spread on toast, mixed in oatmeal, or however suits your fancy. A most delectable way to take your medicine!

Epilogue

In the early morning, when the air is still cool and there is a mist rising from the lake, I often try to get out and run. There's something about the west wind through the leaves, rhythmic breathing, and fast footfalls that makes me feel more alive and engaged—more fully human. Endurance running might be one of our most distinctive skills, at least if you subscribe to the views of Daniel Lieberman, professor of evolutionary biology at Harvard University. His research into the structure of the human body has uncovered many details that, when taken as a whole, lead to the conclusion that our physical frame evolved in the context of a run—a really, really long run. Lieberman takes his study one step further and, based on analysis of runners both barefoot and shod, speculates that we run best when we have no shoes on and are in full contact with the grass and dirt of the trail. In essence, he concludes, we should think about movement from an evolutionary vantage point: our bodies are used to running, and they're used to running with very little between them and nature.

But isn't this exactly what we've found in our exploration of plants? It seems that, as much as the prodigious strength of the Achilles tendon is a direct response to the patterns of movement of early humans, our internal physiology is a direct response to the plant-based xenobiome those same humans experienced in their quest for nutrition. In running, in eating, in medicine (and more), we have been flexing our technological muscle in order to improve our lives. And in many ways we have succeeded beyond all expectations. But a growing chorus of voices, from Lieberman to Richard Louv to those who feel too much hygiene and antiseptics are hurting our species, is rising with one simple message: sometimes it is better to stay just a little more wild, just a little closer to the soil, with less technology between us and nature. In the context of what we ingest, advocates of real food, such as Michael Pollan, remind us that this means eating unprocessed plants and animals that lived more like their wild counterparts. But I would like to take this just a little further. Vegetables, though fantastic for our health, are relatively tame species. It is the wild plants that are essential for the function of our internal physiology. Their richer, more challenging chemistry allows us to achieve our maximum potential. They provide a strong dose of xenobiotic chemicals, the lack of which has left us like fish out of water. They interact with our beings at all levels—many of which we have yet to discover.

Kevin Spelman is working on this process of discovery. His research focus is on the interconnections between plants and human physiology. He has explored the activities of botanicals on sirtuins—those important modulators of epigenetic activity. He has helped to characterize how traditional herbal medicines like echinacea affect the production of immune system chemicals. But despite his research focus, Dr. Spelman began as an herbalist, and still is. Nadja Cech, who grew up on a huge and diverse herb farm in Williams, Oregon, now publishes research on immune-active polyphenols from plants and studies the complex synergy of chemicals in herbs like goldenseal. Her eye turns to how complexity in the botanical world yields unexpected positive results when it interfaces with human physiology. In both these cases, and in many more across the planet, I see research and scientific inquiry driven by an underlying passion for plants. I see the tools of technology, grounded in a relationship with nature and a process of discovery inspired by the green world.

When we study plants, we realize how interwoven they are with our physiology. What can this realization teach us? I believe it comes down to this simple lesson: we turn to our technologies for handling short-term concerns and for making our lives easier. But just as technological medicine may be excellent at eliminating disease but has little to say about how to make us well, all our modern advances still fall short when it comes to building meaning, connection, passion, and purpose in our lives. The net result is a culture that is excellent at quickly pushing back against challenge but is also characterized by a creeping malaise, mental health disturbances, imbalances in metabolism, and a chronic, simmering inflammation that may be at the root of it all. How did this happen?

When we developed the method at the heart of science, somewhere in the sixteenth century, we began a systematic, rapid, and effective process of sorting the accumulated knowledge of the human species into two columns: on one side, the stuff that works; on the other, the stuff that doesn't. Of course, reality is sometimes more nuanced. Some things work often, but not always; others work only in certain contexts; still others may never yield their secrets because simply observing them changes their essential nature (trying to gauge the speed and position of an electron or understanding the interactions of preschoolers are but two examples). Yes, the scientific method has allowed for a rapid pace of progress, and the discoveries it catalyzes change the world every day. But it remains powerless until someone is willing to ask a question. Then all it can do is disprove the hypothesis. You cannot get at truth by removing untruth; all you can do is approximate. Of course, there's nothing wrong with this: our approximations become more and more detailed over time. Nevertheless, I contend that there can be no "gestalt," no "theory of everything," at the end of this process. And this leaves everyone unsatisfied.

What we need is a method for framing questions, a guide for the scientific process that is similar to what guides researchers like Kevin Spelman and Nadja Cech. Just as we follow our heart but use our brain to validate the heart's intuitions, so, too, we can begin research with a system-based understanding that emphasizes connection more than component, that looks at whole ecosystems rather than isolated constituents. The experience of the numinous should be the driver of our search for knowledge, not a desire for a reductionist understanding of the parts and pieces of reality. After all, as Einstein said, "Science without religion is lame. Religion without science is blind." *Religion,* in this context, may not be the best word (it has such a polarizing meaning nowadays). So perhaps we can say that observing reality without being inspired yields little understanding, while being inspired without being observant can run you off a cliff. In the end, we need both—but our connection to nature and the inspiration it yields should probably be the starting point.

My argument is that this lesson is clearly evident when examining how plants work in concert with human beings. Technological medicine, often focused on short-term gains, is having a difficult time with the epidemics of mental health and malaise, diabetes and obesity, cardiovascular inflammation and cancer. Yet when you look at traditional herbal medicine, you find that aromatic, bitter, and tonic plants consumed in a habitual, cultural context are the precise prescription for these ills. This is neither a miracle nor some act of design. In fact, the explanation is much more mundane. Our minds, our guts, our immune systems all evolved in the context of consuming wild plants, and we have eradicated this context quite effectively (though perhaps not consciously) over the last two hundred years. So if, in the case of medicine, we discover that unsolved problems find their solution in nature-based, cuisinelike traditions, I can't help but wonder where else such an approach might yield results. Urban planning? Waste management? Educational models? Food production and distribution? Perhaps even energy generation?

The case for herbal medicine is clear, almost obvious in retrospect. But just as bringing wild plants back into our xenobiome allows us to function at our peak, I believe that a blending of modern technology and the best of nature-based tradition is the synthesis that will bring us to the next phase of evolution and understanding. Neither way is enough alone, as both are incomplete. But in the end, it gives me such great joy to think that humble, weedy, wild botanicals like the common dandelion might be the ones to lead us down this trail, into this new turn of the human spiral. Their lessons might reach far beyond the field of medicine, catalyzing change throughout the culture. These herbs provide positive evidence that we are deeply, inextricably, intertwined with nature. Plants are part of us—or, to put it more gratefully, we are their children. So let us turn our ears toward these ancestors. They speak softly, but their words ring true.

Notes

CHAPTER 1. A CUISINE FOR MEDICINE

1. "World Health Organization Fact Sheet," 2008.
2. Wooltorton, "Several Chinese Herbal Products," 449.
3. Mills and Bone, *Principles and Practices of Phytotherapy*, 111.
4. Weaver, "Science and Complexity," 540.
5. von Bertalanffy, "The Theory of Open Systems in Physics and Biology."
6. Edgar, *Measure, Topology, and Fractal Geometry*, 1.
7. Dobbs, "Newton's Commentary on the Emerald Tablet of Hermes Trismegistus."
8. Capra, *The Web of Life*, 42.
9. Wachs, "Reflections on the Planning Process," 141–61.
10. Barabási and Albert, "Emergence of Scaling in Random Networks."
11. Bateson, *Steps to an Ecology of Mind*. Though Bateson referred to it as *mind*, he was describing consciousness as an emergent quality of a living ecology.
12. Jones and Quinn, *Textbook of Functional Medicine*, 37.
13. Kagan, *Galen's Prophecy*, 2–4.
14. Kaviratna, *The Charaka Samhita*.
15. Wa, *Zhongguo Yixue Shi (A History of Chinese Medicine)*.
16. Tama, Worcel, and Wyllie, "Yohimbine: A Clinical Review."
17. Tierra, *Planetary Herbology*, 303.
18. Chen et al., "Analysis of Yohimbine Alkaloid."
19. Veltmann et al., "Response to Intravenous Ajmaline."

20. Blumenthal et al., "Effects of Exercise and Stress Management."

21. Basta, Schmidt, and De Caterina, "Advanced Glycation End Products and Vascular Inflammation."

22. Alberti, Simmet, and Shaw, "The Metabolic Syndrome."

CHAPTER 2. AROMATICS

1. Dharani and Yenesew, *Medicinal Plants of East Africa,* 265.

2. Ni, *The Yellow Emperor's Classic of Medicine,* 100–101.

3. Avicenna, *The Canon of Medicine,* 297.

4. Hales, *Statical Essays.*

5. Berntson et al., "Heart Rate Variability."

6. Donders, *"Zür Physiologie des Nervus Vagus."*

7. Grossman, "Repiratory and Cardiac Rhythms."

8. Berntson et al., "Heart Rate Variability." Gives an excellent historical overview of the subject of HRV.

9. Hon, "The Electronic Evaluation of Fetal Heart Rate."

10. Hon and Lee, "The Electronic Evaluation of Fetal Heart Rate. VIII."

11. American College of Obstetricians and Gynecologists, "ACOG Practice Bulletin #70: Intrapartum Fetal Heart Rate Monitoring."

12. Burns et al., "An Investigation into the Use of Aromatherapy in Intrapartum Midwifery Practice."

13. Ewing, "Heart Rate Variability."

14. Gill et al., "RR Variability and Baroreflex Sensitivity"; Huikuri, "Frequency Domain Measures of Heart Rate Variability"; Kleiger, "Decreased Heart Rate Variability"; Saul, "Assessment of Autonomic Regulation."

15. Ewing et al., "Differing Patterns of Cardiac Parasympathetic Activity."

16. Ewing et al., "Measurement of Parasympathetic Activity."

17. Zuanetti et al., "Prognostic Significance of Heart Rate Variability."

18. Buccelletti et al., "Heart Rate Variability and Myocardial Infarction."

19. Singh et al., "Reduced Heart Rate Variability and New-Onset Hypertension."

20. Buchanan et al., "Measurement of Recovery from Myocardial Infarction." R. M. Carney's team at Washington University in St. Louis continued to expand on the research into the twenty-first century, addressing the

connection between emotional health, heart disease, and HRV but also focusing on mortality risk. See the bibliography for more of Carney's work. Additionally, see Singh et al., "Brain-Heart Connection and the Risk of Heart Attack." Finally, for an excellent review of the development of the heart/mind/HRV link as expressed in heart disease, see Pizzi et al., "Analysis of Potential Predictors of Depression."

21. McCraty et al., "The Effects of Emotions on Short-Term Power Spectrum Analysis."

22. McCraty et al., "The Effects of Different Types of Music"; McCraty and Childre, "Psychophysiological Correlates of Spiritual Experience"; McCraty, "Heart Rhythm Coherence"; McCraty and Childre, "The Grateful Heart."

23. McCraty et al., "The Impact of a New Emotional Self-Management Program on Stress"; McCraty et al., "Analysis of Twenty-Four Hour Heart Rate Variability."

24. McCraty and Childre, "Coherence." This article builds on previous work, including McCraty and Tomasino, "Emotional Stress, Positive Emotions"; McCraty, "Heart Rhythm Coherence"; McCraty, Atkinson, and Tiller, "Cardiac Coherence."

25. Thayer et al., "Heart Rate Variability, Prefrontal Neural Function."

26. Baddeley, "Working Memory."

27. Masterman and Cummings, "Frontal-Subcortical Circuits."

28. Friedman and Thayer, "Anxiety and Autonomic Flexibility"; Friedman, "Autonomic Balance Revisited"; Thayer and Friedman, "The Heart of Anxiety."

29. Ahern et al., "Heart Rate and Heart Rate Variability Changes"; Lane et al., "Neural Correlates of Heart Rate Variability during Emotion"; Lane et al., "Activity in Medial Prefrontal Cortex"; Lane et al., "Subgenual Anterior Cingulate (BA25)"; Nugent et al., "Anatomical Correlates of Autonomic Control"; Nugent et al., "Alterations in Neural Correlates."

30. Hansen, Johnsen, and Thayer, "Relationship between Heart Rate Variability and Cognitive Function."

31. Thayer et al., "Heart Rate Variability Is Inversely Related to Cortisol Reactivity."

32. Hansen, Johnsen, and Thayer, "Vagal Influence in the Regulation of Attention."

33. Thayer et al., "Heart Rate Variability and Its Relation to Prefrontal Cognitive Function."

34. Macht and Ting, "Experimental Inquiry."

35. Cavanagh and Wilkinson, "Biological Activities of Lavender Essential Oil"; Diego et al., "Aromatherapy Positively Affects Mood."

36. Kubota et al., "Odor and Emotion-Effects of Essential Oils."

37. Galetta et al., "Lifelong Physical Training Prevents the Age-Related Impairment of Heart Rate Variability"; Nesvold et al., "Increased Heart Rate Variability during Nondirective Meditation"; Peressutti et al., "Heart Rate Dynamics in Different Levels of Zen Meditation"; Nakahara et al., "Emotion-Related Changes in Heart Rate."

38. Bradley et al., "Effects of Orally Administered Lavender Essential Oil"; Xu et al., "Pharmaco-physio-psychologic Effect"; Lewith, Godfrey, and Prescott, "A Single-Blinded, Randomized Pilot Study"; Chien, Cheng, and Liu, "The Effect of Lavender Aromatherapy"; Peng, Koo, and Yu, "Effects of Music and Essential Oil"; Wu, *The Effect of Inhalation of Lavender Essential Oils.*

39. Manley, "Psychophysiological Effects of Odor"; Lis-Balchin, "A Preliminary Study."

40. Chang, "Aromatherapy Benefits Autonomic Nervous System."

41. Matsubara, "The Essential Oil of *Abies sibirica*"; Matsubara, "(–)–Bornyl Acetate Induces Autonomic Relaxation."

42. Matsubara et al., "Volatiles Emitted"; Chen, *Effects of Inhalation of Mint Extracts*; Arizono et al., "Reminiscence Therapy"; Cha, Lee, and Yoo, "Effects of Aromatherapy."

43. Mezzacappa et al., "Coconut Fragrance and Cardiovascular Response to Laboratory Stress."

44. Park et al., "The Physiological Effects of Shinrin-yoku."

45. Tsunetsugu, Park, and Miyazak, "Trends in Research Related to 'Shinrin-yoku.'"

46. Della Loggia, Tubaro, and Lunder, "Evaluation of Some Pharmacological Activities."

47. Liu et al., "Enteric-Coated Peppermint-Oil Capsules"; Göbel, Schmidt, and Soyka, "Effect of Peppermint."

48. Göbel et al., "Effectiveness of Oleum Menthae Piperitae."

49. Singh and Singh, "An Ethnobotanical Study of Medicinal Plants."

50. Uri and Felter, *King's American Dispensatory.*

51. Rushforth, *Trees of Britain and Europe.*

52. Houghton, *Valerian: The Genus Valeriana.*

53. Sarris et al., "The Kava Anxiety Depression Spectrum Study."

54. Hoffmann, *Medical Herbalism.*

55. Hoffmann, *The New Holistic Herbal*; Tierra, *The Way of Chinese Herbs.*

56. Hoffmann, *The New Holistic Herbal.*

57. Hoffmann, lecture on "Herbs for Cardiovascular Health."

58. Kaptchuck, *The Web That Has No Weaver.*

59. Manniche, *Sacred Luxuries.*

60. Chevallier, *The Encyclopedia of Medicinal Plants.*

61. Classen, Howe, and Synnott, *Aroma.*

62. Rimmel, *The Book of Perfumes;* Wilson, *The Plague Pamphlets of Thomas Decker.*

63. Culpeper, *Culpeper's Complete Herbal.*

64. Tainter, "The Rise of Synthetic Drugs."

65. Kirk-Smith and Booth, "Chemoreception in Human Behavior."

66. Kirk-Smith and Booth, "Effect of Androstenone on Choice of Location."

67. Lis-Balchin, *Aromatherapy Science.* See the chapters on pharmacological and clinical research as well as appendices 11–15 for collated research on activity organized by specific essential oil.

68. Lall and Meyer, "In Vitro Inhibition of Drug-Resistant"; Yarnell, "Botanical Medicines"; Fang et al., "Experimental Study on the Antibacterial Effect"; Weckesser et al., "Screening of Plant Extracts."

69. Abdel-Tawab, "Boswellia Serrata."

70. Cuaz-Pérolin et al., "Anti-inflammatory and Anti-atherogenic Effects."

71. Hoffmann, *Medical Herbalism.*

72. Lixandru et al., "Antimicrobial Activity of Plant Essential Oils."

73. Hoffmann, *Medical Herbalism.*

74. Gladstar, *Herbal Healing for Women.*

75. Culpeper, *Culpeper's Complete Herbal;* Ciganda, "Herbal Infusions," 235–39.

76. Juergens et al., "Anti-inflammatory Activity of 1.8-Cineol."

77. Franova, Nosalova, and Mokry, "Phytotherapy of Cough."

78. Duke, *The Green Pharmacy Herbal Handbook.* This features garlic, which is aromatic, but tonic, too, as a primary agent for treating Raynaud's.

79. Kohlert et al., "Bioavailability and Pharmacokinetics."

80. Izzo et al., "Spasmolytic Activity of Medicinal Plants."

81. Lis-Balchin and Hart, "Spasmolytic Activity of the Essential Oils."

82. Vuorela et al., "Calcium Channel Blocking Activity."

83. Lis-Balchin, Deans, and Hart, "Bioactivity of New Zealand."

84. Van Toller et al., *Ageing and the Sense of Smell.*

85. Kandel, Schwartz, and Jessell, *Principles of Neural Science.*

86. Ibid.

87. Toller, "Assessing the Impact of Anosmia."

88. Morley et al., "Olfactory Dysfunction."

89. Wysocki and Pelchat, "The Effects of Aging."

CHAPTER 3. BITTERS

1. Pliny, *Natural History*, XXV 4.

2. Scarborough and Nutton, "The Preface of Dioscorides' Materia Medica."

3. Watson, *Theriac and Mithridatium;* Norton, "The Pharmacology of Mithridatum"; Kürschner, Raus, and Venter, *Pflanzen der Türkei.*

4. Citová et al., "Determination of Gentisin, Isogentisin, and Amarogentin."

5. Behrens et al., "The Human Bitter Taste Receptor."

6. Hooper, "How Host-Microbial Interactions."

7. Dobzhansky, "Nothing in Biology Makes Sense."

8. Carpenter, *The History of Scurvy and Vitamin C*; Blencowe et al., "Folic Acid to Reduce Neonatal Mortality"; Oh and Brown, "Vitamin B_{12} Deficiency."

9. Sigma-Aldrich, "Williams' Medium E Formulation."

10. Heiser, *Seed to Civilization;* Schoeninger, "The Agricultural 'Revolution'"; Cordain et al., "Origins and Evolution of the Western Diet."

11. Danielson, "The Cytochrome P450 Superfamily"

12. Rosenthal, "Herbivores."

13. Guengerich, "Influence of Nutrients."

14. Danielson, "The Cytochrome P450 Superfamily."

15. Bennett and Wallsgrove, "Secondary Metabolites in Plant Defense Mechanisms."

16. Singletary and Rokusek, "Tissue-Specific Enhancement."

17. Ming-Shun, "Inducible Direct Plant Defense."

18. Seery, Holman, and Silver, "Whatever Does Not Kill Us."

19. Li et al., "Human Receptors for Sweet and Umami Taste."

20. Nelson et al., "An Amino-Acid Taste Receptor."

21. Huang et al., "The Cells and Logic for Mammalian Sour Taste Detection."

22. Laguerette et al., "Do We Taste Fat?"; Lindemann, "Receptors and Transduction in Taste."

23. Behrens et al., "Bitter Taste Receptors."

24. Meyerhof et al., "The Molecular Receptive Ranges."

25. Sternini, "Taste Receptors in the Gastrointestinal Tract."

26. Rozengurt, "Taste Receptors in the Gastrointestinal Tract."

27. Sternini, "Taste Receptors in the Gastrointestinal Tract."

28. Deshpande et al., "Bitter Taste Receptors"; Singh, "Functional Bitter Taste Receptors."

29. Rolls, Roe, and Meengs, "Salad and Satiety."

30. Schier, Davidson, and Powley, "Ongoing Ingestive Behavior"; Geraedts, "Gastrointestinal Targets."

31. Wicks et al., "Impact of Bitter Taste on Gastric Motility."

32. Little et al., "Sweetness and Bitterness Taste of Meals."

33. Dotson et al., "Bitter Taste Receptors."

34. Dotson, Vigues, and Munger, "T1R and T2R Receptors."

35. Bassoli et al., "Chlorogenic Acid."

36. Cordain et al., "Plant-Animal Subsistence Ratios."

37. Ibid.

38. Wein et al., "Use of and Preference for Traditional Foods."

39. Gadsby, "The Inuit Paradox."

40. Galen, *Opera Omnia,* 60.

41. Gladstar, *Herbal Healing for Women,* 112.

42. "Avena Botanicals Store, Bitter Tonics."

43. Van Loon, Gabriel, *Charaka Samhita: Handbook on Ayurveda,* 28.

44. Edvell and Lindstrom, "Vagotomy in Young Obese Hyperglycemic Mice."

45. Dockaray, "Luminal Sensing in the Gut."

46. Hao, Sternini, and Raybould, "Role of CCK1 and Y2 Receptors."

47. Bradwejn, "Neurobiological Investigations."

48. Chen et al., "Bitter Stimuli Induce Ca2+ Signaling."

49. Liddle, "Physiological Role for Cholecystokinin."

50. Sternini, "Taste Receptors in the Gastrointestinal Tract"; Dotson, "Bitter Taste Receptors."

51. Batterham et al., "Inhibition of Food Intake."

52. Toft-Nielsen, Madsbad, and Holst, "Determinants of the Effectiveness of Glucagon-like Peptide-1."

53. Wegener, "*Anwendung eines Trockenextraktes Augentianae* (Application of a Dry Extract of the Root of Gentiana)."

54. Glatzel and Hackenberg, "*Röntgenologische Untersuchungen der Wirkungen* (Radiographic studies on the feed-forward effects)."

55. Guthrie, "A Clinical Lecture on Colic."

56. Saller et al., "An Updated Systematic Review."

57. Sannia, "Phytotherapy with a Mixture of Dry Extracts."

58. You et al., "In Vitro and In Vivo."

59. Gerard, *The Herbalor General History of Plants;* Fuangchan, "Hypoglycemic Effect of Bitter Melon."

60. Bassoli et al., "Chlorogenic Acid Reduces the Plasma Glucose Peak."

61. Prabhakar and Doble, "A Target-Based Therapeutic Approach to Diabetes Mellitus."

62. Bakhshaee et al., "Effect of Silymarin"; Ross, "An Integrative Approach to Rhinosinusitis in Children"; Bielory and Lupoli, "Herbal Interventions in Asthma and Allergy"; Chan et al., "A Review of Pharmacological Effects of *Arctium lappa*."

63. Louv, *Last Child in the Woods;* Dunn, *The Wild Life of Our Bodies;* Lowry et al., "Identification of an Immune-Responsive Mesolimbocortical Serotonergic System."

CHAPTER 4. TONICS

1. Macalister, "*Lebor Gabála Érenn* (The Book of the Taking of Ireland)."

2. Suh et al., "Pharmacokinetic Study of an Iridoid Glucoside."

3. Waddington, "The Epigenotype."

4. Carey, *The Epigenetics Revolution,* 127.

5. Campbell et al., *Biology,* 309–10.

6. Fraser et al., "Active Genes Dynamically Colocalize."

7. Kuo et al., "Transcription-linked Acetylation."

8. Weaver, "Science and Complexity."

9. Shore et al., "Characterization of Two Genes."

10. Thiagalingam et al., "Histone Deacetylases."

11. Rajendran et al., "Sirtuins."

12. Finkel, Deng and Mostoslavsky, "Recent Progress in the Biology."

13. Carey, *The Epigenetics Revolution*, 67. Or, to use Nessa Carey's analogy, if DNA is the script, methylation of nucleotides is the director's typed instructions to the actors, and acetylation of histones the scribbled-in-pencil notes.

14. Anway et al., "Epigenetic Transgenerational Actions."

15. Taberlay and Jones, "DNA Methylation and Cancer."

16. Jenuwein and Allis, "Translating the Histone Code."

17. Yuan, Minter-Dykhouse, and Lou, "A c-Myc-SIRT1 Feedback Loop."

18. Rajendran et al., "Sirtuins."

19. Lee et al., "A Role for the NAD-Dependent Deacetylase Sirt1."

20. Alcaín and Villalba, "Sirtuin Activators."

21. Chung et al., "Regulation of SIRT1."

22. Ramiro et al., "Flavonoids from Theobroma"; Rigelsky and Sweet, "Hawthorn"; Cho, "Flavonoid Glycosides"; Wang, Provan and Helliwell, "Tea Flavonoids"; Wu, Ng, and Lin, "Antioxidant Activities"; Li et al., "Research on Ultrasonic-Assisted Extraction of Flavonoid."

23. Graf, Mibury, and Blumberg, "Flavonols, Flavones, Flavanones, and Human Health."

24. Yochum et al., "Dietary Flavonoid Intake."

25. Pérez-Vizcaíno and Duarte, "Flavonols."

26. Kirakosyan et al., "Antioxidant Capacity"; Kirakosyan et al., "Applied Environmental Stresses."

27. Iwashina, "Flavonoid Function."

28. Gilbert, "The Genome."

29. Janeway and Medzhitov, "Innate Immune Recognition"; Hoffmann et al., "Phylogenetic Perspectives."

30. Bengtson, "The Controversial 'Cambrian' Fossils."

31. Alexander and Rietschel, "Bacterial Lipopolysaccharides and Innate Immunity."

32. Janeway and Medzhitov, "Innate Immune Recognition."

33. Notarangelo et al., "Primary Immunodeficiencies."

34. Panda et al., "Human Innate Immunosenescence."

35. Pier, Lyczak, and Wetzler, *Immunology, Infection, and Immunity.*

36. Belkaid and Rouse, "Natural Regulatory T Cells."

37. Mosmann and Coffman, "TH1 and TH2 Cells."

38. Belkaid and Rouse, "Natural Regulatory T Cells."

39. Romagnani, "The Th1/Th2 Paradigm."

40. Kidd, "Th1/Th2 Balance."

41. Chan et al., "Interferon-Producing Killer Dendritic Cells."

42. Schneider, "Human Defensins"; Li-Zhen and Zhi-Bin, "Regulation on Maturation and Function of Dendritic Cells."

43. Janeway and Medzhitov, "Innate Immune Recognition."

44. Lin et al., "Polysaccharide Purified from Ganoderma Lucidum."

45. Strachan, "Hay Fever, Hygiene, and Household Size."

46. Folkerts, Walzl, and Openshaw, "Do Common Childhood Infections 'Teach'?"

47. Correale and Farez, "Association between Parasite Infection and Immune Responses."

48. von Mutius and Radon, "Living on a Farm."

49. Remes et al., "Which Factors Explain the Lower Prevalence of Atopy"; Loss et al., "The Protective Effect of Farm Milk."

50. Perkin and Strachan, "Which Aspects of the Farming Lifestyle."

51. Sadako, "The Effects of Gardening Therapy."

52. Louv, *The Nature Principle,* 5.

53. Kelly-Pieper et al., "Safety and Tolerability"; Matkovic et al., "Efficacy and Safety of Astragalus"; Li et al., "Safety and Efficacy of Ganoderma Lucidum."

54. Gao et al., "Effects of Ganopoly"; Tang et al., "A Randomized, Double-Blind and Placebo-Controlled Study."

55. Pollan, *In Defense of Food,* 142.

56. Teeguarden, *The Ancient Wisdom of Chinese Tonic Herbs,* 96.

57. Duke, *Ginseng: A Concise Handbook,* 112.

58. Zhu, *Chinese Materia Medica,* 555.

59. Ibid., 562.

60. McMeekin, "The Perception of Ganoderma Lucidum."

61. Winston and Maimes, *Adaptogens,* 17.

62. Lazarev, "General and Specific Effects of Drugs," 81–86.

63. Brekhman and Dardymor, "New Substances of Plant Origin," 410–26.

64. Selye, *The Physiology and Pathology of Exposure to Stress.*

65. Schar, "Adaptogens in the Eclectic Materia Medica."

66. Brekhman, *Man and Biologically Active Substances,* 58.

67. Grieve, *A Modern Herbal,* 385.

68. Tyler, *Herbs of Choice,* 166.

69. Hoffmann, *Medical Herbalism,* 501.

70. von Bingen, *Hildegard von Bingen's Physica,* 80.

71. Gerard, *The Herbal or General History of Plants,* 1001.

72. Schar, "Adaptogens in the Eclectic Materia Medica."

73. Haller, *Medical Protestants.*

74. Scudder, *The Eclectic Physician,* 49.

75. Jones, *The American Eclectic Materia Medica and Therapeutics,* 203.

76. Scudder, *The Eclectic Physician,* 53.

77. Fox, "ACTH and Cortisone."

78. Larkin, "Cortisone."

79. Schlotz et al., "Perceived Work Overload."

80. Ho et al., "Septic Shock and Sepsis."

81. Yehuda et al., "Low Urinary Cortisol Excretion"; Cleare et al., "Hypothalamo-Pituitary-Adrenal Axis"; Badanes, Watamura, and Hankin, "Hypocortisolism as a Potential Marker."

82. Buske-Kirschbaum et al., "Altered Responsiveness."

83. Dimsdale, "Short Term Catecholamine"; Gusenoff et al., "Cortisol and GH Secretory Dynamics."

84. Seckl and Walker, "Minireview."

85. Culpeper, *Culpeper's Complete Herbal.*

86. Cohn et al., "Reduction in Intestinal Cholesterol Absorption.

87. Park et al., "Biotransformation of Ginsenosides."

88. Ploeger et al., "The Pharmacokinetics of Glycyrrhizic Acid."

89. Olukoga and Donaldson, "Liquorice and its Health Implications."

90. Ghosh et al., "Molecular Mechanism of Inhibition."

91. Zhu, *Chinese Materia Medica,* 572.

92. Francis et al., "The Biological Action of Saponins."

93. Cox, Sjölander, and Barr, "ISCOMs and Other Saponin Based Adjuvants."

94. Kensil et al., "Structure/Function Studies on QS-21."

95. Zhu, *Chinese Materia Medica*, 550.

96. Mills and Bone, *Principles and Practices of Phytotherapy*, 421–22.

97. Schepetkin and Quinn, "Botanical Polysaccharides"; Gordon, "Pattern Recognition Receptors."

98. Babineau et al., "Randomized Phase I/II Trial of a Macrophage-Specific Immune-Modulator"; Tang et al., "A Randomized, Double-Blind and Placebo-Controlled Study"; Gao et al., "Effects of Ganopoly."

99. Usui, Asari, and Mizuno, "Preparation and Antitumor Activities of h-(1Y6) Branched (1Y3)-h-d-glucan Derivatives."

100. Tsukagoshi et al., "Krestin."

101. Ueda et al., "Immunochemo-Therapy Study Group—Gastric Cancer"; Ohwada et al., "Beneficial Effects of Protein-bound Polysaccharide K"; Ohwada, "Adjuvant Therapy"; Toil et al., "Randomized Adjuvant Trial"; Hayakawa et al., "Effect of Krestin as Adjuvant Treatment."

102. Sanderson, "Dietary Modulation of GALT."

103. Schepetkin and Quinn, "Botanical Polysaccharides," 327.

104. Moorman et al., "National Surveillance for Asthma."

105. Chung et al., "Regulation of SIRT1."

106. Rajendran et al., "Sirtuins."

107. Tuteja and Kaestner, "SnapShot."

108. Gilmore, "Introduction to NF-κB."

109. Graf, Milbury, and Blumberg, "Flavonols, Flavones, Flavanones, and Human Health."

110. Kawaii et al., "Antiproliferative Activity of Flavonoids."

111. Greer and Brunet, "FOXO Transcription Factors."

112. Singh and Agarwal, "Natural Flavonoids."

113. Cherniack, "A Berry Thought-Provoking Idea"; Middleton, "The Effects of Plant Flavonoids on Mammalian Cells."

114. Wilhelm and Baynes, *The I Ching*, 24.

115. Cannon, "Can the Polypill Save the World?"

Bibliography

Abdel-Tawab, M. "Boswellia Serrata: An Overall Assessment of in Vitro, Preclinical, Pharmacokinetic and Clinical Data." *Clinical Pharmacokinet* 50, no. 6 (2011): 349–69.

Ahern, G. L., J. J. Sollers, R. D. Lane, et al. "Heart Rate and Heart Rate Variability Changes in the Intracarotid Sodium Amobarbital (ISA) Test." *Epilepsi* 42 (2001): 912–21.

Alberti, K. G., P. Zimmet, and J. Shaw. "The Metabolic Syndrome: A New Worldwide Definition." *Lancet* 366, no. 9491 (September 24, 2005): 301059–62.

Alcaín, F. J., and J. M. Villalba. "Sirtuin Activators." *Expert Opinion on Therapeutic Patents* 19, no. 4 (April 2009): 403–14.

Alexander, C., and E. T. Rietschel. "Bacterial Lipopolysaccharides and Innate Immunity." *Innate Immunity* 7, no. 3 (June 2001): 167–202.

American College of Obstetricians and Gynecologists (ACOG). "ACOG Practice Bulletin #70: Intrapartum Fetal Heart Rate Monitoring." *Obstetrics and Gynecology* 106, no. 6 (2005): 1453–60.

Anda, R., D. Williamson, D. Jones, et al. "Depressed Affect, Hopelessness, and the Risk of Ischemic Heart Disease in a Cohort of U.S. Adults." *Epidemiology* 4, no. 4 (1993): 285–94.

Anway, M. D., A. S. Cupp, M. Uzumcu, et al. "Epigenetic Transgenerational Actions of Endocrine Disruptors and Male Fertility." *Science* 308, no. 5727 (June 3, 2005): 1466–69.

Arizono, H., N. Morita, S. Iizuka, et al. "Reminiscence Therapy Using Odor in Alcohol-Dependent Patients—Psychophysiological Evaluation and Psychological Evaluation; Power Spectral Analysis of Heart Rate Variability." *Nihon Arukoru Yakubutsu Igakkai Zasshi (Japanese Journal of Alcohol Studies and Drug Dependence)* 35, no. 6 (2000): 373–87.

Avena Botanicals. "Avena Botanicals Store, Bitter Tonics." www.avenabotanicals .com/store/bitters-tonic.html.

Avicenna, *The Canon of Medicine (al-Qānūn fī'l-tibb)*. Volume 1. Translated by Kazi Publications Laleh Bakhtiar. Chicago: Kazi Publications, 1999.

Babineau, T. J., P. Marcello, W. Swails, et al. "Randomized Phase I/II Trial of a Macrophage-Specific Immune-Modulator (PGG-glucan) in High-Risk Surgical Patients." *Annals of Surgery* 220 (1994): 601–9.

Badanes, L. S., S. E. Watamura, and B. L. Hankin. "Hypocortisolism as a Potential Marker of Allostatic Load in Children: Associations with Family Risk and Internalizing Disorders." *Developmental Psychopathology* 23, no. 3 (August 2011): 881–96.

Baddeley, A. "Working Memory: Looking Back and Looking Forward; Nature Reviews." *Neuroscience* 4, no. 10 (2003): 829–39.

Bakhshaee, M., F. Jabbari, S. Hoseini, et al. "Effect of Silymarin in the Treatment of Allergic Rhinitis." *Otolaryngology—Head and Neck Surgery* 145, no. 6 (December 2011): 904–9.

Barabási, Albert-László. *Linked: How Everything Is Connected to Everything Else and What It Means for Business, Science, and Everyday Life*. New York: Plume Books, 2002.

Barabási, Albert-László, and Réka Albert. "Emergence of Scaling in Random Networks." *Science* 286 (October 15, 1999): 509–12.

Bassoli, B. K., P. Cassolla, G. R. Borba-Murad, et al. "Chlorogenic Acid Reduces the Plasma Glucose Peak in the Oral Glucose Tolerance Test: Effects on Hepatic Glucose Release and Glycaemia." *Cell Biochemical Function* 26, no. 3 (April 2008): 320–28.

Basta, G., A. M. Schmidt, and R. De Caterina. "Advanced Glycation End Products and Vascular Inflammation: Implications for Accelerated Atherosclerosis in Diabetes." *Cardiovascular Research* 63, no. 4 (September 1, 2004): 582–92.

Bateson, Gregory. *Steps to an Ecology of Mind: Collected Essays in Anthropology, Psychiatry, Evolution, and Epistemology*. Chicago: University of Chicago Press, 2000.

Batterham, R. L., M. A. Cohen, S. M. Ellis, et al. "Inhibition of Food Intake in

Obese Subjects by Peptide YY3-36." *New England Journal of Medicine* 349, no. 10 (September 2003): 941–48.

Behrens, M., A. Brockhoff, C. Batram, et al. "The Human Bitter Taste Receptor hTAS2R50 Is Activated by the Two Natural Bitter Terpenoids Andrographolide and Amarogentin." *Journal of Agricultural Food Chemistry* 57, no. 21 (November 11, 2009): 9860–66.

Behrens, M., and W. Meyerhof. "Bitter Taste Receptors and Human Bitter Taste Perception." *Cellular and Molecular Life Science* 63, no. 13 (July 2006): 1501–9.

Belkaid, Yasmine, and Barry T. Rouse. "Natural Regulatory T Cells in Infectious Disease." *Nature Immunology* 6 (2005): 353–60.

Benarroch, E. E. "The Central Autonomic Network: Functional Organization, Dysfunction, and Perspective." *Mayo Clinic Proceedings* 68 (1993): 988–1001.

Benedict, R. B., and J. M. Evans. "Second-Degree Heart Block and Wenckebach Phenomenon Associated with Anxiety." *American Heart Journal* 43, no. 4 (1952): 626–33.

Bengtson, S. "The Controversial 'Cambrian' Fossils of the Vindhyan Are Real But More Than a Billion Years Older." *Proceedings of the National Academy of Sciences USA* 106, no. 19 (May 2009): 7729–34.

Bennett, Richard N., and Roger M. Wallsgrove. "Secondary Metabolites in Plant Defense Mechanisms." *New Phytologist* 127, no. 4 (August 1994): 617–33.

Berntson, Gary, J. Bigger, D. Eckberg, et al. "Heart Rate Variability: Origins, Methods, and Interpretive Caveats." *Psychophysiology* 34 (1997): 623–48.

Berthoud, H. R. "The Vagus Nerve, Food Intake and Obesity." *Regulatory Peptides* 7:149, nos. 1–3 (August 2008): 15–25.

Bielory, L., and K. Lupoli. "Herbal Interventions in Asthma and Allergy." *Journal of Asthma* 36, nos. 1 (1999): 1–65.

Blencowe, H., S. Cousens, B. Modell, and J. Lawn. "Folic Acid to Reduce Neonatal Mortality from Neural Tube Disorders." *International Journal of Epidemiology* 39 no. 1 (April 2010): S110–S121.

Blumenthal, J. A., A. Sherwood, M. A. Babyak, et al. "Effects of Exercise and Stress Management Training on Markers of Cardiovascular Risk in Patients with Ischemic Heart Disease: A Randomized Controlled Trial." *Journal of the American Medical Association* 293, no. 13 (April 6, 2005): 1626–34.

Bradley, B. F., S. L. Brown, S. Chu, et al. "Effects of Orally Administered

Lavender Essential Oil on Responses to Anxiety-Provoking Film Clips." *Human Psychopharmacology* no. 4 (June 24, 2009): 319–30.

Bradwejn, J. "Neurobiological Investigations into the Role of Cholecystokinin in Panic Disorder." *Journal of Psychiatry and Neuroscience* 18, no. 4 (July 1993): 178–88.

Brekhman, Israel. *Man and Biologically Active Substances: The Effect of Drugs, Diet and Pollution on Health.* Translated by J. H. Appleby and Stephen Fudder. New York: Pergamon Press, 1980.

Brekhman, Israel, and I. V. Dardymov. "New Substances of Plant Origin Which Increase Nonspecific Resistance." *Annual Review of Pharmacology* 9 (1969): 410–26.

Buccelletti, E., E. Gilardi, E. Scaini, et al. "Heart Rate Variability and Myocardial Infarction: Systematic Literature Review and Metanalysis." *European Review for Medical and Pharmacological Science* 13, no. 14 (July–August 2009): 299–307.

Buchanan, L. M., M. Cowan, R. Burr, and C. Waldron. "Measurement of Recovery from Myocardial Infarction Using Heart Rate Variability and Psychological Outcomes." *Nursing Research* 42, no. 2 (1993): 74–78.

Burns, E., C. Blamey, S. J. Ersser, et al. "An Investigation into the Use of Aromatherapy in Intrapartum Midwifery Practice." *Journal of Alternative and Complementary Medicine* 6 (2000): 1141–47.

Buske-Kirschbaum, A., A. Geiben, H. Höllig, et al. "Altered Responsiveness of the Hypothalamus-Pituitary-Adrenal Axis and the Sympathetic Adrenomedullary System to Stress in Patients with Atopic Dermatitis." *Journal of Clinical Endocrinology and Metabolism* 87, no. 9 (September 2002): 4245–51.

Campbell, Neil A., Jane B. Reece, Lawrence G. Mitchell, and Martha R. Taylor. *Biology: Concepts and Connections,* 4th ed. San Francisco: Benjamin/ Cummings, 1996.

Cannon, C. P. "Can the Polypill Save the World from Heart Disease?" *Lancet* 373, no. 9672 (April 2009): 1313–14.

Capra, Fritjof. *The Web of Life.* New York: Anchor Books, 1996.

Cárdenas, M., M. Marder, V. C. Blank, and L. P. Roguin. "Antitumor Activity of Some Natural Flavonoids and Synthetic Derivatives on Various Human and Murine Cancer Cell Lines." *Bioorganic and Medicinal Chemistry* 14, no. 9 (May 2006): 2966–71.

Carey, Nessa. *The Epigenetics Revolution*. London: Icon Books, 2011.

Carmichael, Alexander. *Carmina Gadelica*. Edinburgh: T. and A. Constable, 1900.

Carney, R. M., K. E. Freedland, P. K. Stein, et al. "Change in Heart Rate and Heart Rate Variability during Treatment for Depression in Patients with Coronary Heart Disease." *Psychosomatic Medicine* 62, no. 5 (2000): 639–47.

Carney, R. M., K. E. Freedland, G. E. Miller, et al. "Depression As a Risk Factor for Cardiac Mortality and Morbidity: A Review of Potential Mechanisms." *Journal Psychosomatic Research* 53, no. 4 (2002): 897–902.

Carney, R. M., J. A. Blumenthal, K. E. Freedland, et al. "Low Heart Rate Variability and the Effect of Depression on Post-myocardial Infarction Mortality." *Archives of Internal Medicine* 165, no. 13 (2005): 1486–91.

Carpenter, Kenneth J. *The History of Scurvy and Vitamin C*. Cambridge: Cambridge University Press, 1988.

Cavanagh, H. M., and J. M. Wilkinson. "Biological Activities of Lavender Essential Oil." *Phytotherapy Research* 16, no. 4 (2002): 301–8.

Celsus, Aulus Cornelius. *De Medicina,* vol. 2 (Book V), Ch. XXIII. Trans. G. F. Collier. London: Simpkin and Marshall, 1831.

Cha, J. H., S. H. Lee, and Y. S. Yoo. "Effects of Aromatherapy on Changes in the Autonomic Nervous System, Aortic Pulse Wave Velocity and Aortic Augmentation Index in Patients with Essential Hypertension." *Journal of Korean Academy Nursing* 40, no. 5 (2010): 705–13.

Chan, Y. S., L. N. Cheng, J. H. Wu, et al. "A Review of the Pharmacological Effects of *Arctium lappa* (Burdock)." *Inflammopharmacology* (October 28, 2010): 245–54.

Chan, C. W., E. Crafton, H. N. Fan, et al. "Interferon-Producing Killer Dendritic Cells Provide a Link between Innate and Adaptive Immunity." *Nature Medicine* 12 (2006): 207–13.

Chang, K. "Aromatherapy Benefits Autonomic Nervous System Regulation for Elementary School Faculty in Taiwan." *Evidence-Based Complementary and Alternative Medicine*, 2011, Article ID 946537: 1–7.

Chen, M. C., V. Wu, J. R. Reeve, and E. Rozengurt. "Bitter Stimuli Induce Ca2+ Signaling and CCK Release in Enteroendocrine STC-1 Cells: Role of L-type Voltage-Sensitive Ca2+ Channels." *American Journal of Physiology— Cell Physiology* 291 (2006): C726–C739.

Chen, Q., P. Li, Z. Zhang, et al. "Analysis of Yohimbine Alkaloid from Pausinystalia Yohimbe by Non-Aqueous Capillary Electrophoresis and Gas

Chromatography-Mass Spectrometry." *Journal of Separation Science* 31, no. 12 (July 2008): 2211–18.

Chen, Wen-wen. *Effects of Inhalation of Mint Extracts on Heart Rate Variability.* Taiwan, R.O.C.: Nanhua University, 2008.

Cherniack, E. P. "A Berry Thought-Provoking Idea: The Potential Role of Plant Polyphenols in the Treatment of Age-Related Cognitive Disorders." *British Journal of Nutrition* (April 5, 2012): 1–7.

Chevallier, Andrew. *The Encyclopedia of Medicinal Plants: A Practical Reference Guide to Over 550 Key Herbs and Their Medicinal Uses.* London: Dorling Kindersley, 1999.

Chien, L. W., S. L. Cheng, and C. F. Liu. "The Effect of Lavender Aromatherapy on Autonomic Nervous System in Midlife Women with Insomnia." *Evidence-Based Complementary and Alternative Medicine*, 2012, Article ID 740813: 1–8.

Chin-Ming, Huang, H. C. Chang, S. T. Kao, et al. "Radial Pressure Pulse and Heart Rate Variability in Normotensive and Hypertensive Subjects." *Journal of Alternative and Complementary Medicine* 17, no. 10 (2011): 945–52.

Cho, M. J., L. R. Howard, R. L. Prior, et al. "Flavonoid Glycosides and Antioxidant Capacity of Various Blackberry, Blueberry and Red Grape Genotypes Determined by High-Performance Liquid Chromatography/Mass Spectrometry." *Journal of the Science of Food and Agriculture* 84, no. 13 (October 2004): 1771–82.

Chung, S., H. Yao, S. Caito, et al. "Regulation of SIRT1 in Cellular Functions: Role of Polyphenols." *Archives of Biochemistry and Biophysics* 501, no. 1 (September 1, 2010): 79–90.

Ciganda, C., and A. Laborde. "Herbal Infusions Used for Induced Abortion." *Journal of Toxicology Clinical Toxicology* 41, no. 3 (2003): 235–39.

Citová, I., M. Ganzera, H. Stuppner, and P. Solich. "Determination of Gentisin, Isogentisin, and Amarogentin in Gentiana lutea L. by Capillary Electrophoresis." *Journal of Separation Science* 31, no. 1 (January 2008): 195–200.

Clark-Kennedy, Archibald Edmund. *Stephen Hales: An Eighteenth Century Biography.* Ridgewood, N.J.: University Press, 1929.

Classen, Constance, David Howes, and Anthony Synnott. *Aroma: The Cultural History of Smell.* London: Routledge, 1994.

Cleare, A. J., J. Miell, E. Heap, et al. "Hypothalamo-Pituitary-Adrenal Axis Dysfunction in Chronic Fatigue Syndrome, and the Effects of Low-Dose

Hydrocortisone Therapy." *Journal of Clinical Endocrinology and Metabolism* 86, no. 8 (August 2001): 3545–54.

Cohn, J. S., A. Kamili, E. Wat, et al. "Reduction in Intestinal Cholesterol Absorption by Various Food Components: Mechanisms and Implications." *Atherosclerosis Supplements* 11, no. 1 (June 2010): 45–48.

Cordain, L., J. B. Miller, S.B. Eaton, et al. "Plant-Animal Subsistence Ratios and Macronutrient Energy Estimations in Worldwide Hunter-Gatherer Diets." *American Journal of Clinical Nutrition* 71, no. 3 (March 2000): 682–92.

Cordain, Loren, S. B. Eaton, A. Sebastian, et al., "Origins and Evolution of the Western Diet: Health Implications for the 21st Century." *American Journal of Clinical Nutrition* 81 (2005): 341–54.

Correale, J., and M. Farez. "Association between Parasite Infection and Immune Responses in Multiple Sclerosis." *Annals of Neurology* 61, no. 2 (2007): 97–108.

Cosgrove, J. J. *History of Sanitation.* Pittsburgh: Standard Sanitary Manufacturing Co., 1909.

Cox, J. C., A. Sjölander, and I. G. Barr. "ISCOMs and Other Saponin Based Adjuvants." *Advanced Drug Delivery Reviews* 32, no. 3 (July 6, 1998): 247–71.

Craig, W. J. "Health-Promoting Properties of Common Herbs." *American Journal of Clinical Nutrition* 70, Supplement 3 (September 1999): 491S–499S.

Cuaz-Pérolin, C., L. Billiet, E. Bauge, et al. "Anti-inflammatory and Anti-atherogenic Effects of the NF-κB Inhibitor Acetyl-11-keto-beta-boswellic Acid in LPS-Challenged ApoE-/-Mice." *Arteriosclerosis, Thrombosis and Vascular Biology,* no. 2 (February 28, 2008): 272–77.

Culpeper, Nicholas. *Culpeper's Complete Herbal.* Whitefish, Mont.: Kessinger Publishing, , 2010. First published in 1653.

Danielson, P. B. "The Cytochrome P450 Superfamily: Biochemistry, Evolution and Drug Metabolism in Humans." *Current Drug Metabolism* 3, no. 6 (December 2002): 561–97.

Della Loggia, R., A. Tubaro, and T. L. Lunder. "Evaluation of Some Pharmacological Activities of a Peppermint Extract." *Fitoterapia* 61, no. 3 (1990): 215–21.

DeLuca, Diana. *Botanica Erotica: Herbal Aphrodisiacs for Body, Mind and Spirit.* Portland, Ore.: Viriditas Press, 1997.

Deshpande, D. A., W. C. Wang, E. L. McIlmoyle, et al. "Bitter Taste Receptors on Airway Smooth Muscle Bronchodilate by Localized Calcium Signaling and Reverse Obstruction." *Nature Medicine* 16, no. 11 (November 2010): 1299–1304.

Dharani, Najma, and Abiy Yenesew. *Medicinal Plants of East Africa: An Illustrated Guide.* Nairobi, Kenya: Drongo Editing & Publishing, 2010.

Diego, M. A., N. A. Jones, T. Field, et al. "Aromatherapy Positively Affects Mood, EEG Patterns of Alertness, and Math Computations." *International Journal of Neuroscience* 96 (1998): 217–24.

Dimsdale, J. E. "Short Term Catecholamine Response to Psychological Stress." *Psychosomatic Medicine* 42 (1980): 493–97.

Dioscorides, Pedanius, and Kurt Sprengel, *De Materia Medica.* Lipsiae, Germany: Knobloch, 1829.

Dobbs, B. J. "Newton's Commentary on the Emerald Tablet of Hermes Trismegistus." In *Hermeticism and the Renaissance,* edited by I. Merkel and A. G. Debus, 178–91 Washington: Folger. 1988.

Dobzhansky, T. "Nothing in Biology Makes Sense Except in the Light of Evolution." *American Biology Teacher* 35 (1973): 125–29.

Dockaray, G. J. "Luminal Sensing in the Gut: An Overview." *Journal of Physiology and Pharmacology* 54, Supplement 4 (2003): 9–17.

Donders, F. C. *"Zür Physiologie des Nervus Vagus* (On the Physiology of the Vagus Nerve)." *Pflüger Archiv für die Gesammte Physiologie des Menschen und der Thiere* (Pflüger's Journal of the Whole Physiology of Man and Beast) 1 (1868): 331–61.

Dotson, C. D., L. Zhang, H. Xu, et al. "Bitter Taste Receptors Influence Glucose Homeostasis." *PLOS ONE* 3, no. 12 (2008): e3974.

Dotson, C. D., S. Vigues, and S. D. Munger. "T1R and T2R Receptors: Modulation of Incretin Hormones and Potential Targets for Treatment of Type 2 Diabetes Mellitus." *Current Opinions on Investigational Drugs* 11, no. 4 (2010): 447–54.

Duke, James A. *Ginseng: A Concise Handbook.* Algonac, Mich.: Reference Publications, 1989.

———. *The Green Pharmacy Herbal Handbook.* New York: St. Martin's Paperbacks, 2002.

———. "Dr. Duke's Phytochemical and Ethnobotanical Databases." www.ars-grin.gov/duke/ (accessed October 27, 2011).

Dunn, Robert. *The Wild Life of Our Bodies*. London: HarperCollins Publishers, 2011.

Edgar, Gerald. *Measure, Topology, and Fractal Geometry*. New York: Springer-Verlag, 2008.

Edris, A. E. "Pharmaceutical and Therapeutic Potentials of Essential Oils and Their Individual Volatile Constituents: A Review." *Phytotherapy Research* 21, no. 4 (2007): 308–23.

Edvell, A., and P. Lindström. "Vagotomy in Young Obese Hyperglycemic Mice: Effects on Syndrome Development and Islet Proliferation, Part 1." *American Journal of Physiology* 274, no. 6 (June 1998): E1034–9.

Ellis, R. J., and J. F. Thayer. "Music and Autonomic Nervous System (Dys)function." *Music Perception* 27, no. 4 (2010): 317–26.

Ewing, D. J. "Heart Rate Variability: An Important New Risk Factor in Patients Following Myocardial Infarction." *Clinical Cardiology* 14, no. 8 (1991): 683–85.

Ewing, D. J., A. D. Flapan, R. A. Wright, et al. "Differing Patterns of Cardiac Parasympathetic Activity and Their Evolution in Selected Patients with a First Myocardial Infarction." *Journal of the American College of Cardiology* 21, no. 4 (1993): 926–31.

Ewing, D. J., J. Nolan, A. D. Flapan, et al. "Measurement of Parasympathetic Activity from 24-hour Ambulatory Electrocardiograms and Its Reproducibility and Sensitivity in Normal Subjects, Patients with Symptomatic Myocardial Ischemia, and Patients with Diabetes Mellitus." *American Journal of Cardiology* 77, no. 2 (1996): 154–58.

Fang, L., H. Qinghua, Y. Zhende, et al. "Experimental Study on the Antibacterial Effect of Origanum Volatile Oil on Dysentery Bacilli in Vivo and in Vitro." *Journal of Huazhong University of Science and Technology Medical Sciences* 24, no. 4 (2004): 400–403.

Ferrini, Jean-Bernard, Lydiane Pichard, Jacques Domergue, and Patrick Maurel. "Long-Term Primary Cultures of Adult Human Hepatocytes." *Chemico-Biological Interactions* 107, nos. 1–2 (1997): 31–45.

Fiedorowicz, J. G., J. He, and K. R. Merikangas. "The Association between Mood and Anxiety Disorders with Vascular Diseases and Risk Factors in a Nationally Representative Sample." *Journal of Psychosomatic Research* 70, no. 2 (2011): 145–54.

Finkel, T., C. X. Deng, and R. Mostoslavsky. "Recent Progress in the Biology and Physiology of Sirtuins." *Nature* 460, no. 7255 (2009): 587–91.

Folkerts, G., G. Walzl, and P. J. Openshaw. "Do Common Childhood Infections 'Teach' the Immune System Not to Be Allergic?" *Immunology Today* 21, no. 3 (March 2000): 118–20.

Fox, J. D. "ACTH and Cortisone—Miracle Therapy or Medical Tool." *American Academy of General Practice* 3, no. 2 (February 1951): 33–38.

Francis, G., Z. Kerem, H. P. S. Makkar, et al. "The Biological Action of Saponins in Animal Systems: A Review." *British Journal of Nutrition* 88, no. 6 (December 2002): 587–605.

Franova, S., G. Nosalova, J. Mokry. "Phytotherapy of Cough." *Advances in Phytomedicine* 2 (2006): 111–31.

Fraser, P., S. Lopes, W. Reik, et al. "Active Genes Dynamically Colocalize to Shared Sites of Ongoing Transcription." *Nature Genetics* 36 (2004): 1065–71.

Friedman, B. H., and J. F. Thayer. "Anxiety and Autonomic Flexibility: A Cardiovascular Approach." *Biological Psychology* 49 (1998): 303–23.

———. "Autonomic Balance Revisited: Panic Anxiety and Heart Rate Variability." *Journal Psychosomatic Research* 44 (1998): 133–51.

Fuangchan, A., P. Sonthisombat, T. Seubnukarn, et al. "Hypoglycemic Effect of Bitter Melon Compared with Metformin in Newly Diagnosed Type 2 Diabetes Patients." *Journal of Ethnopharmacology* 134, no. 2 (March 24, 2011): 422–28.

Gabaix, X., P. Gopikrishnan, V. Plerou, et al. "A Theory of Power-Law Distributions in Financial Market Fluctuations." *Nature* 423 (2003): 267–70.

Gadsby, Patricia. "The Inuit Paradox." *Discover,* October 1, 2004. http://discov ermagazine.com/2004/oct/inuit-paradox (accessed April 2, 2012).

Galeni, Claudii. *Opera Omnia Book 2.* Edited by George Olms. Hildesheim, Germany: 1827. Reprint edited and translated by C. G. Kuhn. Cambridge: Cambridge Library Collection, 1965.

Galetta, F., F. Franzoni, F. R. Femia, et al. "Lifelong Physical Training Prevents the Age-Related Impairment of Heart Rate Variability and Exercise Capacity in Elderly People." *Journal of Sports Medicine and Physical Fitness* 45, no. 2 (2005): 217–21.

Gao, Y., S. Zhou, W. Jiang, et al. "Effects of Ganopoly (A Ganoderma Lucidum Polysaccharide Extract) on the Immune Functions in Advanced-Stage Cancer Patients." *Immunology Investigations* 32, no. 3 (August 2003): 201–15.

Gatefossé, René-Maurice. *Gatefossé's Aromatherapy.* Edited by Robert B. Tisserand. Saffron Walden, England: CW Daniel Co., 1993. First published in 1937.

Geraedts, M. C., F. J. Troost, and W. H. Saris. "Gastrointestinal Targets to Modulate Satiety and Food Intake." *Obesity Reviews* 12, no. 6 (June 2011): 470–77.

Gerard, John. *The Herbalor General History of Plants.* London: Dover Publications, 1975. First published in 1633.

Ghorbani, A., G. Langenberger, L. Feng, et al. "Ethnobotanical Study of Medicinal Plants Utilized by Hani Ethnicity in Naban River Watershed National Nature Reserve, Yunnan, China." *Journal of Ethnopharmacology* 134, no. 3 (2011): 651–67.

Ghosh, D., R. Gonzalez-Duarte, J. Jeffery, et al. "Molecular Mechanism of Inhibition of Steroid Dehydrogenases by Licorice-Derived Steroid Analogs in Modulation of Steroid Receptor Function." *Annals of the New York Academy of Science* 12, no. 761 (June 1995): 341–43.

Gilbert, S. F. "The Genome in Its Ecological Context: Philosophical Perspectives on Interspecies Epigenesis." *Annals of New York Academy of Science* 981 (2002): 202–18.

Gill, J. S., T. Farrell, A. Baszko, et al. "RR Variability and Baroreflex Sensitivity in Patients with Ventricular Tachycardia Associated with Normal Heart and Patients with Ischemic Heart Disease, Part 2." *Pacing and Clinical Electrophysiology* 14, no. 11 (1991): 2016–21.

Gilmore, T. D. "Introduction to NF-κB: Players, Pathways, Perspectives." *Oncogene* 25, no. 51 (2006): 6680–84.

Gladstar, Rosemary. *Herbal Healing for Women.* Clearwater, Fla.: Touchstone, 1993.

———. *Rosemary Gladstar's Family Herbal.* North Adams, Mass.: Storey Publishing, 2001.

———. *Rosemary Gladstar's Herbal Recipes for Vibrant Health.* North Adams, Mass.: Storey Publishing, 2008.

Glatzel, H., and K. Hackenberg. "*Röntgenologische Untersuchungen der Wirkungen von Bittermitteln auf die Verdauungsorgane* (Radiographic studies on the feed-forward effects of bitter tastants on the digestive organs)." *Planta Medica* 3 (1967): 223–32.

Göbel, H., G. Schmidt, and D. Soyka. "Effect of Peppermint and Eucalyptus

Oil Preparations on Neurophysiological and Experimental Algesimetric Headache Parameters." *Cephalalgia* 14, no. 3 (1994): 228–34.

Göbel, H., J. Fresenius, A. Heinze, et al. "Effectiveness of Oleum Menthae Piperitae and Paracetamol in Therapy of Headache of the Tension Type." *Nervenarzt* 67, no. 8 (1996): 672–81.

Gordon, S. "Pattern Recognition Receptors: Doubling Up for the Innate Immune Response." *Cell* 111 (2002): 927–30.

Graf, B. A., P. E. Milbury, and J. B. Blumberg. "Flavonols, Flavones, Flavanones, and Human Health: Epidemiological Evidence." *Journal of Medicinal Food* 8, no. 3 (Fall 2005): 281–90.

Green, James. *The Male Herbal: Health Care for Men and Boys.* 2nd ed. Berkeley, Calif.: Crossing Press, 2007.

Greer, E. L., and A. Brunet. "FOXO Transcription Factors at the Interface between Longevity and Tumor Suppression." *Oncogene* 24 (2005): 7410–25.

Grieve, M., *A Modern Herbal.* New York: Barnes and Noble Books, 1996.

Grossinger, Richard. *Planet Medicine: Origins.* 6th ed. Berkeley, Calif.: North Atlantic Books, 1995.

Grossman, P. "Respiratory and Cardiac Rhythms as Windows to Central and Autonomic Biobehavioral Regulation: Selection Frames, Keeping the Panes Clean and Viewing Neural Topography." *Biological Psychology* 34 (1992): 131–61.

Grossman, P., and M. Kollai. "Respiratory Sinus Arrhythmia, Cardiac Vagal Tone, and Respiration: Within- and Between-Subject Relations." *Psychophysiology* 28 (1993): 201–16.

Guengerich, F. P. "Influence of Nutrients and Other Dietary Materials on Cytochrome P450 Enzymes." *American Journal of Clinical Nutrition* 61, no. 3 (1995): S651–S658.

Gusenoff, J. A., S. M. Harman, J. D. Veldhuis, et al. "Cortisol and GH Secretory Dynamics, and Their Interrelationships, in Healthy Aged Women and Men." *American Journal of Physiology—Endocrinology and Metabolism* 280, no. 4 (April 2001): E616–E625.

Guthrie, Rankin. "A Clinical Lecture on Colic." *British Medical Journal* 1, no. 12686 (June 22, 1912): 1409–12.

Hales, Stephen. *Statical Essays: Containing Haemostaticks; or, An Account of Some Hydraulik and Hydrostatical Experiments Made on the Blood and Blood-Vessels of Animals.* London: W. Innys, R. Manby, T. Woodward, 1733.

Haller, John S. *Medical Protestants: The Eclectics in American Medicine, 1825–1939.* Carbondale: Southern Illinois University Press, 1994.

Hansen, A. L., B. H. Johnsen, and J. F. Thayer. "Vagal Influence in the Regulation of Attention and Working Memory." *International Journal of Psychophysiology* 48 (2003): 263–74.

———. "Relationship between Heart Rate Variability and Cognitive Function during Threat of Shock." *Anxiety Stress Coping* 22 (2009): 77–89.

Hao, S., C. Sternini, and H. E. Raybould. "Role of CCK1 and Y2 Receptors in Activation of Hindbrain Neurons Induced by Intragastric Administration of Bitter Taste Receptor Ligands." *American Journal of Physiology—Regulatory, Integrative and Comparative Physiology* 294, no. 1 (January 2008): R33–R38.

Hayakawa, K., N. Mitsuhashi, Y. Sait, et al. "Effect of Krestin as Adjuvant Treatment Following Radical Radiotherapy in Non-small Cell Lung Cancer Patients." *Cancer Detection and Prevention* 21, no. 1 (1997): 71–77.

Heiser, Charles B. *Seed to Civilization: The Story of Food.* Cambridge, Mass.: Harvard University Press, 1990.

Herz, R. S. "Aromatherapy Facts and Fictions: A Scientific Analysis of Olfactory Effects on Mood, Physiology and Behavior." *International Journal of Neuroscience* 119, no. 2 (2009): 263–90.

Ho, J. T., H. Al-Musalhi, M. J. Chapman, et al. "Septic Shock and Sepsis: A Comparison of Total and Free Plasma Cortisol Levels." *Journal of Clinical Endocrinology and Metabolism* 91, no. 1 (January 2006): 105–14.

Hoffmann, David. *The New Holistic Herbal.* Rockport, Mass.: Element Books, 1991.

———. *Medical Herbalism: The Science Principles and Practices of Herbal Medicine.* Rochester, Vt.: Healing Arts Press, 2003.

———. "Herbs for Cardiovascular Health." Lecture at the 9th International Herb Symposium, Norton, Mass., 2009.

Hoffmann, J. A., F. C. Kafatos, C. A. Janeway Jr., et al. "Phylogenetic Perspectives in Innate Immunity." *Science* 284 (1999): 1313–18.

Hon, Edward H. "The Electronic Evaluation of Fetal Heart Rate." *American Journal of Obstetrics and Gynecology* 75 (1958): 1215–30.

Hon, Edward H., and S. T. Lee, "The Electronic Evaluation of Fetal Heart Rate. VIII. Patterns Preceding Fetal Death: Further Observations." *American College of Obstetrics and Gynecology* 87 (1963): 814.

Hood, R. "Anxiety Neurosis and the Prognosis of Heart Disease." *Journal of the Arkansas Medical Society* 49, no. 6 (1952): 93–96.

Hooper, L. V. "How Host-Microbial Interactions Shape the Nutrient Environment of the Mammalian Intestine." *Annual Review of Nutrition* (2002): 283–307.

Houghton, Peter, ed. *Valerian: The Genus Valeriana*. New York: CRC Press, 1997.

Huang, A. L., X. Chen, M. A. Hoon, et al. "The Cells and Logic for Mammalian Sour Taste Detection." *Nature* 442 (2006): 934–38.

Huikuri, H. V., J. O. Valkama, K. E. Airaksinen, et al. "Frequency Domain Measures of Heart Rate Variability before the Onset of Nonsustained and Sustained Ventricular Tachycardia in Patients with Coronary Artery Disease." *Circulation* 87, no. 4 (1993): 1220–28.

"Institute of HeartMath Research Library." www.heartmath.org/research/research-library/research-library.html (accessed October 27, 2011).

Iwashina, T. "Flavonoid Function and Activity to Plants and Other Organisms." *Biological Sciences in Space* 17, no. 1 (2003): 24–44.

Izzo, A. A., R. Capasso, F. Senatore, et al. "Spasmolytic Activity of Medicinal Plants Used for the Treatment of Disorders Involving Smooth Muscle." *Phytotherapy Research* 10 (1996): S107–S108.

Janeway, C. A., and Ruslan Medzhitov. "Innate Immune Recognition." *Annual Review of Immunology* 20 (2002): 197–216.

Jenuwein, T., and C. D. Allis. "Translating the Histone Code." *Science* 293, no. 5532 (August 10, 2001): 1074–80.

John, A. J., R. Cherian, H. S. Subhash, et al. "Evaluation of the Efficacy of Bitter Gourd (*Momordica Charantia*) as an Oral Hypoglycemic Agent: A Randomized Controlled Clinical Trial." *Indian Journal of Physiology and Pharmacology* 47, no. 3 (July 2003): 363–65.

Jones, David S., and Shiela Quinn, eds. *Textbook of Functional Medicine*. Gig Harbor, Wash.: Institute for Functional Medicine, 2005.

Jones, Lorenzo E., and John Milton Scudder. *The American Eclectic Materia Medica and Therapeutics*. 2 vols. Cincinnati: Medical Publishing Company, 1874.

Juergens, U. R., U. Dethlefsen, G. Steinkamp, et al. "Anti-inflammatory Activity of 1.8-Cineol (Eucalyptol) in Bronchial Asthma: A Double-Blind Placebo-Controlled Trial." *Respiratory Medicine* 97, no. 3 (2003): 250–56.

Justinus, Marcus Junianus. *Epitome of the Philippic History of Pompeius Trogus.* Translated by the Rev. John Selby Watson. London: Henry G. Bohn, 1853.

Kagan, Jerome. *Galen's Prophecy: Temperament in Human Nature.* New York: Basic Books, 1998.

Kalsbeek, J. K., and J. H. Ettema. "Scored Irregularity of the Heart Pattern and the Measurement of Perceptual or Mental Load." *Ergonomics* 6 (1963): 306–7.

Kamata, Y. "The Practicability of Horticultural Therapy for Asthmatic Children: Program Description." *Acta Horticolturae* (International Society for Horticultural Science) 790 (2008): 75–82.

Kandel, Eric R., James H. Schwartz, and Thomas M. Jessell, eds., *Principles of Neural Science.* 4th ed. New York: McGraw-Hill, 2000.

Kaptchuck, Ted J. *The Web That Has No Weaver.* Chicago: Contemporary Books, 2000.

Kaviratna, A. C. *The Charaka Samhita.* 5 vols. Indian Medical Science Series. Translated by P. V. Sharma. Delhi, India: Sri Satguru Publications, a Division of Indian Books Centre, 1997.

Kawaii, S., Y. Tomono, E. Katase, et al. "Antiproliferative Activity of Flavonoids on Several Cancer Cell Lines." *Bioscience, Biotechnology and Biochemistry* 63, no. 5 (May 1999): 896–99.

Kelly-Pieper, K., S. P. Patil, P. Busse, et al. "Safety and Tolerability of an Antiasthma Herbal Formula (ASHMI™) in Adult Subjects with Asthma: A Randomized, Double-Blinded, Placebo-Controlled, Dose-Escalation Phase I Study." *Journal of Alternative and Complementary Medicine* 15, no. 7 (July 2009): 735–43.

Kensil, C. R., S. Soltysik, D. A. Wheeler, et al. "Structure/Function Studies on QS-21, a Unique Immunological Adjuvant from Quillaja Saponaria." *Advances in Experimental Medicine and Biology* 404 (1996): 165–72.

Kessler, D., MD. *The End of Overeating: Taking Control of the Insatiable American Appetite.* Emmaus, PA: Rodale Press, 2009.

Kidd, P. "Th1/Th2 Balance: The Hypothesis, Its Limitations, and Implications for Health and Disease." *Alternative Medical Review* 8, no. 3 (August 2003): 223–46.

Kinnamon, S. C., and T. A. Cummings. "Chemosensory Transduction Mechanisms in Taste." *Annual Review of Physiology* 54 (1992): 715–31.

Kirakosyan, A., E. Seymour, P. B. Kaufman, et al. "Antioxidant Capacity of Polyphenolic Extracts from Leaves of Crataegus Laevigata and Crataegus

Monogyna (Hawthorn) Subjected to Drought and Cold Stress." *Journal of Agricultural and Food Chemistry* 51, no. 14 (2003): 3973–76.

Kirakosyan, A., P. Kaufman, S. Warber, et al. "Applied Environmental Stresses to Enhance the Levels of Polyphenolics in Leaves of Hawthorn Plants." *Physiologia Plantarum* 121, no. 2 (2004): 182–6.

Kirk-Smith, M., and D. Booth. "Effect of Androstenone on Choice of Location in Others' Presence." In *Olfaction and Taste VII,* edited by H. Van Der Starre, 397–400. London: IRL Press, 1980.

———. "Chemoreception in Human Behavior: An Analysis of the Social Effects of Fragrance." *Chemical Senses* 12 (1987): 159–66.

Kleiger, R. E., and J. P. Miller. "Decreased Heart Rate Variability and Its Association with Increased Mortality after Acute Myocardial Infarction." *American Journal of Cardiology* 59 (1987): 256–62.

Kohlert, C., I. Van Rensen, R. März, et al. "Bioavailability and Pharmacokinetics of Natural Volatile Terpenes in Animals and Humans." *Planta Medica* 66 (2000): 495–505.

Kubota, M., T. Ikemoto, R. Komaki, et al. "Odor and Emotion-Effects of Essential Oils on Contingent Negative Variation." In *Proceedings of the 12th International Congress on Flavors, Fragrances and Essential Oils,* October 4–8, 1992, edited by H. and G.Woidlich & Buchbauer, 456–61. Vienna, Austria: Fachzeitschriftenverlags, 1992.

Kuo, M. H., J. E. Brownell, R. E. Sobel, et al. "Transcription-Linked Acetylation by Gcn5p of Histones H3 and H4 at Specific Lysines." *Nature* 383, no. 6597 (September 19, 1996): 269–72.

Kürschner, H., T. Raus, and J. Venter. *Pflanzen der Türkei; Ägäis, Taurus, Inneranatolien (Plants of Turkey: Agains, Taurus, inner Anatolia).* Wiesbaden, Germany: Quelle & Meyer, 1995.

Lacey, J. I. "Somatic Response Patterning and Stress: Some Revisions of Activation Theory." In *Psychological Stress: Issues in Research,* edited by M. H. Appley and R. Trumbull, 14–44. New York: Appleton-Century-Crofts, 1967.

Lad, Vasant. *Textbook of Ayurveda, Volume 1: Fundamental Principles.* Albuquerque: Ayurvedic Press, 2011.

Laguerette, F., D. Gaillard, P. Passilly-Degrace, et al. "Do We Taste Fat?" *Biochimie* 89 (2007): 265–69.

Lall, N., and J. J. Meyer. "In Vitro Inhibition of Drug-Resistant and Drug-Sensitive Strains of Mycobacterium Tuberculosis by Ethnobotanically

Selected South African Plants." *Journal of Ethnopharmacology* 66, no. 3 (1999): 347–54.

Lane, R. D., K. McRae, E. M. Reiman, et al. "Neural Correlates of Heart Rate Variability during Emotion." *Neuroimage* 44 (2009): 213–22.

Lane, R. D., E. M. Reiman, G. L. Ahern, and J. F. Thayer. "Activity in Medial Prefrontal Cortex Correlates with Vagal Component of Heart Rate Variability During Emotion." *Brain and Cognition* 47 (2001): 97–100.

Lane, R. D., H. Weidenbacher, C. L. Fort, et al. "Subgenual Anterior Cingulate (BA25) Activity Covaries with Changes in Cardiac Vagal Tone During Affective Set Shifting in Healthy Adults." *Psychosomatic Medicine* 70 (2008): A–42.

Larkin, Tim. "Cortisone: The Limits of a Miracle." *Nutrition Health Review: The Consumer's Medical Journal,* no. 60 (Autumn 1991): 12.

Lazarev, N. V. "General and Specific Effects of Drugs." *Farmacol Toxicol* 21, no. 3 (1958): 81–86.

Lee, H. I., L. Cao, R. Mostoslavsky, et al. "A Role for the NAD-Dependent Deacetylase Sirt1 in the Regulation of Autophagy." *Proceedings of the National Academy of Sciences USA* 105, no. 9 (March 4, 2008): 3374–79.

Lewith, G. T., A. D. Godfrey, and P. Prescott. "A Single-Blinded, Randomized Pilot Study Evaluating the Aroma of Lavandula Augustifolia as a Treatment for Mild Insomnia." *Journal of Alternative and Complementary Medicine* 11, no. 4 (2005): 631–37.

Li, E. K., L. S. Tam, C. K. Wong, et al. "Safety and Efficacy of Ganoderma Lucidum (Lingzhi) and San Miao San Supplementation in Patients with Rheumatoid Arthritis: A Double-Blind, Randomized, Placebo-Controlled Pilot Trial." *Arthritis and Rheumatism* 57, no. 7 (October 15, 2007): 1143–50.

Li, X., L. Staszewski, H. Xu, et al. "Human Receptors for Sweet and Umami Taste." *Proceedings of the National Academy of Sciences USA* 99 (2002): 4692–96.

Li, Xia, N. Ma, H. Guo, et al. "Research on Ultrasonic-Assisted Extraction of Flavonoid from Schizandra Chinensis (Turcz) Baill." *Contemporary Eco-Agriculture* Z2 (2010): 47–48.

Li-Zhen, Cao, and Lin Zhi-Bin. "Regulation on Maturation and Function of Dendritic Cells by Ganoderma Lucidum Polysaccharides." *Immunology Letters* 83, no. 3 (October 1, 2002): 163–69.

Liddle, R. A. "Physiological Role for Cholecystokinin in Reducing Postprandial Hyperglycemia in Humans." *Journal of Clinical Investigation* 81, no. 6 (June 1988): 1675–81.

Lin, Y. L., S. S. Lee, S. M. Hou, et al. "Polysaccharide Purified from Ganoderma Lucidum Induces Gene Expression Changes in Human Dendritic Cells and Promotes T Helper 1 Immune Response in BALB/c Mice." *Molecular Pharmacology* 70, no. 2 (August 2006): 637–44.

Lindemann, B. "Chemoreception: Tasting the Sweet and the Bitter." *Current Biology* 6, no. 10 (October 1996): 1234–47.

———. "Receptors and Transduction in Taste." *Nature* 413 (2001): 219–25.

Lis-Balchin, Maria. "Comparison of the Pharmacological and Antimicrobial Action of Commercial Plant Essential Oils." *Journal of Herbs, Spices and Medicinal Plants* 4 (1996): 69–86.

———. *Aromatherapy Science*. New York: Pharmaceutical Press, 2006.

Lis-Balchin, Maria, and S. Hart. "The Effect of Essential Oils on the Uterus Compared to That on Other Muscles." In *Proceedings of the 27th International Symposium on Essential Oils,* edited by C. H. Franz, et al., 29–32. Carol Stream, Ill.: Allured Publishing, 1996.

———. "A Preliminary Study on the Effects of Essential Oils on Skeletal and Smooth Muscle in Vitro." *Journal of Ethnopharmacology* 58 (1997): 183–87.

———. "Spasmolytic Activity of the Essential Oils of Scented Pelargoniums (Geraniaceae)." *Phytotherapy Research* 11 (1997): 583–84.

Lis-Balchin, Maria, S. Deans, and S. Hart. "Bioactivity of New Zealand Medicinal Plant Essential Oils." In *Proceedings of the International Symposium on Medicinal and Aromatic Plants,* edited by L. E. Cracker, et al., 13–27. New York: Haworth Press, 1996.

Little, T. J., N. Gupta, R. M. Case, et al. "Sweetness and Bitterness Taste of Meals Per Se Does Not Mediate Gastric Emptying in Humans." *American Journal of Physiology—Regulatory, Integrative and Comparative Physiology* 297, no. 3 (September 2009): R632–R639.

Liu, J. H., G. H. Chen, H. Z. Yeh, et al. "Enteric-Coated Peppermint-Oil Capsules in the Treatment of Irritable Bowel Syndrome: A Prospective, Randomized Trial." *Journal of Gastroenterology* 32, no. 6 (1997): 765–68.

Lixandru, B. E., N. O. Drăcea, C. C. Dragomirescu, et al. "Antimicrobial Activity of Plant Essential Oils against Bacterial and Fungal Species Involved in

Food Poisoning and/or Food Decay." *Roumanian Archives of Microbiology and Immunology* 69, no. 4 (2010): 224–30.

Loss, G., S. Apprich, M. Waser, et al. "The Protective Effect of Farm Milk Consumption on Childhood Asthma and Atopy: The GABRIELA Study." *Journal of Allergy and Clinical Immunology* 128, no. 4 (October 2008): 766–73.

Louv, Richard. *Last Child in the Woods: Saving Our Children from Nature-Deficit Disorder.* Chapel Hill, N.C.: Algonquin Books, 2008.

———. *The Nature Principle: Human Restoration and the End of Nature-Deficit Disorder.* Chapel Hill, N.C.: Algonquin Books, 2011.

Lovelock, James E., and C. E. Giffen. "Planetary Atmospheres: Compositional and Other Changes Associated with the Presence of Life, Advanced Space Experiments." *Advances in the Astronautical Sciences* 25 (1969): 179–93.

Lovelock, James, and Lynn Margulis. "Atmospheric Homeostasis by and for the Biosphere: The Gaia Hypothesis." *Tellus* 26 (1974): 2–10.

Lowry, C. A., J. H. Hollis, A. De Vries, et al. "Identification of an Immune-Responsive Mesolimbocortical Serotonergic System: Potential Role in Regulation of Emotional Behavior." *Neuroscience* 146, no. 2 (May 2007): 756–72.

Macalister, Robert A. S., ed. and trans. *"Lebor Gabála Érenn* (The Book of the Taking of Ireland)." Dublin: Irish Texts Society by the Educational Company of Ireland, 1938. www.archive.org/details/leborgablare00macauoft (accessed May 5, 2012).

Macht, D. I., and G. C. Ting. "Experimental Inquiry into the Sedative Properties of Some Aromatic Drugs and Fumes." *Journal of Pharmacology and Experimental Therapeutics* 18 (1921): 361–72.

Maholick, L., and R. B. Logue. "Psychosomatic Aspects of Heart Disease: Anxiety Hysteria in a Patient with Patent Ductus Arteriosus." *Annals of Internal Medicine* 30, no. 5 (1949): 1043–49.

Manley, C. H. "Psychophysiological Effects of Odor." *Critical Reviews in Food Science and Nutrition* 33 (1993): 57–62.

Manniche, L. *Sacred Luxuries: Fragrance, Aromatherapy and Cosmetics in Ancient Egypt.* London: Opus Publishing, 1999.

Masterman, D. L., and J. L. Cummings. "Frontal-Subcortical Circuits: The Anatomical Basis of Executive, Social and Motivated Behaviors." *Journal of Psychopharmacology* 11 (1997): 107–14.

Matkovic, Z., V. Zivkovic, M. Korica, et al. "Efficacy and Safety of Astragalus

Membranaceus in the Treatment of Patients with Seasonal Allergic Rhinitis." *Phytotherapy Research* 24, no. 2 (February 2010): 175–81.

Matsubara, E., M. Fukagawa, T. Okamoto, et al. "The Essential Oil of *Abies sibirica* (Pinaceae) Reduces Arousal Levels After Visual Display Terminal Work." *Flavor and Fragrance Journal* 26, no. 3 (2011): 204–10.

———."Volatiles Emitted from the Leaves of Laurus Nobilis L. Improve Vigilance Performance in Visual Discrimination Task." *Biomedical Research* 32, no. 1 (2011): 19–28.

———."(–)–Bornyl Acetate Induces Autonomic Relaxation and Reduces Arousal Level After Visual Display Terminal Work without Any Influences of Task Performance in Low-Dose Condition." *Biomedical Research* 32, no. 2 (2011): 151–57.

Mayor, A. *The Poison King: The Life and Legend of Mithridates*. Princeton, N.J.: Princeton University Press, 2010.

McCraty, Rollin. "Heart Rhythm Coherence—An Emerging Area of Biofeedback." *Biofeedback* 30, no. 1 (2002): 23–25.

McCraty, Rollin, and Doc Childre. "Psychophysiological Correlates of Spiritual Experience." *Biofeedback* 29, no. 4 (2001): 13–17.

———. "The Grateful Heart: The Psychophysiology of Appreciation." In *The Psychology of Gratitude*, edited by Robert A. Emmons and Michael E. McCullough, 230–55. New York: Oxford University Press, 2004.

———. "Coherence: Bridging Personal, Social, and Global Health." *Alternative Therapies in Health and Medicine* 16, no. 4 (2010): 10–24.

McCraty, Rollin, and Dana Tomasino. "Emotional Stress, Positive Emotions, and Psychophysiological Coherence." In *Stress in Health and Disease*, edited by Bengt B. Arnetz and Rolf Ekman, 342–65. Weinheim, Germany: Wiley-VCH, 2006.

McCraty, Rollin, M. Atkinson, and W. A. Tiller. "Cardiac Coherence: A New, Noninvasive Measure of Autonomic System Order." *Alternative Therapies in Health and Medicine* 2, no. 1 (1996): 52–65.

McCraty, Rollin, M. Atkinson, D. Tomasino, and W. P. Stuppy. "Analysis of Twenty-Four Hour Heart Rate Variability in Patients with Panic Disorder." *Biological Psychology* 56, no. 2 (2001): 131–50.

McCraty, Rollin, M. Atkinson, W. A. Tiller, et al. "The Effects of Emotions on Short-Term Power Spectrum Analysis of Heart Rate Variability." *American Journal of Cardiology* 76, no. 14 (1995): 1089–93.

McCraty, Rollin, M. Atkinson, D. Tomasino, et al. "The Impact of an Emotional Self-Management Skills Course on Psychosocial Functioning and Autonomic Recovery to Stress in Middle School Children." *Integrative Physiological and Behavioral Science* 34, no. 4 (1999): 246–68.

McCraty, Rollin, B. Barrios-Choplin, M. Atkinson, and D. Tomasino. "The Effects of Different Types of Music on Mood, Tension, and Mental Clarity." *Alternative Therapies in Health and Medicine* 4, no. 1 (1998): 75–84.

McCraty, Rollin, B. Barrios-Choplin, D. Rozman, et al. "The Impact of a New Emotional Self-Management Program on Stress, Emotions, Heart Rate Variability, DHEA and Cortisol." *Integrative Physiological and Behavioral Science* 33, no. 2 (1998): 151–70.

McMeekin, D. "The Perception of Ganoderma Lucidum in Chinese and Western Culture." *Mycologist* 18 (2004): 165–69.

Mensah, J. K., R. I. Okoli, A. A. Turay, et al. "Phytochemical Analysis of Medicinal Plants Used for the Management of Hypertension by Esan People of Edo State, Nigeria." *Ethnobotanical Leaflets* no. 10 (2009): 7.

Meyerhof, W., C. Batram, C. Kuhn, et al. "The Molecular Receptive Ranges of Human TAS2R Bitter Taste Receptors." *Chemical Senses* 35, no. 2 (2010): 157–70.

Mezzacappa, E., U. Arumugam, S. Y. Chen, et al. "Coconut Fragrance and Cardiovascular Response to Laboratory Stress: Results of Pilot Testing." *Holistic Nursing Practice* 24, no. 6 (2010): 322–32.

Middleton, E., C. Kandaswami, and T. C. Theoharides. "The Effects of Plant Flavonoids on Mammalian Cells: Implications for Inflammation, Heart Disease, and Cancer." *Pharmacological Reviews* 52, no. 4 (December 1, 2000): 673–751.

Mills, Simon, and Kerry Bone. *Principles and Practices of Phytotherapy*. Edinburgh, UK: Elsevier Churchill Livingstone, 2000.

———. *The Essential Guide to Herbal Safety*. Edinburgh, UK: Elsevier Churchill Livingstone, 2005.

Ming-Shun, Chen. "Inducible Direct Plant Defense against Insect Herbivores: A Review." *Insect Science* 15, no. 2 (April 2008): 101–14.

Moorman, J. E., R. A. Rudd, C. A. Johnson, et al. "National Surveillance for Asthma—United States, 1980–2004." *Surveillance Summaries* 56, no. S S08 (October 19, 2007): 1–14; 18–54.

Morley, J. F., D. Weintraub, E. Mamikonyan, et al. "Olfactory Dysfunction Is

Associated with Neuropsychiatric Manifestations in Parkinson's Disease." *Movement Disorders* 26, no. 11 (2011): 2051–57.

Moskalenko, S. A. "Slavic Ethnomedicine in the Soviet Far East. Part I: Herbal Remedies Among Russians/Ukrainians in the Sukhodol Valley, Primorye." *Journal of Ethnopharmacology* 21, no. 3 (1987): 231–51.

Mosmann, T. R., and R. L. Coffman. "TH1 and TH2 Cells: Different Patterns of Lymphokine Secretion Lead to Different Functional Properties." *Annual Review of Immunology* 7 (1989): 145–73.

Nakahara, H., S. Furuya, S. Obata, et al. "Emotion-Related Changes in Heart Rate and Its Variability During Performance and Perception of Music." *Annals of the New York Academy of Sciences* 1169 (2009): 359–62.

Nelson, G., J. Chandrashekar, M. A. Hoon, et al. "An Amino-Acid Taste Receptor." *Nature* 416 (2002): 199–202.

Nesvold, A., M. W. Fagerland, S. Davanger, et al. "Increased Heart Rate Variability during Nondirective Meditation." *European Journal of Cardiovascular Prevention and Rehabilitation* (June 21, 2011): 773–80.

Ni, Maoshing, trans. *The Yellow Emperor's Classic of Medicine: A New Translation of the Neijing Suwen with Commentary*. Boston: Shambhala Publications, 1995.

Norton, S. "The Pharmacology of Mithridatum: A 2000-Year-Old Remedy." *Molecular Intervention* 6, no. 2 (April 2006): 60–66.

Notarangelo, L. D., A. Fischer, R. S. Geha, et al. "Primary Immunodeficiencies: 2009 Update: The International Union of Immunological Societies (IUIS) Primary Immunodeficiencies (PID) Expert Committee." *Journal of Allergy and Clinical Immunology* 124, no. 6 (December 2009): 1161–78.

Nugent, A. C., E. E. Bain, J. F. Thayer, et al. "Alterations in Neural Correlates of Autonomic Control in Females with Major Depressive Disorder." *Psychosomatic Medicine* 70 (2008): A–99.

Nugent, A. C., E. E. Bain, J. F. Thayer, and W. C. Drevets. "Anatomical Correlates of Autonomic Control During a Motor Task." *Psychosomatic Medicine* 69 (2007): A–74.

Oh, R., and D. L. Brown. "Vitamin B_{12} Deficiency." *American Family Physician* 67, no. 5 (March 2003): 979–86.

Ohwada, S. "Adjuvant Therapy with Protein-Bound Polysaccharide K and Tegafur Uracil in Patients with Stage II or III Colorectal Cancer: Randomized, Controlled Trial." *Diseases of the Colon and Rectum* 46, no. 8 (August 2003): 1060–68.

Ohwada S., T. Ogawa, F. Makita, et al. "Beneficial Effects of Protein-Bound Polysaccharide K Plus Tegafur/Uracil in Patients with Stage II or III Colorectal Cancer: Analysis of Immunological Parameters." *Oncology Report* 15, no. 4 (April 2006): 861–68.

Olukoga, A., and D. Donaldson. "Liquorice and Its Health Implications." *Journal of the Royal Society for the Promotion of Health* 120, no. 2 (June 2000): 83–89.

Panda, A., A. Arjona, E. Sapey, et al. "Human Innate Immunosenescence: Causes and Consequences for Immunity in Old Age." *Trends in Immunology* 30, no. 7 (July 2009): 325–33.

Park, B. J., Y. Tsunetsugu, T. Kasetani, et al. "The Physiological Effects of Shinrin-yoku (Taking in the Forest Atmosphere or Forest Bathing): Evidence from Field Experiments in 24 Forests across Japan." *Environmental Health and Preventative Medicine* 15, no. 1 (2010): 18–26.

Park, C. S., M. H. Yoo, K. H. Noh, et al. "Biotransformation of Ginsenosides by Hydrolyzing the Sugar Moieties of Ginsenosides Using Microbial Glycosidases." *Applied Microbiology and Biotechnology* 87, no. 1 (June 2010): 9–19.

Pendelton, J. "Hawthorn Herbal Extract and Cardiac Health: Crataegus Species Protect and Support the Heart." 2009. http://jamespendleton.suite101.com/hawthorn-extract-and-cardiac-health-a131747#ixzz1smIuHvYj (accessed May 12, 2012).

Peng, S. M., M. Koo, and Z. R. Yu. "Effects of Music and Essential Oil Inhalation on Cardiac Autonomic Balance in Healthy Individuals." *Journal of Alternative and Complementary Medicine* 15, no. 1 (2009): 53–57.

Peressutti, C., J. M. Martín-González, M. García-Manso, et al. "Heart Rate Dynamics in Different Levels of Zen Meditation." *International Journal of Cardiology* 145, no. 1 (2010): 142–46.

Pérez-Vizcaíno, F., and J. Duarte. "Flavonols: Biochemistry behind Cardiovascular Effects, in Plant Phenolics and Human Health." In *Plant Phenolics and Human Health: Biochemistry, Nutrition, and Pharmacology,* edited by Cesar G. Fraga, 197–214. Hoboken, N.J.: John Wiley & Sons, 2009.

Perkin, M. R., and D. P. Strachan. "Which Aspects of the Farming Lifestyle Explain the Inverse Association with Childhood Allergy?" *Journal of Allergy and Clinical Immunology* 117, no. 6 (2006): 1374–81.

Petersen, F. J. *Materia Medica and Clinical Therapeutics.* Los Olivos, Calif.: F. J. Petersen, M.D., 1905.

Pier, Gerald B., Jefferey B. Lyczak, and Lee M. Wetzler. *Immunology, Infection, and Immunity.* Herndon, Va.: American Society for Microbiology Press, 2004.

Pillai, A. K., K. K. Sharma, Y. K. Gupta, et al. "Anti-emetic Effect of Ginger Powder Versus Placebo as an Add-on Therapy in Children and Young Adults Receiving High Emetogenic Chemotherapy." *Pediatric Blood and Cancer* 56, no. 2 (2011): 234–38.

Pizzi, C., L. Manzoli, S. Mancini, et al. "Analysis of Potential Predictors of Depression among Coronary Heart Disease Risk Factors Including Heart Rate Variability, Markers of Inflammation, and Endothelial Function." *European Heart Journal* 29, no. 9 (2008): 1110–17.

Pliny. *Natural History.* Translated by H. Rackham. Cambridge, Mass: Harvard University Press, Loeb Classical Library, 1938.

Ploeger, B., T. Mensinga, A. Sips, et al. "The Pharmacokinetics of Glycyrrhizic Acid Evaluated by Physiologically Based Pharmacokinetic Modeling." *Drug Metabolism Review* 33, no. 2 (May 2001): 125–47.

Pollan, Michael. *The Botany of Desire.* New York: Random House, 2001.

———. *The Omnivore's Dilemma.* London: The Penguin Press, 2006.

———. *In Defense of Food.* London: The Penguin Press, 2008.

Prabhakar, P. K., and M. Doble. "A Target-Based Therapeutic Approach to Diabetes Mellitus Using Medicinal Plants." *Current Diabetes Reviews* 4 (2008): 291–308.

Proville, J. J., and Will Blunt. "Spring Medicinals from Apothéke's Chemist-Mixologists." March 2009. www.starchefs.com/features/spring_medicinal_cocktails/index.shtml (accessed March 7, 2012).

Rajendran, R., R. Garva, M. Krstic-Demonacos, et al. "Sirtuins: Molecular Traffic Lights in the Crossroad of Oxidative Stress, Chromatin Remodeling, and Transcription." *Journal of Biomedicine and Biotechnology,* 2011, Article ID 368276: 1–17.

Ramiro, E., À. Franch, C. Castellote, et al. "Flavonoids from Theobroma Cacao Down-Regulate Inflammatory Mediators." *Journal of Agricultural and Food Chemistry* 53, no. 22 (November 2, 2005): 8506–11.

Remes, S. T., K. Iivanainen, H. Koskela, et al. "Which Factors Explain the Lower Prevalence of Atopy Amongst Farmers' Children?" *Clinical and Experimental Allergy* 33, no. 4 (2003): 427–34.

Rigelsky, J. M., and B. V. Sweet, "Hawthorn: Pharmacology and Therapeutic Uses." *American Journal of Health-System Pharmacy* 59, no. 5 (2002): 417–22.

Rimmel, Eugene. *The Book of Perfumes*. London: Chapman and Hall, 1865.

Roberts, A., and J. M. G. Williams. "The Effect of Olfactory Stimulation on Fluency, Vividness of Imagery and Associated Mood: A Preliminary Study, Part 2." *British Journal of Medical Psychology* 65 (1992): 197–99.

Rolls, B. J., L. S. Roe, and J. S. Meengs. "Salad and Satiety: Energy Density and Portion Size of a First-Course Salad Affect Energy Intake at Lunch." *Journal of the American Dietetic Association* 104, no. 10 (October 2004): 1570–76.

Romagnani, S. "The Th1/Th2 Paradigm." *Immunology Today* 18, no. 6 (1997): 263–66.

Rosenthal, Gerald A., and May Berenbaum. In *Herbivores, Their Interactions with Secondary Plant Metabolites: Ecological and Evolutionary Processes*, edited by G.A. Rosenthal and M. Berenbaum, 221–49. New York: Academic Press, 1992.

Ross, S. M. "An Integrative Approach to Rhinosinusitis in Children." *Holistic Nurse Practice* 23, no. 5 (September–October 2009): 302–4.

Rozengurt, E. "Taste Receptors in the Gastrointestinal Tract. I. Bitter Taste Receptors and Alpha-gustducin in the Mammalian Gut." *American Journal of Physiology—Gastrointestinal and Liver Physiology* 291, no. 2 (August 2006): G171–G177.

Rushforth, Keith. *Trees of Britain and Europe*. London: Collins, 1999.

Ryan, J. L., C. E. Heckler, J. A. Roscoe, et al. "Ginger (Zingiber Officinale) Reduces Acute Chemotherapy-Induced Nausea: A URCC CCOP Study of 576 Patients." *Support Care Cancer* (2011): 1479–89.

Sadako, N. "The Effects of Gardening Therapy for Asthmatic Children." *Allergy in Practice* 286 (2002): 150–53.

Saller, R., R. Brignoli, J. Melzer, et al. "An Updated Systematic Review with Meta-analysis for the Clinical Evidence of Silymarin." *Forschende Komplementärmedizin (Research-based Complementary Medicine)* 15, no. 1 (February 2008): 9–20.

Sanderson, I. R. "Dietary Modulation of GALT." *Journal of Nutrition* 137, no. 11 (November 2007): S2557–S2562.

Sannia, A. "Phytotherapy with a Mixture of Dry Extracts with Hepato-Protective Effects Containing Artichoke Leaves in the Management of

Functional Dyspepsia Symptoms." *Minerva Gastroenterologica e Dietologica* 56, no. 2 (June 2010): 93–99.

Sarris, J., D. J. Kavanagh, G. Byrne, et al. "The Kava Anxiety Depression Spectrum Study (KADSS): A Randomized, Placebo-Controlled Crossover Trial Using an Aqueous Extract of Piper Methysticum." *Psychopharmacology* (Berlin) 205, no. 3 (2009): 399–407.

Saul, P., Y. Arai, R. D. Berger, et al. "Assessment of Autonomic Regulation in Congestive Heart Failure by Heart Rate Spectral Analysis." *American Journal of Cardiology* 61 (1988): 1292–99.

Scarborough, J., and V. Nutton. "The Preface of Dioscorides' Materia Medica: Introduction, Translation, and Commentary." *Transactions and Studies of the College of Physicians of Philadelphia* 4, no. 3 (1982): 187–227.

Schar, D. D. "Adaptogens in the Eclectic Materia Medica." Advanced Study in Complementary Health Studies thesis, University of Exeter, May 11, 2006.

Schepetkin, I. A., and M. T. Quinn. "Botanical Polysaccharides: Macrophage Immunomodulation and Therapeutic Potential." *International Immunopharmacology* 6 (2006): 317–33.

Schier, L. A., T. L. Davidson, and T. L. Powley. "Ongoing Ingestive Behavior Is Rapidly Suppressed by a Preabsorptive, Intestinal 'Bitter Taste' Cue." *American Journal of Physiology—Regulatory, Integrative and Comparative Physiology* 301, no. 5 (November 2011): R1557–R1568.

Schlotz, W., J. Hellhammer, P. Schulz, et al. "Perceived Work Overload and Chronic Worrying Predict Weekend-Weekday Differences in the Cortisol Awakening Response." *Psychosomatic Medicine* 66, no. 2 (March–April 2004): 207–14.

Schneider, J. J. "Human Defensins." *Journal of Molecular Medicine* 83, no. 8 (2005): 587–95.

Schoeninger, M. J. "The Agricultural 'Revolution': Its Effect on Human Diet in Prehistoric Iran and Israel." *Paléorient* 7, no. 1 (1981): 73–91.

Scott, T. R., and J. V. Verhagen. "Taste as a Factor in the Management of Nutrition." *Nutrition* 16, no. 10 (October 2000): 874–85.

Scudder, John Milton. *The Eclectic Physician.* 21st ed. Cincinnati: John K. Scudder, 1887.

Seckl, J. R., and B. R. Walker. "Minireview: 11Beta-Hydroxysteroid Dehydrogenase Type 1—A Tissue-Specific Amplifier of Glucocorticoid Action." *Endocrinology* 142, no. 4 (April 2001): 1371–76.

Seery, M. D., E. A. Holman, and R. C. Silver. "Whatever Does Not Kill Us: Cumulative Lifetime Adversity, Vulnerability, and Resilience." *Journal of Personality and Social Psychology* 99 (2010): 1025–41.

Selye, Hans. *The Physiology and Pathology of Exposure to Stress: A Treatise Based on the Concepts of the General Adaptation Syndrome and the Diseases of Adaptation.* Montreal: Acta Inc. Medical Publishers, 1950.

Shimamura, A. P. "The Role of the Prefrontal Cortex in Dynamic Filtering." *Psychophysiology* 28 (2000): 207–18.

Shore, D., M. Squire, and K. A. Nasmyth. "Characterization of Two Genes Required for the Position-Effect Control of Yeast Mating-Type Genes." *European Molecular Biology Organization Journal* 3, no. 12 (1984): 2817–23.

Sigma-Aldrich. "Williams' Medium E Formulation." *Aldrich's Catalog of Fine Chemicals*, 2012, www.sigmaaldrich.com/life-science/cell-culture/learning-center/media-formulations/williams.html# (accessed March 17, 2012).

Singh, A., and P. K. Singh. "An Ethnobotanical Study of Medicinal Plants in Chandauli District of Uttar Pradesh." *Indian Journal of Ethnopharmacology* 121, no. 2 (2009): 324–29.

Singh, J. P., M. G. Larson, H. Tsuji, et al. "Reduced Heart Rate Variability and New-Onset Hypertension: Insights into Pathogenesis of Hypertension: The Framingham Heart Study." *Hypertension* 32, no. 2 (1998): 293–97.

Singh, N., M. Vrontakis, F. Parkinson, et al. "Functional Bitter Taste Receptors Are Expressed in Brain Cells." *Biochemical and Biophysical Research Communications* 406 (2001): 146–51.

Singh, R. B., C. Kartik, K. Otsuka, et al. "Brain-Heart Connection and the Risk of Heart Attack." *Biomedical Pharmacotherapy* 56, no. 2 (2002): S257–S265.

Singh, R. P., and R. Agarwal. "Natural Flavonoids Targeting Deregulated Cell Cycle Progression in Cancer Cells." *Current Drug Targets* 7, no. 3 (March 2006): 345–54.

Singh, Simon, and Edzard Ernst. *Trick or Treatment?: The Undeniable Facts About Alternative Medicine.* New York: W.W. Norton and Co., 2008.

Singletary, K. W., and J. T. Rokusek. "Tissue-Specific Enhancement of Xenobiotic Detoxification Enzymes in Mice by Dietary Rosemary Extract." *Plant Foods for Human Nutrition* (formerly *Qualitas Plantarum*) 50, no. 1 (1997): 47–53.

Smith, C. "Ginger Reduces Severity of Nausea in Early Pregnancy Compared with Vitamin B$_6$, and the Two Treatments Are Similarly Effective for Reducing Number of Vomiting Episodes." *Evidence-Based Nursing* 13, no. 2 (2010): 40.

Sternini, C. "Taste Receptors in the Gastrointestinal Tract. IV. Functional Implications of Bitter Taste Receptors in Gastrointestinal Chemosensing." *American Journal of Physiology* 292, no. 2 (2007): G457–G461.

Strachan, D. P. "Hay Fever, Hygiene, and Household Size." *British Medical Journal* 299, no. 6710 (November 1989): 1259–60.

Suh, Nan-Joo, C. K. Shim, M. H. Lee, et al. "Pharmacokinetic Study of an Iridoid Glucoside: Aucubin." *Pharmaceutical Research* 8, no. 8 (1991): 1059–63.

Taberlay, P. C., and P. A. Jones. "DNA Methylation and Cancer." *Epigenetics and Disease, Progress in Drug Research* 67 (2011): 1–23.

Tainter, M. "The Rise of Synthetic Drugs in the American Pharmaceutical Industry." *Bulletin of the New York Academy of Medicine* 35, no. 6 (1959): 387–405.

Tama, S. W., M. Worcel, and M. Wyllie. "Yohimbine: A Clinical Review." *Pharmacology and Therapeutics* 91, no. 3 (September 2001): 215–43.

Tang, W., Y. Gao, G. Chen, et al. "A Randomized, Double-Blind and Placebo-Controlled Study of a Ganoderma Lucidum Polysaccharide Extract in Neurasthenia." *Journal of Medicinal Food* 8, no. 1 (Spring 2005): 53–58.

Teeguarden, Ron. *The Ancient Wisdom of Chinese Tonic Herbs.* New York: Warner Books, 1998.

Thayer, J. F., B. H. Johnsen, A. L. Hansen, et al. "Heart Rate Variability Is Inversely Related to Cortisol Reactivity during Cognitive Stress." *Psychosomatic Medicine* 64 (2002): 289.

———. "Heart Rate Variability and Its Relation to Prefrontal Cognitive Function: The Effects of Training and Detraining." *European Journal of Applied Physiology* 93 (2004): 263–72.

Thayer, J. F., A. L. Hansen, E. Saus-Rose, et al. "Heart Rate Variability, Prefrontal Neural Function, and Cognitive Performance: The Neurovisceral Integration Perspective on Self-Regulation, Adaptation, and Health." *Annals of Behavior Medicine* 37, no. 2 (2009): 141–53.

Thayer, J. F., C. S. Weber, M. Rudat, et al. "Low Vagal Tone Is Associated with Impaired Post Stress Recovery of Cardiovascular, Endocrine, and Immune Markers." *European Journal of Applied Physiology* 109, no. 2 (2010): 201–11.

Thayer, J. F., B. Verkuil, J. F. Brosschot, et al. "Effects of Momentary Assessed Stressful Events and Worry Episodes on Somatic Health Complaints." *Psychological Health* 28 (2010): 1–18.

Thayer, J. F., S. S. Yamamoto, and J. F. Brosschot. "The Relationship of Autonomic Imbalance, Heart Rate Variability and Cardiovascular Disease Risk Factors." *International Journal of Cardiology* 141, no. 2 (2010): 122–31.

Thayer, J. F., L. Taylor, A. Loerbroks, et al. "Depression and Smoking: Mediating Role of Vagal Tone and Inflammation." *Annals of Behavioral Medicine* 42, no. 3 (2011): 334–40.

Thayer, J. F., T. W. Smith, M. R. Cribbet, et al. "Matters of the Variable Heart: Respiratory Sinus Arrhythmia Response to Marital Interaction and Associations with Marital Quality." *Journal of Personal and Social Psychology* 100, no. 1 (2011): 103–19.

Thayer, J. F., and B. H. Friedman. "The Heart of Anxiety: A Dynamical Systems Approach." In *The (Non) Expression of Emotions in Health and Disease,* edited by A. Vingerhoets, 39–48. Amsterdam, Netherlands: Springer, 1997.

Thayer, Julian F. *Zaku.* Union City, NJ: KSJAZZ Label, 2007. Compact Disc.

Thiagalingam, S., K. H. Cheng, H. J. Le, et al. "Histone Deacetylases: Unique Players in Shaping the Epigenetic Histone Code." *Annals of the New York Academy of Science* 983 (March 2003): 84–100.

Tierra, Michael. *Planetary Herbology.* Twin Lakes, WI: Lotus Press, 1988.

———. *The Way of Chinese Herbs.* New York: Pocket Books, 1998.

Toft-Nielsen, M., S. Madsbad, and J. Holst. "Determinants of the Effectiveness of Glucagon-like Peptide-1 in Type 2 Diabetes." *Journal of Clinical Endocrinology and Metabolism* 86, no. 8 (2001): 3853–60.

Toil, M., T. Hattori, M. Akagi, et al. "Randomized Adjuvant Trial to Evaluate the Addition of Tamoxifen and PSK to Chemotherapy in Patients with Primary Breast Cancer. 5-Year Results from the Nishi-Nippon Group of the Adjuvant Chemoendocrine Therapy for Breast Cancer Organization." *Cancer* 70, no. 10 (November 15, 1992): 2475–83.

Toller, S. V. "Assessing the Impact of Anosmia: Review of a Questionnaire's Findings." *Chemical Senses* 24, no. 6 (1999): 705–12.

Torii, S., H. Fukuda, H. Kanemoto, et al. "Contingent Negative Variation and the Physiological Effects of Odor." In *Perfumery: The Psychology and Biology of Fragrance,* edited by Steve Van Toller and G. H. Dodd, 235–46. New York: Chapman and Hall, 1988.

Trickey, R. *Women, Hormones and the Menstrual Cycle*. Sydney, Australia: Allen and Unwin, 2004.

Tsuji, P. A., and T. Walle. "Cytotoxic Effects of the Dietary Flavones Chrysin and Apigenin in a Normal Trout Liver Cell Line." *Chemico-Biological Interactions* 171, no. 1 (January 2008): 37–44.

Tsukagoshi, S., Y. Hashimoto, G. Fujii, et al. "Krestin (PSK)." *Cancer Treatment Reviews* 11, no. 2 (June 1984): 131–55.

Tsunetsugu, Y., B. J. Park, and Y. Miyazak. "Trends in Research Related to 'Shinrin-yoku' (Taking in the Forest Atmosphere or Forest Bathing) in Japan." *Environmental Health and Preventive Medicine* 15, no. 1 (2010): 27–37.

Tuteja, G., and K. H. Kaestner. "SnapShot: Forkhead Transcription Factors I." *Cell* 130, no. 6 (September 2007): 1160.

Tyler, Varro E. *Herbs of Choice: The Therapeutic Use of Phytomedicinals*. Binghamton, N.Y.: Pharmaceutical Products Press, 1994.

Ueda, Y., T. Fujimura, S. Kinami, et al. "Immunochemo-Therapy Study Group—Gastric Cancer (HKIT-GC): A Randomized Phase III Trial of Postoperative Adjuvant Therapy with S-1 Alone Versus S-1 Plus PSK for Stage II/IIIA Gastric Cancer." *Japanese Journal of Clinical Oncology* 36, no. 8 (August 2006): 519–22.

Uglow, Jenny. *The Lunar Men: Five Friends Whose Curiosity Changed the World*. New York: Farrar, Straus and Giroux, 2002.

Uri, Lloyd J., and H. Felter. *King's American Dispensatory*. Cincinnati: Cincinnatti Valley Company, 1918.

Usui, S., K. Asari, and T. Mizuno. "Preparation and Antitumor Activities of h-(1Y6) Branched (1Y3)-h-d-glucan Derivatives." *Biological and Pharmaceutical Bulletin* 18 (1995): 1630–36.

Van Laar, Judith, M. M. Porath, C. H. L. Peters, et al. "Spectral Analysis of Fetal Heart Rate Variability for Fetal Surveillance: Review of the Literature." *Acta Obstetrica et Gynecologica* 87 (2008): 300–306.

Van Loon, Gabriel, ed. *Charaka Samhita: Handbook on Ayurveda*. Vol. 1. Varanasi, Uttar Pradesh, India: Chaukhambha Orientalia, 2003.

Van Toller, Steve, C. Van Toller, G. H. Dodd, and Anne Billing. *Ageing and the Sense of Smell*. Springfield, Ill.: Charles C. Thomas, 1985.

Veltmann, C., C. Wolpert, F. Sacher, et al. "Response to Intravenous Ajmaline: A Retrospective Analysis of 677 Ajmaline Challenges." *Europace* 11, no. 10 (October 2009): 1345–52.

Von Bertalanffy, Ludwig. "The Theory of Open Systems in Physics and Biology." *Science* 111, no. 2872 (January 13, 1950): 23–29.

von Bingen, Hildegard. *Heavenly Revelations.* Performed by Oxford Camerata, Robert Evans, Michael McCarthy, Sterence Rice, Carys-Anne Lane. Hong Kong: Naxos, 1995. Compact Disc.

———. *Hildegard von Bingen's Physica: The Complete English Translation of Her Classic Work on Health and Healing.* Translated by Priscilla Throop. Rochester, Vt.: Healing Arts Press, 1998.

von der Vogelweide, Walter. *Die Gedichte Walthers von der Vogelweide (Poems of Walter von der Vogelweide), Besorgt von Albert Leitzmann (Collected by Albert Leitzmann).* 6th ed. Edited by Paul Hermann. Halle, Germany: Niemeyer Verlag, 1945.

von Mutius, E., and K. Radon. "Living on a Farm: Impact on Asthma Induction and Clinical Course." *Immunology Allergy Clinics of North America* 28, no. 3 (August 2008): 631–47.

Vuorela, H., P. Vuorela, K. Törnquist, et al. "Calcium Channel Blocking Activity: Screening Method for Plant Derived Compounds." *Phytomedicine* 4 (1997): 167–81.

Wa, Zhiya, ed. *Zhongguo Yixue Shi (A History of Chinese Medicine).* Beijing: Renmin Weisheng, 1991.

Wachs, M. "Reflections on the Planning Process." In *The Geography of Urban Transportation,* 3rd ed., edited by Susan Hansen and Genevieve Guliano, 141–61. New York: The Guilford Press, 2004.

Waddington, C. H. "The Epigenotype." *Endeavour* 1 (1942): 18–20.

Wang, H., G. J. Provan, and K. Helliwell. "Tea Flavonoids: Their Functions, Utilisation and Analysis." *Trends in Food Science and Technology* 11, nos. 4–5 (2000): 152–60.

Watson, Gilbert. *Theriac and Mithridatium: A Study in Therapeutics.* London: Wellcome Historical Medical Library, 1966.

Weaver, W. "Science and Complexity." *American Scientist* 36 (1948): 536–44.

Weckesser, S., K. Engel, B. Simon-Haarhaus, et al. "Screening of Plant Extracts for Antimicrobial Activity against Bacteria and Yeasts with Dermatological Relevance." *Phytomedicine* 14, nos. 7–8 (2007): 508–16.

Weed, Susun. *Healing Wise.* Woodstock, N.Y.: Ash Tree Publishing, 1989.

Wegener, D. *"Anwendung eines Trockenextraktes Augentianae luteae radix bei dyspeptischem Symptomcomplex.* (Application of a Dry Extract of the

Root of Gentiana lutea in Dyspeptic Symptom Complex)." *Zeitschrift für Phytotherapie (Phytotherapy Journal)* 19 (1998): 164.

Wein, E. E., M. Milton, R. Freeman, and Jeanette C. Makus. "Use of and Preference for Traditional Foods among the Belcher Island Inuit." *Arctic* 49, no. 3 (September 1996): 256–64.

Wicks, D., J. Wright, P. Rayment, and R. Spiller. "Impact of Bitter Taste on Gastric Motility." *European Journal of Gastroenterology Hepatology* 17, no. 9 (September 2005): 961–65.

Wilhelm, R., and C. F. Baynes, trans. *The I Ching: Or Book of Change Book 24.* London: Routledge and Kegan Paul, 1983.

Wilson, Frank Percy. *The Plague Pamphlets of Thomas Decker.* Oxford, UK: Clarendon Press, 1925.

Winston, David, and Steven Maimes. *Adaptogens: Herbs for Strength, Stamina, and Stress Relief.* Rochester, Vt.: Healing Arts Press, 2007.

Wooltorton, E. "Several Chinese Herbal Products May Contain Toxic Aristolochic Acid." *Canadian Medical Association Journal* 171, no. 5 (August 31, 2004): 449.

"World Health Organization Fact Sheet." Fact Sheet no. 134, December 2008. www.who.int/mediacentre/factsheets/fs134/en/ (accessed January 24, 2012).

Wu, H. *The Effect of Inhalation of Lavender Essential Oils on Autonomic Nervous System Function of the Shift-Working Nurses.* Taiwan, R.O.C.: Nanhua University, 2009.

Wu, S. J., L. T. Ng, and C. C. Lin. "Antioxidant Activities of Some Common Ingredients of Traditional Chinese Medicine, Angelica Sinensis, Lycium Barbarum and Poria Cocos." *Phytotherapy Research* 18, no. 12 (2004): 1008–12.

Wysocki, C. J., and M. L. Pelchat. "The Effects of Aging on the Human Sense of Smell and its Relationship to Food Choice." *Critical Review of Food Science and Nutrition* 33, no. 1 (1993): 63–82.

Xu, F., K. Uebaba, H. Ogawa, et al. "Pharmaco-physio-psychologic Effect of Ayurvedic Oil-Dripping Treatment Using an Essential Oil from Lavendula Angustifolia." *Journal of Alternative and Complementary Medicine* 14, no. 8 (2008): 947–56.

Yarnell, E. "Botanical Medicines for the Urinary Tract." *World Journal of Urology* 20, no. 5 (2002): 285–93.

Yehuda, R., S. M. Southwick, G. Nussbaum, et al. "Low Urinary Cortisol Excretion in Patients with Posttraumatic Stress Disorder." *Journal of Nervous and Mental Disorders* 178, no. 6 (June 1990): 366–69.

Yochum, L., L. H. Kushi, K. Meyer, and F. Aaron. "Dietary Flavonoid Intake and Risk of Cardiovascular Disease in Postmenopausal Women." *American Journal of Epidemiology* 149 (1999): 943–49.

You, Y., S. Yoo, H. G. Yoon, et al. "In Vitro and In Vivo Hepatoprotective Effects of the Aqueous Extract from Taraxacum Officinale (Dandelion) Root against Alcohol-induced Oxidative Stress." *Food and Chemical Toxicology* 48, no. 6 (June 2010): 1632–37.

Yuan, J., K. Minter-Dykhouse, and Z. Lou. "A c-Myc-SIRT1 Feedback Loop Regulates Cell Growth and Transformation." *Journal of Cell Biology* 185, no. 2 (April 20, 2009): 203–11.

Zhu, You-Ping. *Chinese Materia Medica*. Florence, Ky.: CRC Press, 1998.

Zuanetti, G., J. M. M. Neilson, D. J. Ewing, et al. "Prognostic Significance of Heart Rate Variability in Post-myocardial Infarction Patients in the Fibrinolytic Era: The GISSI-2 Results. Gruppo Italiano per lo Studio della Sopravvivenza nell' Infarto Miocardico (Italian Heart Attack Survival Study Group)." *Circulation* 94, no. 3 (1996): 432–36.

Index

BOOKS OF RELATED INTEREST

Herbs: Partners in Life
Healing, Gardening, and Cooking with Wild Plants
by Adele G. Dawson

The Herbal Handbook
A User's Guide to Medical Herbalism
by David Hoffmann, FNIMH, AHG

Adaptogens
Herbs for Strength, Stamina, and Stress Relief
by David Winston and Steven Maimes

Health from God's Garden
Herbal Remedies for Glowing Health and Well-Being
by Maria Treben

The Family Herbal
A Guide to Natural Health Care for Yourself and Your Children
from Europe's Leading Herbalists
by Barbara and Peter Theiss

Adaptogens in Medical Herbalism
Elite Herbs and Natural Compounds for Mastering Stress,
Aging, and Chronic Disease
by Donald R. Yance, CN, MH, RH (AHG)

The Seasonal Detox Diet
Remedies from the Ancient Cookfire
by Carrie L'Esperance

Traditional Foods Are Your Best Medicine
Improving Health and Longevity with Native Nutrition
by Ronald F. Schmid, N.D.

INNER TRADITIONS • BEAR & COMPANY
P.O. Box 388
Rochester, VT 05767
1-800-246-8648
www.InnerTraditions.com

Or contact your local bookseller